AF548593

Ultrasound in Cancer

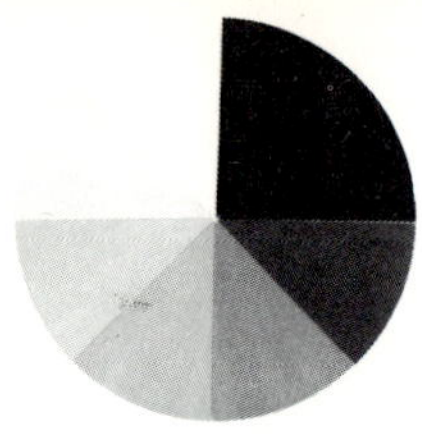

CLINICS IN DIAGNOSTIC ULTRASOUND VOLUME 6

Volumes Already Published

Vol. 1 Diagnostic Ultrasound in Gastrointestinal Disease, Kenneth J. W. Taylor, Guest Editor

Vol. 2 Genitourinary Ultrasonography, Arthur T. Rosenfield, Guest Editor

Vol. 3 Diagnostic Ultrasound in Obstetrics, John C. Hobbins, Guest Editor

Vol. 4 Two-Dimensional Echocardiography, Joseph A. Kisslo, Guest Editor

Vol. 5 New Techniques and Instrumentation, P. N. T. Wells and Marvin Ziskin, Guest Editors

Forthcoming Volumes in the Series

Vol. 7 Ultrasound in Emergency Medicine, Kenneth J. W. Taylor and Gregory N. Viscomi, Guest Editors

Vol. 8 Diagnostic Ultrasound in Pediatrics, Jack O. Haller and Arnold Shkolnik, Guest Editors

Ultrasound in Cancer

Edited by

Barry B. Goldberg, M.D.

Professor of Radiology
Director, Division of Diagnostic Ultrasound
Thomas Jefferson University Hospital
Philadelphia, Pennsylvania

CHURCHILL LIVINGSTONE
NEW YORK, EDINBURGH, LONDON, AND MELBOURNE
1981

Distributed in the United Kingdom by Churchill Livingstone, Robert Stevenson House, 1-3 Baxter's Place, Leith Walk, Edinburgh EH1 3AF and by associated companies, branches and representatives throughout the world.

First published 1981

Printed in USA

ISBN 0-443-08144-1

7 6 5 4 3 2 1

Library of Congress Cataloging in Publication Data
Main entry under title:

Ultrasound in cancer.

(Clinics in diagnostic ultrasound; 6)
Bibliography: p.
Includes index.
1. Cancer. 2. Diagnosis, Ultrasonic. 3. Ultrasonic waves—Therapeutic use. I. Goldberg, Barry B. II. Series. [DNLM:
1. Neoplasms—Diagnosis. 2. Ultrasonics—Diagnostic use.
W1 CL831BC v. 6/QZ241 U464]
RC262.U4 616.99'407543 80-23399
ISBN 0-443-08144-1

Contributors

John W. Breckenridge, M.D.
Clinical Assistant Professor, Department of Radiology, Thomas Jefferson University Hospital, Philadelphia, Pennsylvania; Assistant Radiologist, Abington Memorial Hospital, Abington, Pennsylvania

Barbara A. Carroll, M.D.
Assistant Professor, Chief of Diagnostic Ultrasound, Department of Radiology, Stanford University Medical Center, Stanford, California

Catherine Cole-Beuglet, M.D.
Associate Professor of Radiology, Division of Diagnostic Ultrasound, Thomas Jefferson University Hospital, Philadelphia, Pennsylvania

David O. Cosgrove, M.D.
Consultant, Nuclear Medicine and Ultrasound, The Royal Marsden Hospital, London, ENGLAND

Michael Crade, M.D.
Assistant Director of Diagnostic Ultrasound, Long Beach Memorial Hospital, Long Beach, California

Richard L. Dallow, M.D.
Department of Ophthalmology, Harvard Medical School, Massachusetts Eye and Ear Infirmary, Boston, Massachusetts

Barry B. Goldberg, M.D.
Professor of Radiology, Director, Division of Diagnostic Ultrasound, Thomas Jefferson University Hospital, Philadelphia, Pennsylvania

Alfred Kratochwil, M.D.
Department of Ultrasound, University of Vienna, Frauenklinik Vienna, Vienna, AUSTRIA

Frederick W. Kremkau, Ph.D.
Associate Professor of Medicine (Biophysics), Wake Forest University, Bowman Gray School of Medicine, Winston-Salem, North Carolina

Alfred B. Kurtz, M.D.
Associate Professor of Radiology, Division of Diagnostic Ultrasound, Department of Radiology, Thomas Jefferson University Hospital, Philadelphia, Pennsylvania

George R. Leopold, M.D.
Professor of Radiology, Chief, Division of Diagnostic Ultrasound, University of California at San Diego, University Hospital, San Diego, California

Harvey L. Neiman, M.D.
Associate Professor of Radiology, Director, Angiography and Sectional Imaging, Northwestern University Medical School and Northwestern Memorial Hospital, Chicago, Illinois

Sharyn J. Pussell, M.D., F.R.A.C.P.
Senior Registrar, Department of Nuclear Medicine and Ultrasound, The Royal Marsden Hospital, London, ENGLAND

Roger C. Sanders, M.D.
Associate Professor of Radiology and Urology, Department of Radiology, The Johns Hopkins Hospital, Baltimore, Maryland

Morton Schneider, M.D.
Associate Professor of Clinical Radiology, Department of Radiology, Division of Ultrasound and Computerized Body Tomography, The New York Hospital Cornell Medical Center, New York, New York

Kenneth J. W. Taylor, M.D., Ph.D., F.A.C.P.
Professor of Diagnostic Radiology, Head, Section of Diagnostic Ultrasound, Yale University School of Medicine, New Haven, Connecticut

Barbara J. Weinstein, M.D.
Attending Radiologist, Department of Diagnostic Radiology, St. Francis General Hospital, Pittsburgh, Pennsylvania

David P. Weinstein, M.D.
Attending Radiologist, Department of Radiology, Citizens' General Hospital, New Kinsington, Pennsylvania

Contents

Foreword
Barry B. Goldberg

1. Liver
David O. Cosgrove 1

2. Biliary Tract
Michael Crade and Kenneth J. W. Taylor 22

3. Pancreas
David P. Weinstein and Barbara J. Weinstein 35

4. Lymphoma
Barbara A. Carroll 52

5. Kidneys
Roger C. Sanders 68

6. Retroperitoneum
Harvey L. Neiman 90

7. Gynecology
John W. Breckenridge and Alfred B. Kurtz 104

8. Pediatrics
Morton Schneider 115

9. Superficial Organs
George R. Leopold 123

10. Eye and Orbit
Richard L. Dallow 136

11. Breast
Catherine Cole-Beuglet and Barry B. Goldberg 157

12. Treatment Planning
Alfred Kratochwil 167

13. Therapy
Frederick W. Kremkau 186

CASE STUDIES

NO. 1 Liver Cyst in a Woman with Carcinoma of the Ovary
S.J. Pussell and D.O. Cosgrove 199

NO. 2 Carcinoma of the Gallbladder? What Is Your Diagnosis?
M. Crade and K. Taylor 201

NO. 3 Painless Jaundice
B.J. Weinstein and D.P. Weinstein 205

NO. 4 Fever and Right Inguinal Mass in a Young Man
B. Carroll 207

NO. 5 The Multiple Appearances of Hematomas
R. C. Sanders 209

NO. 6 Increasing Abdominal Girth in a Young Woman
A.B. Kurtz and J.W. Breckenridge 213

NO. 7 Palpable Left Flank Mass
M. Schneider 215

NO. 8 Thyroid Nodule—Benign or Malignant?
G.R. Leopold 217

Index 219

Foreword

This volume of Clinics in Diagnostic Ultrasound is devoted exclusively to the use of ultrasound in tumor evaluation. Not only are all of the major areas covered (with emphasis on diagnoses and differential diagnosis of various abnormalities involving benign and malignant tumors), but also a special chapter is devoted to a newly emerging field—the use of ultrasound in tumor treatment.

The individuals who contributed to this volume have covered the highlights and new advances in their particular field that would be of interest to the ultrasonographer, both physician and technologist. The scope of ultrasound tumor diagnosis is obviously extensive. In considering the subjects of these Clinics, it is likewise obvious that an effort to include all of the information known—techniques, approaches, and differential diagnoses—would result in a book four times this size. However, it is hoped that this overview will enable the reader to appreciate the importance of ultrasound in this area of diagnosis and also to learn of newer uses of and approaches to ultrasound, such as treatment planning. Since many areas of interest are covered, it is also hoped that the physician or sonographer whose interests are of a narrow scope will broaden his knowledge by reading this volume and come to appreciate the full extent of ultrasound tumor diagnosis in the adult and pediatric patient. Some areas have not been covered to any great extent, such as the prostate and heart and aspiration-biopsy techniques, because of in-depth coverage in either earlier or forthcoming volumes in this series. However, all major areas have been discussed, and this has necessitated some overlapping of information available in other Clinics volumes, such as the previous volume on urologic ultrasound. This, unfortunately, is necessary when a broad topic such as tumor diagnosis is covered in this format. In general, this book should be considered an overview of the many potential uses of ultrasound in the diagnosis and treatment of tumors. It is the hope of the editor that this aim has been accomplished. For more in-depth knowledge, individuals should refer to books specifically devoted to areas of their special interest.

Thanks must be given to the numerous secretaries and technologists of the many authors who have contributed to this volume. Special thanks is given to my staff who spent many hours editing this volume, including Dr. Paul Dubbins, Rhoda Porter, and Kathy Bonner, as well as my own personal editor and wife, Phyllis Goldberg.

Barry B. Goldberg

Ultrasound in Cancer

1 Liver

DAVID O. COSGROVE

The application to medical diagnosis of technologies spawned by developments during World War II—first nuclear imaging, then ultrasonography, and lately computed X-ray tomography—has had a major impact on studies of the liver, where previously tissue biopsy was usually required. This is especially true for tumors of the liver. Here noninvasive methods for detecting metastases with minimal disturbance to the patient have improved staging and management. The ultrasonic findings discussed in this chapter are followed by an evaluation of the contribution of the three techniques to the management of patients with possible liver malignancy.

BENIGN TUMORS

Hemangiomata (Table 1.1) are the most common benign tumor of the liver. Foci of high level echoes characterize the capillary type, while the cavernous varieties return a low level of echoes, sometimes with fluid-solid levels representing layering of the contents of the tumor (Fig. 1.1).[1-3] Attenuation is usually equal to that of normal liver, so neither shadowing nor distal enhancement is seen. The tumors are usually solitary and asymptomatic, but when they are large or multiple, they may present as hepatomegaly or with high output heart failure, especially in neonates. Specific diagnosis requires angiography, but sonography may be suggestive when feeding vessels can be shown, and is useful in follow-up; pulsed Doppler devices are promising here. Biopsy should be avoided, but inadvertent puncture with a skinny needle has been performed without catastrophic bleeding. However, if fresh blood is aspirated from a focal lesion, the patient should be admitted for observation and crossmatched. Cystic mesenchymal hamartomas, lymphangiomatous tumors of early childhood, appear as large fluid masses with lacy septae and cause gross displacement of normal liver.[4]

Simple cysts, either single or multiple, display the characteristic triad of a smooth wall, echo-free contents (i.e., echoes at system noise level), and distal enhancement whose intensity relates to the length of fluid path. For this reason, small cysts (< 1 cm) pose diagnostic difficulties (Fig. 1.2).[5] Differentia-

TABLE 1.1. Benign liver "tumors."

True lesions	
Hemangioma	Echogenic—capillary types Echo-poor—cavernous types
Adenoma	Texture ? = liver unless hemorrhagic
Focal nodular hyperplasia	Echogenic (presumed)
Simple cyst	Echo-free with enhancement and smooth walls
Cirrhotic nodule	Texture = normal liver
Ultrasonic pseudotumors	
Normal structures	Echogenic—ligamentum teres diaphragmatic leaflets perinephric fat and fascia Echo-poor—blood vessels upper pole of right kidney shadows behind porta, neck of gall bladder
Abnormalities	Adjacent masses masquerading as hepatic, e.g., adrenal as right lobe lesion, precaval nodes as caudate lesion

tion from hydatid cysts depends on demonstrating developing daughter cysts, which initially appear simply as internal elevations of the capsule wall that later separate out into cysts within the cyst. When the cysts are immature, these features may be too subtle to be detectable by ultrasound.

Benign solid tumors are rare, and experience with their ultrasonic appearance is scanty. Echogenic foci that remain stable on serial scans have been described as incidental findings. Masses that deform the contour of the liver, but produce echoes indistinguishable from those reflected from normal liver tissue have been supposed to represent benign tumors. Complex masses with ultrasonic fluid spaces interspersed between reflective tissue in a disordered fashion have been seen in hemorrhagic adenomas induced by estrogens.[6] Pathologically, two types must be distinguished.[7] The true adenoma is a disease of women of childbearing age, strongly associated with estrogen medication. They are encapsulated, pure hepatocyte tumors, frequently hemorrhagic. Presentation is as a mass or with hemorrhage, and surgical intervention is required. By contrast, focal nodular hyperplasia is asymptomatic, is found at any age, and occurs in both sexes, with females involved four times as often as males. The association with steroids is not as strong. The lobulated lesion characteristically contains a central stellate scar, and the nodules comprise all liver cell elements in an arrangement similar to cirrhosis. The structure suggests a response to some sort of vascular damage. Resection is not required. These lesions may take up colloid, but the true adenomas are always cold on scintigraphy. In principle, one would expect

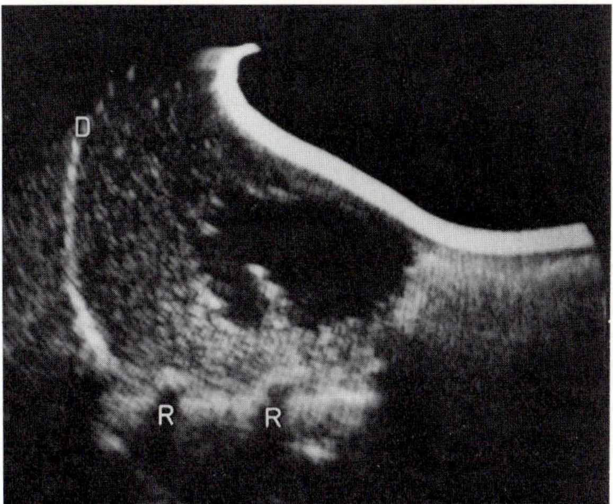

FIGURE 1.1. Cavernous hemangioma. Sagittal section through the right lobe of liver in a 6-year-old. A large echo-poor lesion occupies the lower half of this part of the liver. It has an irregular margin with a suggestion of scalloping and slight distal echo enhancement. D = diaphragm; R = rib and associated shadow.

focal nodular hyperplasia to return high level echoes because of the fibrosis. Likewise, hemorrhagic adenomas should be echogenic because of organization by scarring, while uncomplicated adenomas, with their uniform sheets of hepatocytes, should have low levels of echoes.[8, 9]

The designation *pseudotumors* is used to cover normal but confusing appearances, as well as masses of regenerating tissue, as seen in macronodular cirrhosis.[10] As with adenomas, and presumably for the same reason that the tissue concerned is very similar to normal liver, regenerating nodules are difficult to define ultrasonically unless they distort the surface or vascular architecture of the liver. Since they may be detected as photon-poor regions on scintigraphy, the confirmation that they possess a normal ultrasonic texture is reassuring with respect to the differential diagnosis of hepatocellular carcinoma.

Normal structures that may be confused with focal lesions include the highly reflective round ligament (ligamentum teres) (Fig. 1.3), which always lies close but inferior to the left portal vein; diaphragmatic leaflets lying in "cough furrows" on the dome of the right lobe of the liver, the upper pole of the right kidney, or its perinephric fat and fascia; and shadows distal to the porta and the neck of the gallbladder.

An understanding of the ultrasonic appearances of benign and pseudotumors has obvious importance in the differential diagnosis of focal lesions seen at sonography. In addition, these and many other focal changes will produce photon-deficient areas on colloid scintigraphy, which can often be evaluated by ultrasound.

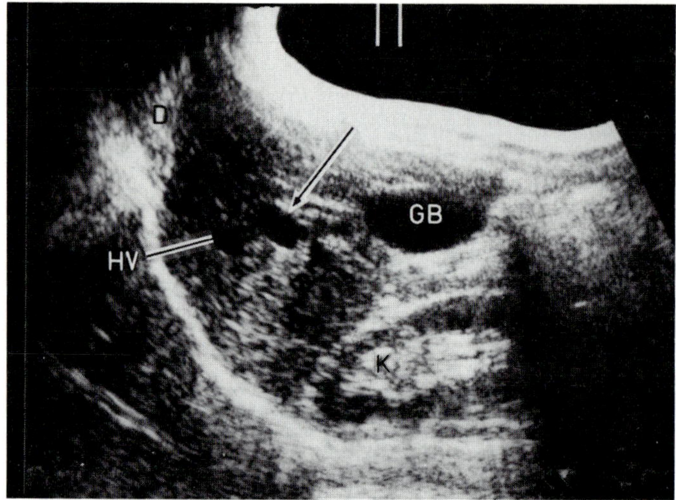

FIGURE 1.2. Simple cyst. Sagittal section, right mid clavicular line. A 1.5 cm cyst (arrow) near the porta shows the diagnostic ultrasound triad of absent echoes (cf. the gall bladder) a smooth wall and distal echo enhancement, not shown by the nearby right hepatic vein. GB = gallbladder, HV = hepatic vein, K = kidney

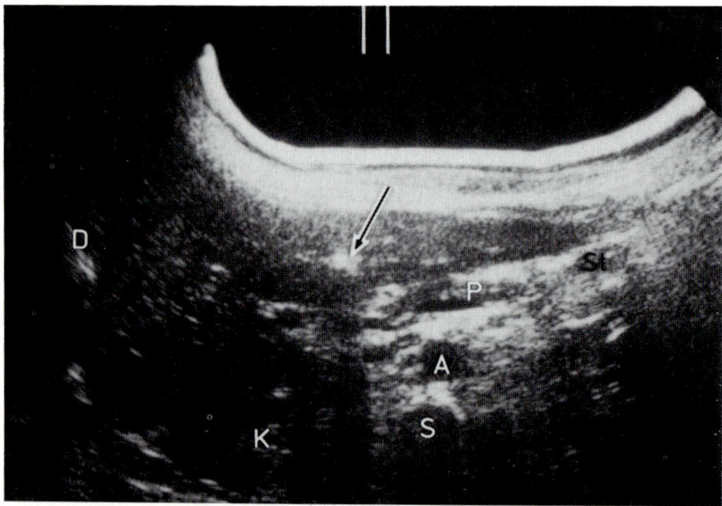

FIGURE 1.3. Round ligament. Transverse epigastric section. The round ligament (ligamentum teres) is seen in cross section in transverse views inferior to the portal vein demarcating the anatomical left and right lobes of the liver. It is prominent on ultrasound due to its fibrotic nature and the associated fat, and may, as in this case, cast an acoustic shadow. It should not be mistaken for an echogenic lesion. A = aorta, P = pancreas, S = spine, St = stomach.

TABLE 1.2. Incidence of liver metastases.

1° tumor	Percent at presentation	Percent in late cases	References
Breast	1	33	11,12
Hodgkin disease	5	66	13,14
Bronchus	15	45	15,16
Colorectal	17	62	16,17
Melanoma	34	75	16,18

MALIGNANT LIVER TUMORS

Hepatocellular carcinoma is a highly malignant disease. Its geographic prevalence varies markedly, ranging from 2 per 100,000 population in most westernized countries to 100 per 100,000 among the Bantus of Southern Africa. Environmental agents, including dietary, have been incriminated in these differences. There is a strong association with cirrhosis of the macronodular type, especially in the West where it is observed in 75 percent of cases. Pathologically, hepatocellular carcinoma may appear as a solitary well-defined lesion, but in some cases tumor is widespread within the liver at presentation. The debate as to whether this is due to early local spread or to multicentric origin under the general influence of a chemical carcinogen remains unresolved. Spread beyond the liver is by local invasion through the capsule and by hematogenous metastasis to the lungs. Serum alpha-fetoprotein (AFP) is raised, often grossly, in up to three-quarters of the cases in areas in which the incidence of hepatocellular carcinoma is high. It is less commonly elevated in countries where the disease has a lower incidence, and is not positive in cholangiocarcinoma. Both hepatocellular carcinoma and the hepatoblastoma of childhood have ultrasonic appearances indistinguishable from secondary liver tumors.[4]

Metastatic tumors far out-number primary tumors of the liver in all parts of the world. The incidence varies with the primary site and the stage of disease (Table 1.2). Metastases can be detected in "early" disease—i.e., at presentation—in over one-third of malignant melanomata but hardly ever in squamous carcinoma of skin, with bronchus, breast, and colon showing an intermediate incidence. At autopsy, liver involvement is found in approximately one-half of the total number of patients with malignant disease who die; interestingly, the proportion is higher (67 percent) for primary sites drained by the portal circulation than for those with a systemic drainage (48 percent).[16] The pattern of metastases, with groups of tumors of similar size, is in keeping with the concept that seeding is an episodic rather than a continuous process, which would produce lesions with an even gradation of sizes. Their number varies between innumerable miliary metastases and the solitary lesions often seen in colorectal metastases.

TABLE 1.3. Ultrasonic features of malignant liver tumors.

	Appearance	Tumor type
Focal	Echogenic	Carcinomas especially UG and GIT including hepatoma
	Echo-poor	Any 1° or 2°
	Target (Bull's eye)	Any 1° or 2°
	Echogenic with shadowing	Calcifying 2° carcinoma especially gut and ovary
	Cystic	Mucin secreting 2°, especially ovary and pancreas
	Necrotic	Any, especially large masses (simulated by some sarcomas)
Generalized	Moth-eaten texture of replaced liver	Any 1° or 2°
	Diffuse fine texture	Miliary 1° or 2°
	Echo-poor liver	Lymphomata

Ultrasound Appearance of Malignant Liver Tumors

The appearances on sonography (Table 1.3) are varied, in keeping with the range of histology found in both primary and secondary liver malignancy. Focal lesions predominate, producing nonspecific mass effects. Hepatomegaly is usual but not invariable and is often associated with a rounding-up of the liver that leads to blunting of the normally sharp anterior margin. The enlargement predominates in the affected portion of the liver and, when superficial, produces localized bumps of the liver contour.[19] These are most easily seen when there is coexistent ascites. They should not be confused with the normal surface projection that may occur on a superior surface of the liver between prominent diaphragmatic leaflets. Distortions of the normal hepatic blood vessels can sometimes be recognized, as can biliary distension of segmental distribution upstream of the obstruction. These features are all nonspecific and may also be due to inflammatory masses and to hematomata.

Characteristic alterations in echo properties often occur in tumors of the liver. The most common are rounded foci of reduced or increased reflectivity with rather ill-defined margins and normal attenuation so that neither shadowing nor distal enhancement is seen (Figs. 1.4 and 1.5).[6, 9, 20-23] The texture of the echoes within these lesions differs little from that of the normal liver, though sometimes it may be slightly coarser (larger, more widely spaced dots). The degree to which the reflectivity of a lesion differs from normal liver constitutes the contrast that allows their detection; differences of only a few decibels are usual, with extremes of +10 dB for intensely echogenic and −15

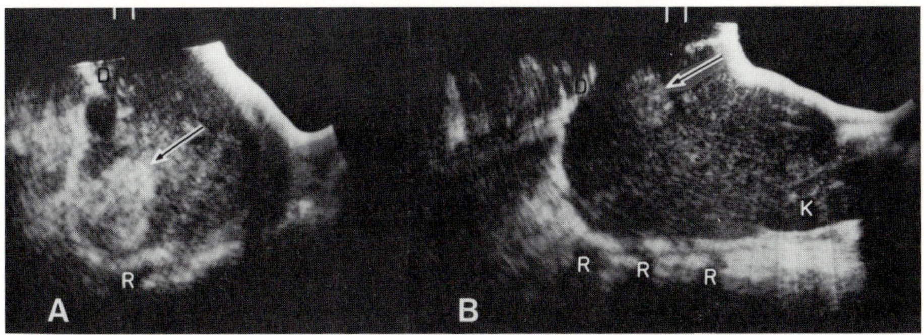

FIGURE 1.4. Echogenic metastases. Sagittal sections through the right lobe of liver. Two examples of echogenic focal metastases (arrowed) in two patients both with colorectal carcinoma. In (a) there is also an echo-poor focus anterior to the echogenic lesion. Note the rounding of the liver's free margin (see Fig. 1.5a).

dB from extremely echo-poor lesions. Apart from the echogenic normal "pseudolesions," echogenic tumors can be confused with capillary hemangiomata, adenomata, and fibrous scars. Multiplicity and growth are features of malignancy. Likewise, relatively anechoic lesions need to be distinguished from pseudotumors by their anatomy, and from blood vessels by their tubular arrangement when sectioned in the appropriate plane. Echo-poor masses that can cause difficulty are cavernous hemangiomata and traumatic hematomata. These may be differentiated by their failure to concentrate gallium and their lack of growth on serial scans.

Combinations of increased and reduced reflectivity occur, sometimes randomly distributed within one lesion but often arranged concentrically with a cortex of relatively anechoic tissue arranged around a more reflective central core. The exact proportion of the two components varies somewhat (Fig. 1.6). This pattern is commonly referred to as the "target" or "bulls-eye" lesion. Abscesses may occasionally give rise to this pattern also.

Calcification produces extremely intense echoes with strong distal shadowing. Gas in abscesses, or in the biliary tree, has the same echo characteristics as calcification; a plain X-ray will differentiate between them.

Tumors with fluid properties are also encountered (Fig. 1.7). When truly cystic, these are echo-free, have smooth walls, and show distal echo enhancement. This pattern is seen in mucin-secreting tumors. Such lesions are indistinguishable on ultrasound from simple cysts or smooth-walled hydatid cysts. Since biopsy in the latter can be hazardous, repeat ultrasound scanning should be performed. Progressive enlargement over weeks or months suggests tumor. Tumor necrosis or hemorrhage also produces fluid properties with distal enhancement, but the lesion walls are usually irregular, sometimes with a well-marked solid component, and the necrotic material may produce irregular low-level echoes (Fig. 1.8).[24] In large necrotic or hemorrhagic lesions, layering of the denser components may occur, producing pos-

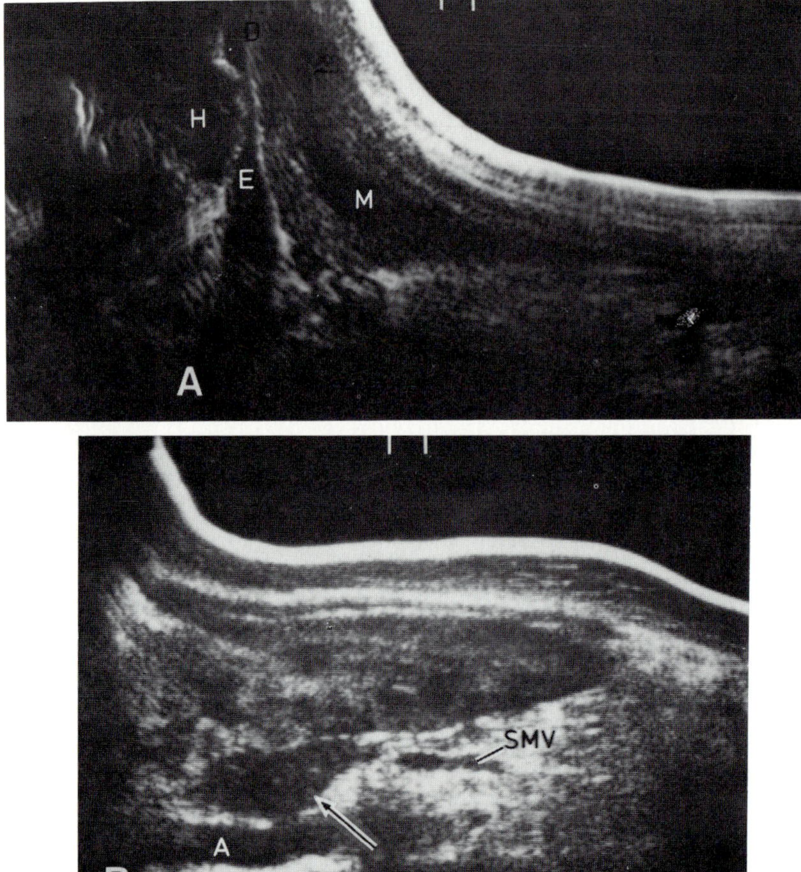

FIGURE 1.5. Echo-poor metastases. (a) Sagittal section through the left lobe of liver. A solitary, centrally placed 2 cm lesion has a low level of echoes, an ill-defined margin and no distal enhancement. This was from a carcinoma of bronchus that had invaded the pericardium producing the pericardial effusion shown. E = pericardial effusion, H = heart, M = metastasis. (b) Sagittal section through the left lobe of liver. The caudate lobe (arrow) is replaced by tumor; confusion with preaortic lymphadenopathy requires careful transverse sections to establish continuity of this lobe with the right lobe. In addition, there are very many 0.5 to 1 cm echo-poor foci in the left lobe, most prominent in a subcapsular position inferiorly. There is hepatomegaly. The primary was carcinoma of the breast. SMV = superior mesenteric vein.

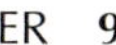

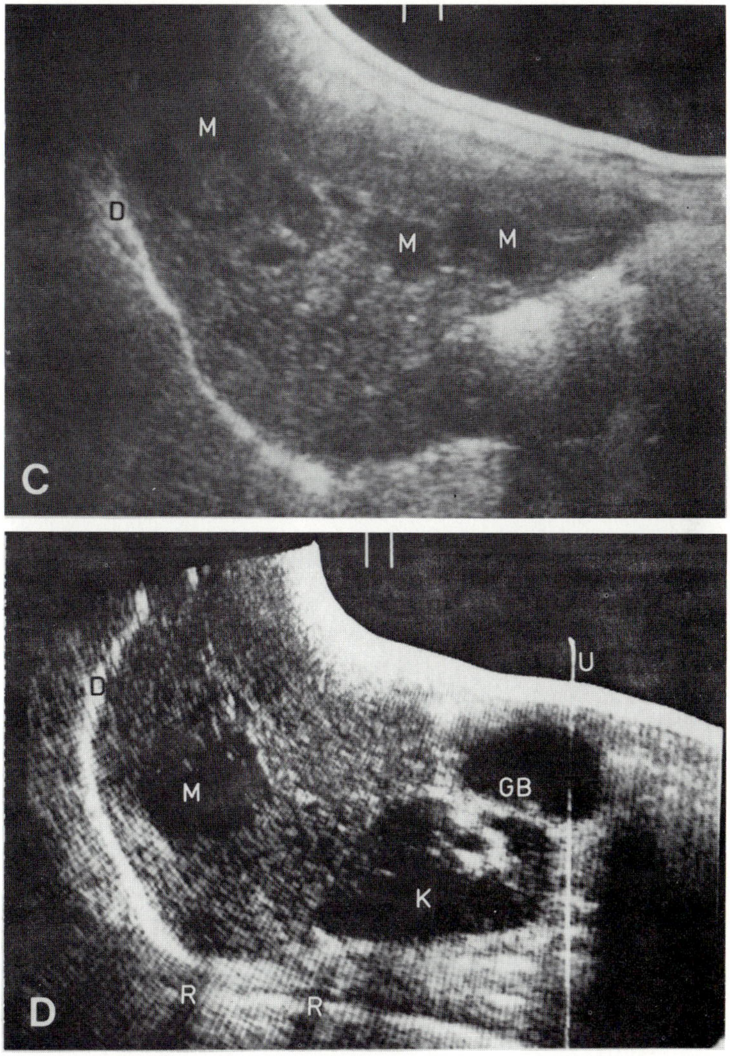

FIGURE 1.5. (c) Sagittal section: right lobe of liver. Several echo-poor deposits between 0.5 and 3 cm diameter are seen in this case. (d) Sagittal section: right lobe of liver. A large focal lesion is seen in this patient with lymphoma (see Fig. 1.10). There is also renal involvement. The gallbladder contains debris.

turally dependent fluid-fluid layers. Degenerating tumors have ultrasonic features identical to those of abscesses. The clinical content is usually distinctive, and guided aspiration of fluid material for culture and cytology is definitive.

Rarely, lesions that are solid but display a degree of enhancement may be encountered. These confusing appearances are a feature of sarcomata.

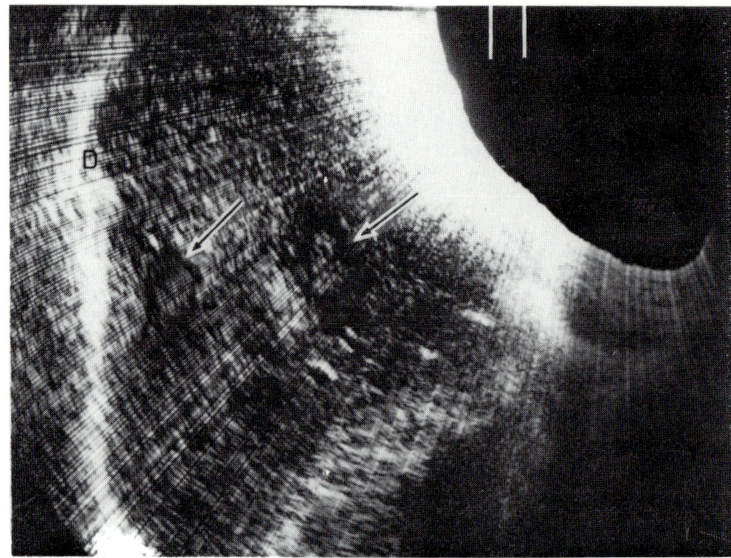

FIGURE 1.6. Target lesions. Sagittal section: right lobe of liver. Two of the lesions (arrows) show the concentric ring pattern in this patient with carcinoma of the bronchus. Note the flat diaphragm.

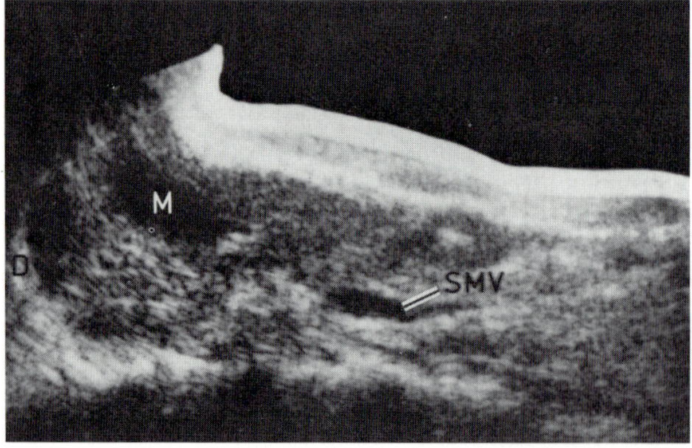

FIGURE 1.7. Cystic metastasis. Sagittal section: midline. There is a 2 cm anechoic lesion showing distal enhancement. Its irregular ill-defined walls allow differentiation from a simple cyst (see Fig. 1.1).

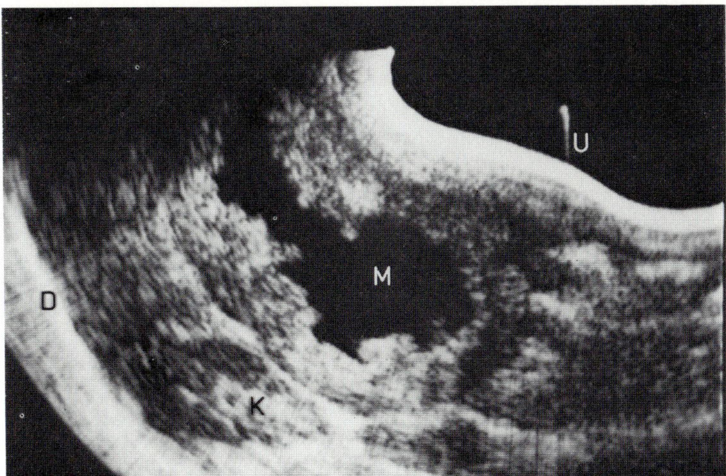

FIGURE 1.8. Necrotic metastasis. Sagittal section: right lobe. The centre of this enormous colonic deposit has undergone necrosis to produce a shaggy edged, echo-free region. This pattern is similar to an abscess; guided aspiration will usually be definitive.

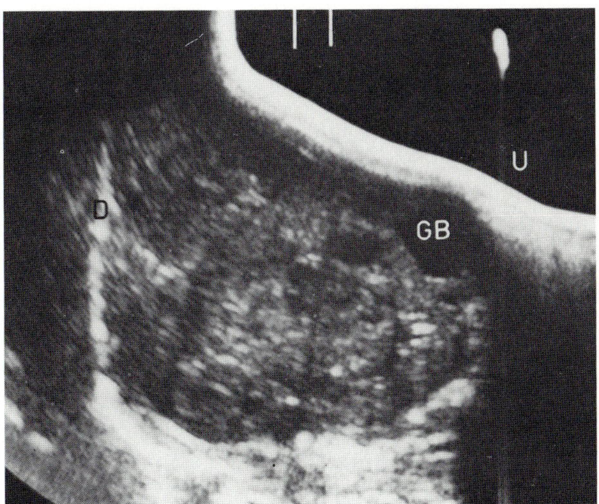

FIGURE 1.9. Widespread liver malignancy. Sagittal section: right lobe. The overall texture of this large liver is uneven; though it is difficult to define any one lesion, this "moth eaten" pattern is due to near replacement of the liver by tumor. The primary was a choroidal melanoma.

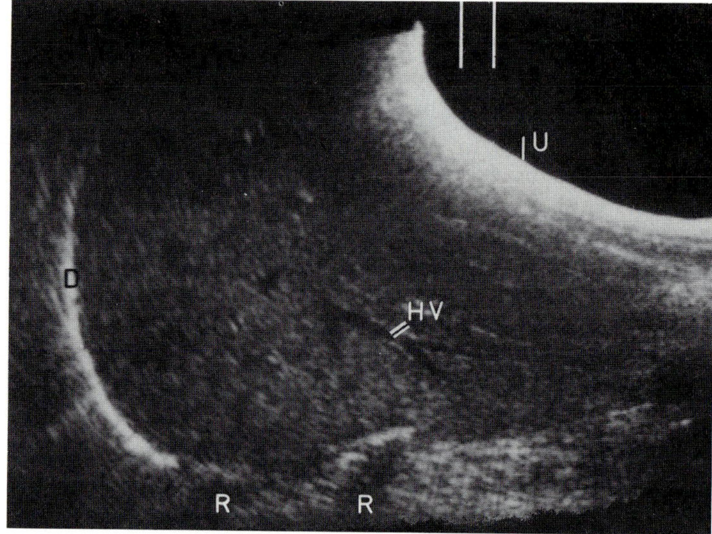

FIGURE 1.10. Hodgkin disease. Sagittal section: right lobe. The liver is greatly enlarged with low level echoes of an even but perhaps slightly altered texture. This appearance in a lymphoma is due to lymphocytic infiltration but ultrasound cannot determine whether this is reactive or lymphomatous.

Where there is massive replacement of liver with tumor, the nodules coalesce and the sonogram develops a widespread patchy texture in which it may be difficult to judge which portions represent normal liver and which are tumor (Fig. 1.9). This appearance can also be produced by toxic processes, giving patchy liver necrosis, such as in alcoholic hepatitis. The appearance of malignant cases is relentless deterioration on serial scans.

Tumor in the liver occasionally takes the form of numerous millimeter-sized foci, which are evenly distributed through the parenchyma and are known as miliary metastases. On ultrasound, this produces a fine echo texture (small spots, closely spaced) similar to that of several nonmalignant diffuse liver diseases, such as the granulomata and fatty change. Usually however, larger focal lesions coexist with the miliary metastases, suggesting the true diagnosis.[25]

In the lymphomas, lympocyte infiltration may produce a uniform reduction in echo level, so that unusually high gain settings are required to image the liver parenchyma (Fig. 1.10). It is not possible to distinguish reactive from diffuse neoplastic lymphocyte infiltration with current technology. Low-level focal lesions may coexist.

Histologic Correlation

Because the sonogram is a map of elasticity differences, it is predictable that tumors with a uniform homogeneous structure will return low-level echoes, and this is indeed typical of the lymphomas and sarcomas. The presence of fibrous tissue (perivascular or reactive) blood vessels themselves, necrosis, and hemorrhage would all be expected to produce the interfaces necessary for echo generation. However, the precise contribution of these factors has not been established. There are suggestions that echogenicity correlates with vascularity[26] and with necrosis. A mechanism has been proposed for the target appearance, with the echo-poor cuff of tissue being due to the "sinus hyperplasia" that surrounds many tumors.[27] This is a result of pressure atrophy, affecting the hepatocytes predominantly, and leading to the condensation of surviving blood vessels to form a sinusoidal margin. It seems clear, from contrast enhancement CT scans of these lesions, that the earlier suggestion of peritumoral edema to account for this pattern can be discounted.

There has been much debate on the frequency with which the various sonographic appearances occur in different types of tumor. Some of the difficulties were due to inadequacies in earlier equipment and some to variations in incidence in the population groups under study.

Hepatocelluar carcinoma can show any of the patterns described, the most common being the echogenic and the echo-poor focal lesions.[23] The widespread "replaced liver" pattern is seen in extensive tumors.

The tumors producing cystic metastases are mucin-secreting adenocarcinomas chiefly from ovary, pancreas, colon, and stomach. Ovarian deposits are notable in that they are often superficially placed. This is due to their characteristic transcoelomic spread pattern. This type of deposit is really a peritoneal lesion and carries a less poor prognosis than the true parenchymal lesion, which may also occur.[24] This same group of tumors may occasionally calcify.

Focal deposits from lymphoma have very low echo levels and, on occasion, may seem to be quite echo free. Sarcomata also return very low levels of echoes and sometimes show distal enhancement, apparently in the absence of necrotic or cystic change. This rare and puzzling phenomenon is not clinically important, since these lesions do not have the clear smooth walls of a typical cyst so that serious diagnostic errors should not occur. All of these tumors may also undergo true necrosis.

Deposits from carcinomata show the whole spectrum of patterns, from echogenic to echo poor, and include admixtures where different lesions within the same liver show different features. However, within this generalization there appear to be correlative trends, which can be identified. Deposits from the breast, bronchus, and melanoma are far more commonly echo poor, whereas deposits from the gastrointestinal and urogenital tracts are quite commonly echogenic, the exact proportion ranging from about one quarter to three quarters, depending on the population studied.[21] Clinically, the distinction is largely academic, except in the occasional problem when a patient presents with metastases. Here the demonstration of echogenic liver lesions should direct further search towards a primary in the gut or urogenital tract. Colorectal metastases additionally are often solitary or sparse, whereas those from breast or bronchus tend to be multiple.

The ultrasonic appearances of focal lesions may change with time; enlargement or, with successful treatment, shrinkage are usual. Necrosis, often leading to the development of irregular, echo-poor zones with variable distal enhancement, is often seen. Apart from necrosis, the echo levels may change, echo-poor lesions becoming echogenic and vice versa. The development of high-level echoes as a feature of response to treatment, perhaps due to scarring, has been reported in a few cases.[28] More often, lesions that respond simply shrink until they are no longer detectable, leaving no trace. Miliary pattern of deposits has been seen in breast, bronchus, melanoma, and primary liver tumors, both hepatocellular and cholangiocarcinomas.

Accuracy of Ultrasound in Liver Malignancy

The resolution of current generation ultrasound equipment (typically < 0.5 mm axially and 1 to 2 mm transverse) enables 1 to 2 mm structures, such as the normal pancreatic and empty common bile duct, to be imaged routinely. However, the minimal focal lesion that can be detected is about 1 to 2 cm. This discrepancy arises partly because the detection of a lesion, such as a tumor, is a pattern recognition process that requires a change in a reasonable number of displayed structural units (in this case the normal liver dot matrix) to be discernible. At least three, and probably five, dots need to be altered in size or intensity before such an irregularity can be confidently detected. An additional factor is the contrast of the lesion; if the change in reflectivity is minor, a larger area must be affected before it is discernible. In practice, 0.5 to 1 cm echogenic lesions can be discerned on high quality scans. Echo-poor lesions are more difficult to detect, both intrinsically and because they simulate blood vessels, and minimal limits are 1 to 2 cm. Optimal scans cannot be obtained in around 5 percent of patients, due to overlying gas or scars, and in obese or muscular subjects. Additionally, certain portions of the liver are difficult to image clearly, even under good conditions. Examples include the anterior surface (due to near field effects and to inaccessibility because of the rib cage), the extreme lateral margin (difficulties of access), and portions of the liver shadowed by the porta hepatis.

Accuracy figures for liver malignancy have been published from several centers using gray scale quipment (Table 1.4) and indicate that 70 to 90 percent of involved livers are correctly predicted, with a small false positive rate. This compares with accuracies of only about 50 percent for older results with bistable equipment.[37] However, these figures should not be taken at face value, partly because of the variable scoring assigned to results. "Accurate results" ranged from a rather vague "clinically useful"[30, 34] to a requirement for precise prediction of histology.[36] Also great difficulties are involved in the assessment of accuracy for any investigative technique in the liver, because there is no acceptable yardstick by which to judge the results. Of the methods that suggest themselves, biopsy is subject to sampling limitations and a negative result is valueless; laparotomy and *a fortiori* laparoscopy are limited to the available surfaces of the liver, and again negative results are unreliable. Angiography, though accurate, is less often performed nowadays.

TABLE 1.4. Accuracy of ultrasound in the detection of focal liver malignancy.

Year	Cases	Fail (%)	TP (%)	TN (%)	FP (%)	FN (%)	Overall accuracy (%)	Note
1973[29]	71	–	63	85	15	26	65	Includes benign focal lesions
1975[30]	120	–	–	–	8		92	
1976[31]	21	–	100	43	57	–		
1976[32]	70	–	93	94	6	7	94	Ca of the breast
1976[9]	350	–	–	–	–	–	90	
1977[33]	30	37	67	93	17	33		Includes benign focal lesions
1978[34]	77	10	–	–	8		87	"Most errors FN"
1978[35]	100	4	83	97	3	11	93	Follow-up for equivocal scintigrams
1979[36]	94	23	75	50	17	10	84	Exact histology* required for TP
1980[24]	26	4	67	100	0	36	92	Ca of the ovary

*TP + FN and TN + FP should = 100%; where this is not true one presumes that failures have been included in the calculation.

Notes:[37] True positive: $\frac{\text{disease detected}}{\text{all diseased cases}}$ = sensitivity

True negative: $\frac{\text{normal result}}{\text{all normal cases}}$ = specificity

False positive: $\frac{\text{disease detected}}{\text{all normal cases}}$

False negative: $\frac{\text{normal result}}{\text{all diseased cases}}$

Overall accuracy: $\frac{\text{TN + TP cases}}{\text{total cases}}$

Autopsy is ultimately reliable but cannot be used for assessing the techniques in early disease where they are most needed. Examiners have been obliged to resort to a combination of techniques to define the abnormals in their series. For normals presumptive diagnostic and clinical follow-up evidence have been used. The other factor to be borne in mind is that metastatic disease is usually multiple; *in vitro* data suggest that ultrasound may correctly detect liver involvement more often than it detects single lesions.[39] Experienced sonographers are familiar with the embarrassing situation of being unable to demonstrate a deposit shown to be present at a recent laparotomy, and comparison with CT shows that, on occasion, even large lesions readily demonstrated with one technique cannot be detected by the other.

The specificity of ultrasound for focal lesions in the liver is considered to be good, but it is by no means perfect.[36] It is usually able to discern confusing normal variants, and it is helpful in differentiating true liver pathology from adjacent mass lesions.[40] It is usually reliable in distinguishing cystic from solid lesions, but some examples of confusing malignancies have been referred to. For solid lesions there are difficult differential diagnostic problems as between abscesses, hematomata, hemangiomata, adenomata, and malignant tumor. The use of guided biopsies with a 23-gauge "skinny needle" for cytology is helpful in many of these problems,[41] but should be used with due caution in any lesion that might be hemorrhagic (hemangioma, estrogen adenoma).

Experience with ultrasound in hepatocellular carcinoma is too limited to assess its accuracy here. Well-defined lesions are easily detected, and their extent within the liver can be defined to assist in planning possible surgical resection. The diffuse varieties are more difficult ultrasonic problems. Ultrasound is helpful in differentiating cold lesions seen on scintigraphy in cirrhosis, since the commoner regenerating nodules are acoustically unremarkable, whereas tumors show textural alteration.

Comparison with Other Investigations

Ultrasound can detect smaller tumors than either scintigraphy or CT scanning. It also offers higher specificity than scintigraphy, but is more labor intensive, fails to produce diagnostic images in some patients, and does not easily image the whole liver. For these reasons, the overall accuracy of scintigraphy in detecting space-occupying lesions is of the same order in practice. Ultrasound is particularly valuable in elucidating equivocal areas on the scintigram; these are often due to normal variations that are obvious on ultrasound. In addition, when the scintigram is normal, subsequent sonography is unlikely to detect focal disease.[35] When a lesion is awkwardly placed (e.g., anterior subcapsular, extreme lateral surface of right lobe), a scintigram is useful in directing the attention of the sonographer to the region of suspicion.

Gallium concentrates slightly in normal liver. It is taken up strongly by inflammatory lesions but not by other nonmalignant diseases.[42] Uptake into malignant tumors is variable, being the rule in hepatocellular carcinoma but less regular in metastases. It has found moderate use in differentiating cold lesions found on colloid scintigraphy and is especially helpful in distinguishing cirrhotic nodules from malignant change.

The demonstration of tumors in the liver using CT requires views before and after contrast enhancement,[40] which makes the examination time-consuming. Computed tomography is properly reserved for problem cases in which ultrasound is of no help, as in technical failures and cases where a major management decision rests on excluding involvement in the liver or in part of it, as to where a solitary metastasis is to be excised. Since some lesions, even large ones, are inapparent on one of these techniques but obvious on the other, critical regions may need to be examined by both ultrasound and

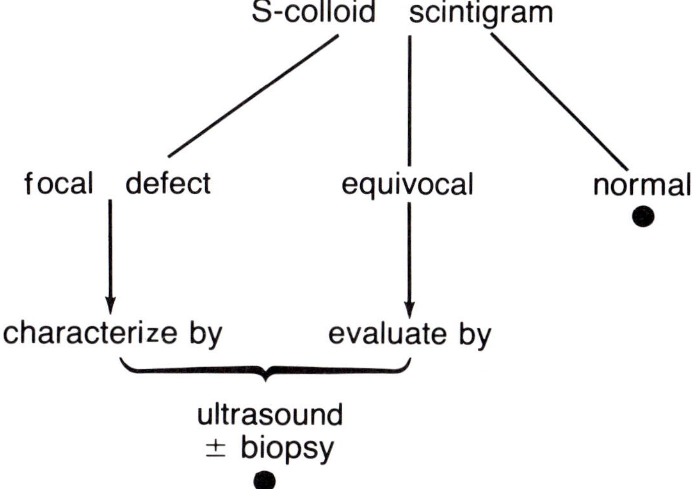

FIGURE 1.11. Algorithm for "liver metastases."
Note 1. A normal scintigram should be followed by an ultrasound or CT exam if the index of suspicion is high.
Note 2. When exclusion of liver metastasis is crucial to management (e.g. consideration for partial resection) a normal ultrasound should be followed up with CT and angiography.

CT. Specificity for CT has been reported as higher than that of ultrasound, enabling more accurate differentiation between benign and malignant focal disease, although a 23 percent failure rate for ultrasound in this series is worse than that currently achieved at most centers.[36]

Arteriography is probably the most sensitive test for liver metastases, but there are difficulties in differentiating regenerating nodules from neoplastic masses. Its invasive nature restricts its value, but it can be used to perfuse lesions. Chemotherapeutic drugs and embolization, using gels or fibrin, have specific uses in pain relief and in bleeding lesions.

Serum biochemistry, though nonspecific, remains most useful in screening. Few cases with liver metastases detectable by noninvasive imaging have normal liver tests, the alkaline phosphatase being the most reliable.[18] Alphafetoprotein has a special role in the diagnosis and monitoring of hepatocellular carcinoma.

CLINICAL ROLE OF ULTRASOUND

In the detection and characterization of focal liver disease of all types, ultrasound is generally regarded as the most sensitive and specific of the available noninvasive techniques. Where a histologic diagnosis is required, ultrasound directed biopsy (using a Menghini needle for a tissue core to give histology or a 23-gauge Chiba needle for cytology) is readily performed and greatly increases the success rate. Nevertheless the labor intensiveness of ultrasound is a handicap for routine screening studies, if only because the sonographer may have difficulty in giving full attention and best services when there is prior assumption that an abnormality is unlikely to be discovered. The difficult-to-image areas of the liver add to this problem. Therefore, ultrasound is better used as a problem-solving technique, leaving routine screening to scintigraphy. Abnormal and equivocal cases are then referred for sonography. When the index of suspicion for liver malignancy is high, the patient should be referred for sonography, even when the scintigram is negative. However, it is recommended that scintigraphy be performed first in any case, since it may provide the sonographer with valuable clues (Fig. 1.11).[35]

Computed tomography, then, is reserved for cases in which ultrasound is not helpful, such as technical failures, or where a strong clinical suspicion is not corroborated by a sonogram. In addition, CT is recommended for those cases in which a critical decision rests on the exclusion of disease and in whom ultrasound is negative.[42-44]

Arteriography is valuable where the precise vascular relationships of a tumor need to be defined before surgery, or where intraarterial chemotherapy or embolization is considered.

References

1. Stanley P, Gates GF, Eto RT, et al: Hepatic cavernous haemangiomas and haemangioendotheliomas in infancy. Am J Roentgenol 129:317–319, 1977.
2. Wiener SN, Parulekar SG: Scintigraphy and ultrasonography of hepatic haemangioma. Radiology 132:149–153, 1979.
3. Freeny PC, Vimont TR, Barnett DC: Cavernous haemangioma of the liver: Ultrasonography, arteriography and CT. Radiology 132:143–145, 1979.
4. Gates GF: Atlas of Abdominal Ultrasonography in Children. Edinburgh, Churchill Livingstone, 1978.
5. Spiegel RM, King DL, Green WM: Ultrasonography of primary cysts of the liver. Am J Radiol, 131:235–238, 1978.
6. Cosgrove DO: Liver tumours. In: Ultrasound in Tumour Diagnosis, eds. Hill CR, McCready VR, Cosgrove DO. London, Pitman Medical, 1978.
7. Casarella WJ, Knowles DM, Wolff M, Johnson PM: Focal nodular hyperplasia and liver cell adenoma: Radiological and pathological differentiation. Am J Roentgenol 131: 393–402, 1978.
8. Miller JH, Gates GF, Stanley P: Radiological investigation of hepatic tumours in childhood. Radiology 124:451–458, 1977.
9. Taylor KJW, Carpenter DA, Hill CR, McCready VR: Grey scale ultrasound imaging-the liver. Radiology 119:415–420, 1976.
10. Prando A, Goldstein HM, Bernadino ME: Ultrasonic pseudolesions in the liver. Radiology 130:403–405, 1979.
11. Sears HF, Gerber FH, Sturtz DL, Fouty WJ: Liver scans and carcinoma of the breat. Surg Gynecol Obstet 140:409–411, 1975.
12. Ariel IM, Molander D, Galey M: Hepatic gamma scanning—an aid in determining treatment policies for carcinoma involving the liver. Am J Surg 118:5–7, 1969.
13. Ultmann JE: The management of lymphoma. Semin Haematol 7:441–460, 1970.

14. Levitan R, Diamond HD, Craver LF: The liver in Hodgkin's disease. Gut 2:60–65, 1961.
15. Bell JW: Abdominal exploration in 100 lung carcinoma suspects prior to thoracotomy. Ann Surg 167:199–203, 1967.
16. Conn HO, Yesner R: A re-evaluation of needle biopsy in the diagnosis of metastatic carcinoma of the liver. Ann Intern Med 59:53–61, 1963.
17. Davies RJ, Vernon M, Croft DN: Liver snaps and the detection of clinically unsuspected liver metastases. Lancet 1:279–280, 1974.
18. Carvalho N, Harbert JC, de Leiva AH, et al: The gastrointestinal system, Ch. 4. In: Textbook of Nuclear Medicine—Clinical Applications, eds. Rocha AFG, Harbert JC. Philadelphia, Lea and Febiger, 1979.
19. Weill FS: Ultrasonography of Digestive Diseases. St Louis, Mosby, 1978.
20. Scheible W, Gosink BB, Leopold GR: Grey scale echographic patterns of hepatic metastatic disease. Am J Roentgenol 129:983–985, 1977.
21. Meire HB: Grey scale echographic appearances of liver metastases. In: Ultrasound in Medicine, vol 3, ed. White DN. New York, Plenum Press, 1977, pp 315–319.
22. Green B, Bree RL, Goldstein HM, Stanley C: Grey scale ultrasound evaluation of hepatic neoplasms. Radiology 124:203–205, 1977.
23. Kamin PD, Bernadino ME, Green B: Ultrasonic manifestations of hepatocellular carcinoma. Radiology 131:459–461, 1979.
24. Pussell SJ, Cosgrove DO, Wiltshaw E, et al: Carcinoma of the ovary: Correlation of ultrasound with second look laparotomy. Br J Obstet Gynaecol, 1980, in press.
25. Cosgrove DO, McCready VR: Diffuse metastatic disease in the liver. In: Ultrasound in Medicine, vol 3a, eds. White DN, Barnes RE. New York, Plenum Press, 1977.
26. Rubatelli L, del Maschio A,: Hepatic metastases: Experimental ultrasound, microradiography and histological study (Abstr). WFUMB, Tokyo, Scimed Publishing Inc, 1979, p 114.
27. Joseph AEA, Dewbury KC, Milward-Sadler GH, Clarke CW: Correlation of histopathology and ultrasonic appearances of liver metastases (abstr). Tenth British Medical Ultrasound Society Annual Meeting, 1978, p 47.
28. Gilby ED, Taylor KJW: Ultrasonic monitoring of hepatic metastases during chemotherapy. Br Med J 1:371–373, 1975.
29. Leyton B, Halpern S, Leopold G, Hagen S: Correlation of ultrasound and colloid scintiscan studies in the liver. J Nuclear Med 14:27–33, 1973.
30. Taylor KJW, Carpenter DA: Comparison of ultrasound and scintigraphy in the diagnosis of hepatobiliary disease. In: Ultrasound in Medicine, vol 1, ed. White DN. New York, Plenum Press, 1975, pp 159–167.
31. McArdle CR: Ultrasonic diagnosis of liver metastases. J Clin Ultrasound 4:265–268, 1976.
32. Smith IE, Taylor KJW, McCready VR, et al: Comparison of grey scale ultrasound with other methods for the detection of liver metastases from breast carcinoma. Clin Oncol 2: 47–53, 1976.
33. Zatz L, Goulding J, Hanley G: Comparison of grey scale ultrasound and radionuclide imaging for the detection of focal hepatic lesions. J Clin Ultrasound 5:178–184, 1977.
34. Cosgrove DO, McCready VR: Diagnosis of liver metastases using ultrasound and isotope scanning techniques. J R Soc Med 71:652–658, 1978.
35. Sullivan DC, Taylor KJW, Gottschalk A: The use of ultrasound to enhance the diagnostic utility of the equivocal liver scintigram. Radiology 128:727–732, 1978.
36. Snow JH, Goldstein HM, Wallace S: Comparison of scintigraphy, sonography and CT in the evaluation of hepatic neoplasms. Am J Roentgenol 132:915–918, 1979.
37. McNeil BJ: Guidelines for evaluating new tests, Ch 13. In: Textbook of Nuclear Medi-

cine—Clinical Applications, eds. Rocha AFG, Harbert JC. Philadelphia, Lea and Febiger, 1979.

38. McCarthy CF, Davies ER, Wells PNT, et al: Comparison of ultrasound and isotope scanning in the diagnosis of liver diseases. Br J Radiol 43:100–109, 1970.
39. King JA, Cosgrove DO, Heyderman E, et al: Post mortem investigation of B scan appearances of malignant liver pathology (abstr). British Medical Ultrasound Society, 10th Annual Meeting, 1978, p 45.
40. Bryan PJ, Dinn WM, Grossman ZD, Wistow BW, McAfee JG, Kieffer SA: Correlation of CT, grey scale ultrasound and radionuclide imaging of the liver in detecting space occupying processes. Radiology 124:387–393, 1977.
41. Ras SN, Holm HH, Kristensen JK, Barlebo H: Ultrasonically guided liver biopsy. Br Med J 2:500–502, 1972.
42. Maze M, Wood J: Uptake of ^{67}Ga in space occupying lesions in the liver. J Nuclear Med 16:443–445, 1975.
43. Baker C, Way LW: Clinical utility of CAT body scans. Am J Surg 136:37–44, 1978.
44. Whalen JP: Radiology of the abdomen: Impact of newer imaging methods. Am J Roentgenol 133:586–619, 1979.

2 Biliary Tract

MICHAEL CRADE
KENNETH J. W. TAYLOR

Tumors of the biliary tract may originate in the gallbladder and cystic duct, or in the bile ducts—intrahepatic, common hepatic, and common bile duct. Most of these tumors are adenocarcinomas, quite unresponsive to therapeutic assaults. Carcinomas of the gallbladder and biliary ducts have distinctive clinical, pathologic, radiologic, and ultrasonic characteristics, which will be considered in the following discussion.

CARCINOMA OF THE GALLBLADDER

Carcinoma of the gallbladder is the fifth most common malignancy of the gastrointestinal tract, comprising 1 to 3 percent of all cancers. The prevalence increases with age, peaking in the 6th or 7th decades, with an age range extending from the fourth to the ninth decades. These tumors occur more frequently in whites than in blacks, and the effective female to male ratio is approximately 4:1. Gallstones are present in 70 to 90 percent of patients with carcinoma of the gallbladder,[1, 2] suggesting a possible etiologic role. Ethnic groups prone to gallstones are also prone to this neoplasm. In view of the apparent association between chronic cholecystitis, gallstones, and carcinoma of the gallbladder, it is interesting that derivatives of cholic acid, a bile component, are some of the most powerful carcinogenic agents known.[3] Other environmental factors, as yet not completely elucidated, appear to increase the prevalence of this tumor in workers in the automotive and rubber industries.[4]

Since stones are found so frequently in patients with gallbladder tumors, prophylactic surgery for cholelithiasis might appear beneficial. However, such a conclusion is contradicted by the study conducted by Wenckert and Robertson.[5] They found abnormal oral cholecystograms (OCGs) in 1,402 patients, only 5 of whom subsequently developed malignancy during the 11 years following. This risk for malignant transformation, which is 0.4 percent, is far less than the overall surgical mortality for acute cholecystitis (1 to 5 percent), but comparable with mortality due to surgery on the asymptomatic patient.[2]

Pathologically, carcinomas of the gallbladder occur in two patterns: infiltrating or fungating. Most involve the fundus or neck of the gallbladder, and only about 20 percent involve the side walls.[3] The infiltrating type is more common, diffusely thickening and indurating the gallbladder wall. If its growth is not checked, it erodes into the liver. Ulceration of the center of the tumor may produce a fistula into an adjacent viscus.

The fungating tumor protrudes into the lumen of the gallbladder as an irregular cauliflower-like mass that invades the underlying walls simultaneously. By the time of diagnosis, most of these tumors have invaded the liver centrifugally, and many have extended to obstruct the cystic duct, common bile duct, and periportal lymph nodes, producing obstructive jaundice. In contrast to many tumors of the extrahepatic biliary tree, tumors of the gallbladder tend to be relatively asymptomatic until an advanced stage of local spread.[2] Most patients present with either nonspecific symptoms, mimicking an exacerbation of chronic cholecystitis, or with a palpable tumor mass in the right upper quadrant, often involving the pancreas, stomach, and adjacent liver. If the cystic duct is occluded by tumor, bile is replaced by a mucinous secretion called white bile and produces a hydrops of the gallbladder. This is a nonspecific occurrence associated with occlusion of the cystic duct by any mechanism.

Histologically over 90 percent of these tumors are adenocarcinomas, most of which are well differentiated; occasionally anaplastic tumors occur. Less commonly (in approximately 5 percent of these patients), squamous cell tumors arise, presumably by metaplastic differentiation of the columnar lining of the gallbladder.[6]

The mean survival of patients with carcinoma of the gallbladder is less than 5 months from the time of diagnosis. Only 3 or 4 percent live for 5 years or more, and virtually all of these patients have tumors that were so small at surgery they were missed on gross examination. Only meticulous histologic sections of the gallbladder specimen reveal the tumor. Even when tumor is found fortuitously and considered to be resectable at the time of surgery, only 3 percent of patients have a significant survival.[7]

Unlike cholangiocarcinomas, with gallbladder cancers metastatic lesions usually spread widely throughout the liver substance even when the primary tumor appears to be well localized. The rich venous and lymphatic channels are said to account for this. While the feasibility of right hepatic lobectomy has been called "illogical" by Bismuth and Malt,[8] Adson reported 10 patients who survived for up to 12 years after the gallbladder, adjacent liver tumor, and involved lymph nodes were successfully resected.[2]

Radiologic studies have been of limited value in making an early diagnosis, which is the only way to improve prognosis in these patients. The finding of a "wall defect" on a contrast study may be due to impacted stones or even benign tumors, so that this finding lacks specificity. Similarly, nonvisualization of the gallbladder by oral cholecystography is a nonspecific finding, not necessarily related to gallbladder pathology. However, with calcification of the gallbladder wall, gallbladder carcinoma develops often enough to merit prophylactic surgery in patients with these so-called porcelain gallbladders. The number of patients developing such gallbladder tumors with this radiographic marker is small.[9]

Ultrasound and Gallbladder Tumors

Whenever a patient is evaluated by ultrasound for gallbladder disease, the possibility of an occult neoplasm should be considered. Recent reports have greatly expanded our appreciation of the varied ultrasonic appearances of this neoplasm. Similar changes may be seen in patients with inflammatory conditions only. Thus, accurate differentiation between inflammatory and neoplastic changes of the gallbladder appears to be impossible by ultrasound.

Olken[10] reported an extremely unusual patient with an intraluminal mass visualized by cholecystography and ultrasound, which proved to be a neoplasm with a local nodal metastasis, correctly predicted by the ultrasonologist. Phillips[11] reported five patients with intraluminal malignant masses that were all imaged by ultrasound and appeared to be more echogenic than the surrounding wall. Yeh's review[12] of 14 patients with such neoplasms included 3 with protruding wall irregularities, and 5 in whom a diffusely thickened wall was demonstrated by ultrasound. These same appearances have been noted repeatedly when inflammatory changes are present,[13-18] and may possibly be mimicked by normal wall contractions after a fatty meal.[18]

When tumor produces gross thickening of the gallbladder wall and obliterates the lumen, a contracted echogenic organ may be imaged. Shadowing from retained stones may also occur.

Case History

A 76-year-old female with a history of right upper quadrant pain was admitted for a routine cholecystectomy. At surgery a thickened gallbladder containing stones was excised and the patient was discharged. Pathologic examination revealed an adenocarcinoma of the gallbladder, which was not apparent at surgery (Fig. 2.1).

Yeh[12] reported two patients with such findings. However, identical appearances are found in patients with chronic cholecystitis and cholelithiasis so that these findings are nonspecific for either condition. As yet, there have been no reported instances where curative cancer surgery has been prompted by the specific findings of ultrasound examination. When tumor growth is advanced, the ultrasonic findings of a complex right upper-quadrant mass have been reported.[11, 12, 19]

Case History

An 80-year-old male presented with a palpable right upper-quadrant mass. A complex tumor mass is seen on ultrasound (Fig. 2.2a), indistinguishable from

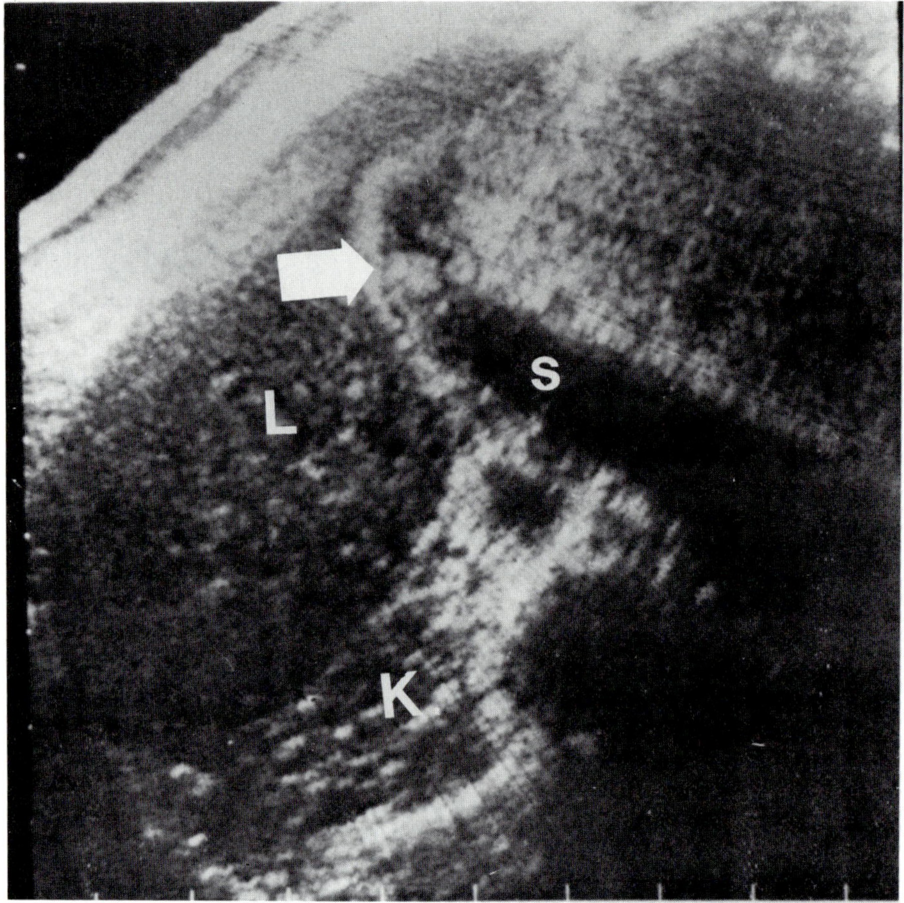

FIGURE 2.1. Shadowing (S) from stones within a small gallbladder (arrow) was noted on this transverse ultrasound section, also demonstrating liver (L) and right kidney (K). Although unrecognized at surgery, and not predictable by ultrasound, an adenocarcinoma was found during pathologic examination of the gallbladder.

an inflammatory mass imaged in another patient (Fig. 2.2b). The pathologic appearance of such a tumor is seen in Figure 2.2(c).

BILE DUCT TUMORS

Cholangiocarcinomas account for about 20 percent of all "primary liver tumors," but unlike the more common hepatocellular carcinomas, association with prior cirrhosis or hepatitis is not evident.[20, 21]

Cholangiocarcinomas are more prevalent in American Indians, Mexicans, and Japanese, than in blacks or whites.[4, 21] Ethnic differences may be related in part to an inherited tendency to form lithogenic bile. However, the relation to gallstone formation is not obvious. Although cholelithiasis occurred in 50 percent of patients with bile duct tumors at the Mayo Clinic,[22] in other reports the association was found in only 29 to 30 percent[23, 24] Most authors report a slight predominance of males in the affected population.[21, 23, 25] The affected age range is the 6th and 7th decade, the same as for carcinoma of the gallbladder.

The possibility that bile contains a carcinogenic agent, which is enhanced by relative stasis, inflammation, or turbulence, is suggested by the more common occurrence of bile duct tumors at the junction of ducts,[8] within bile cysts,[1, 26] and in patients with ulcerative colitis,[27] a disease known to be associated with cholangitis. In addition, after cholecystectomy patients appear to be more prone to biliary tree tumors.[23] Other populations at risk include workers in the automotive and rubber industries,[4] and those infected with liver flukes, particularly in Asia.[8]

These tumors are almost invariably very small, with few metastases because of their early presentation due to obstructive jaundice. Histologically, these lesions are almost invariably adenocarcinomas.

Early clinical misdiagnosis is frequent,[25, 27-29] since symptoms are nonspecific and imitate more common benign diseases afflicting a similar age group (50 to 70 years).[25, 29] Indeed, despite the insidious growth, many such tumors present with acute right upper-quadrant pain, biliary colic, jaundice, and loss of weight. It should be noted that necrosis of the tumor may occur with temporary relief of the jaundice so that the clinical presentation may mimic the presence of gallstones. Although jaundice is present in 80 to 100 percent of reported series;[21, 23, 25] 63 percent of the more peripheral intrahepatic lesions may present prior to the onset of jaundice.[21] At such times, only abnormalities of the liver enzymes may indicate the presence of disease. Pruritis occurs in 28 percent of patients, malaise in 15 percent, abdominal pain in 38 percent, and fever in 17 percent.[24] These may simulate the symptoms of cholecystitis, common duct stones, benign stricture, sclerosing cholangitis, and pancreatic tumors. Since cholangiocarcinomas promote a fibroblastic reaction, misdiagnosis as a benign stricture, or sclerosing cholangitis, may occur, even at surgery, or on histologic diagnosis. Fibrosis may predominate almost to the exclusion of neoplastic cells.[24, 25, 28]

McDermott,[30] summarizing a 15-year experience with tumors of the bile ducts, reported 34 such patients. The anatomic distribution was: hepatic ducts, 15 percent; common hepatic duct, 35 percent; midcommon bile duct, 32 percent; and periampullary, 15 percent. Surgically, the periampullary tumors form a subgroup that is clinically, and even histologically, indistinguishable and comprise tumors derived from the common bile duct, pancreas, and duodenum. Those derived from the common bile duct constitute only 8 percent of this group of tumors. Approximately half of these patients were resectable at the time of diagnosis, and the average survival time after operation was 27 months.

Longmire and his associates classified tumors of the common bile duct into three categories, according to site: lower, middle, and upper thirds.[31] This classification is helpful in many respects. To the surgeon, the location of the

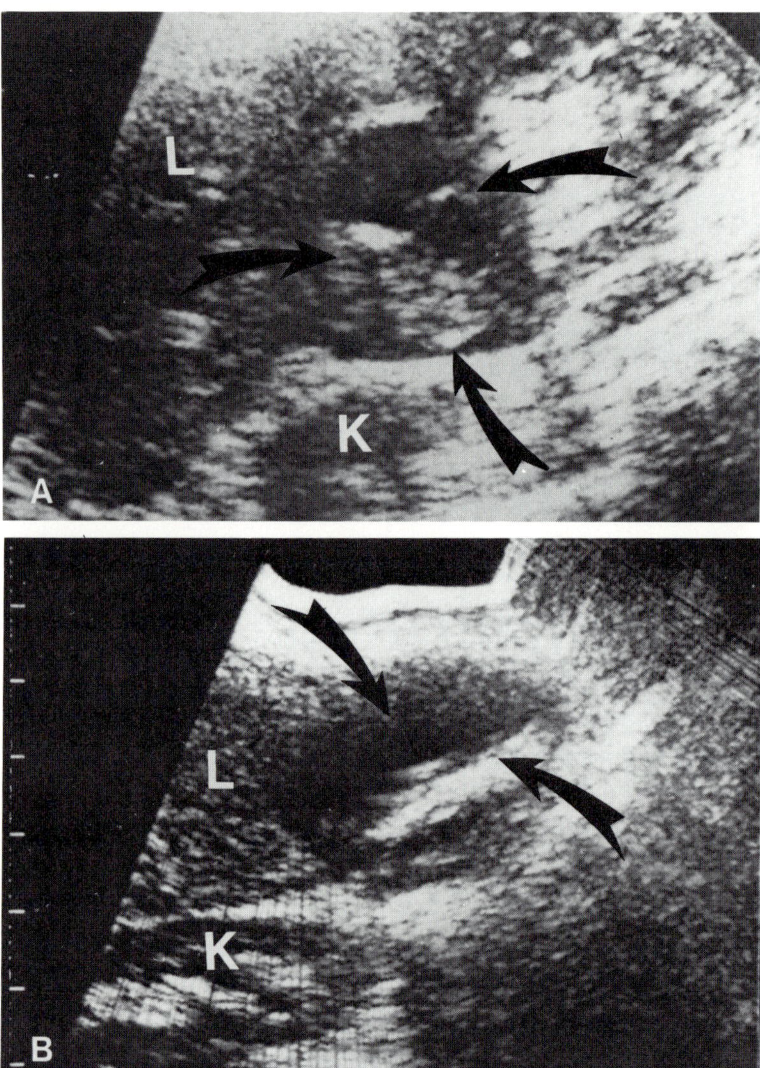

FIGURE 2.2. (a) An adenocarcinoma was imaged as an ultrasonically complex mass (arrows) protruding from the right upper quadrant towards the midline on the transverse scan. Liver = L; right Kidney = K. (b) A similarly complex mass (arrows) replacing the normal boundaries of the gallbladder is seen on this longitudinal scan. This proved to be an abscess, free of tumor. Liver = L; right kidney = K.

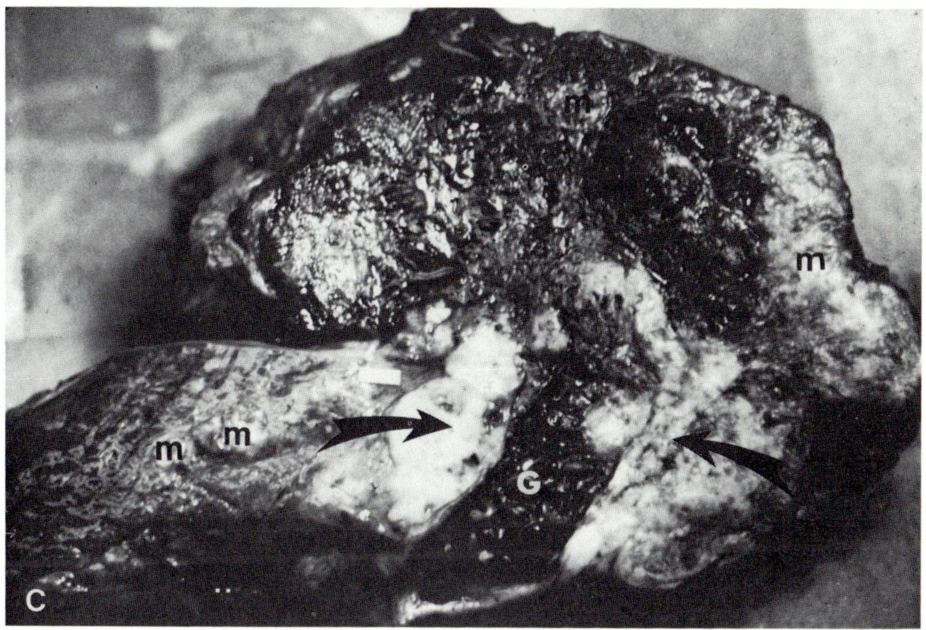

FIGURE 2.2. (c) Pathologic specimen demonstrates the widespread liver metastases (M) from the gallbladder primary adenocarcinoma (arrows) growing into adjacent hepatic parenchyma. Stones fill the gallbladder lumen (G).

tumor is of paramount importance in planning therapy. Tumors in the middle and lower extrahepatic biliary system seem to benefit more from aggressive resection when possible.

Authors have reported a mean survival time of only 11 months, which is only 6 months better than unresectable involvement.[23] Sporadic cures have been reported in this group of patients as well, especially when early lesions are discovered, usually by chance, during routine gallbladder surgery. Ross[24] reported a survival of 5½ years for a patient whose common bile duct tumor was unexpectedly found during cholecystectomy.[6] Tsunekana[32] reviewed 13 similar "survivors" and emphasized the need for compulsive and careful imaging of the biliary tree when elevated serum alkaline phosphatase levels indicate early cholestasis.[32]

When tumors occur in the upper third of the common bile duct, involvement of biliary structures, portal vein, or hepatic artery make resection more difficult, and choledochojejunostomy frequently not feasible.[33]

The most proximal lesions, described by Klatskin, may represent tumors that grow more slowly and are less likely to have metastasized widely. Patients with these tumors benefit from decompression; they survive for approximately 23 months after the obstruction is relieved, but only about 10 months without decompression.[33, 34]

Reports from Japan further emphasize the importance of early diagnosis of

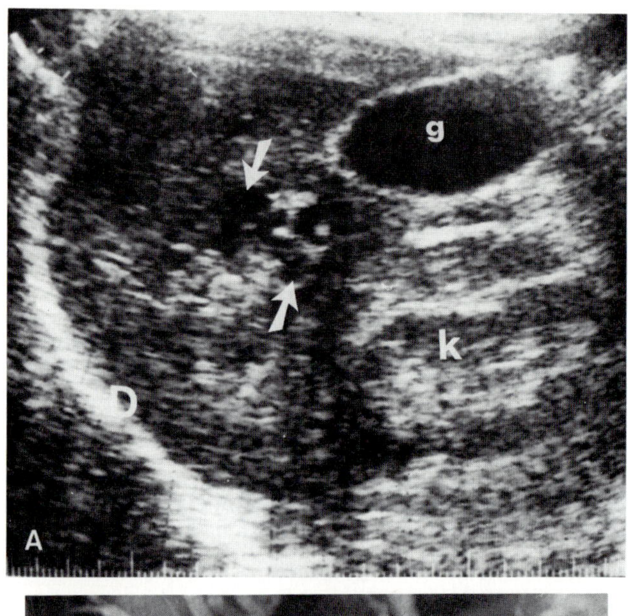

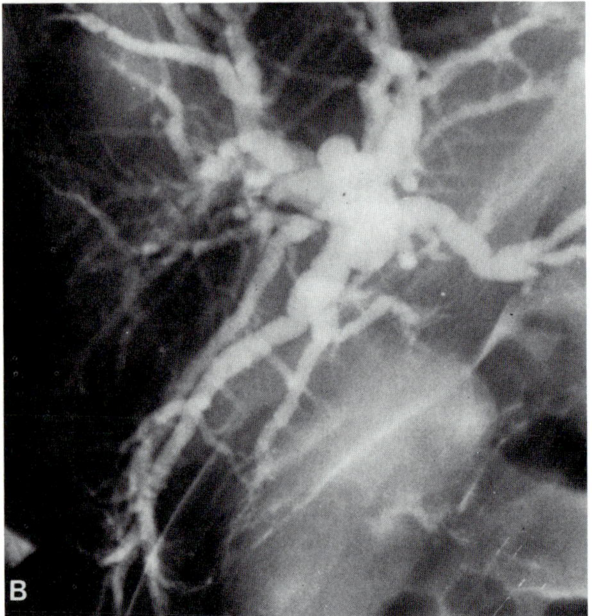

FIGURE 2.3. (a) Longitudinal scan through the right lobe of liver demonstrates proximal biliary tree dilatation (arrows), while other scans through the left lobe were normal. Gallbladder = G; right kidney = K; diaphram = D. (b) Transhepatic cholangiogram demonstrates the dilated and obstructed right hepatic ducts.

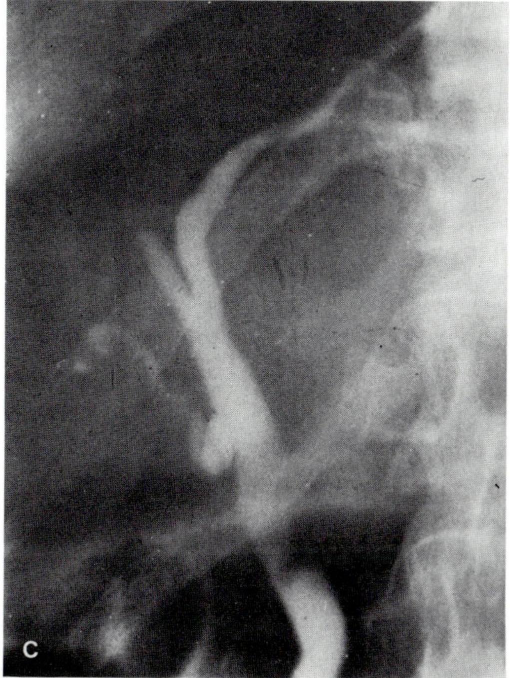

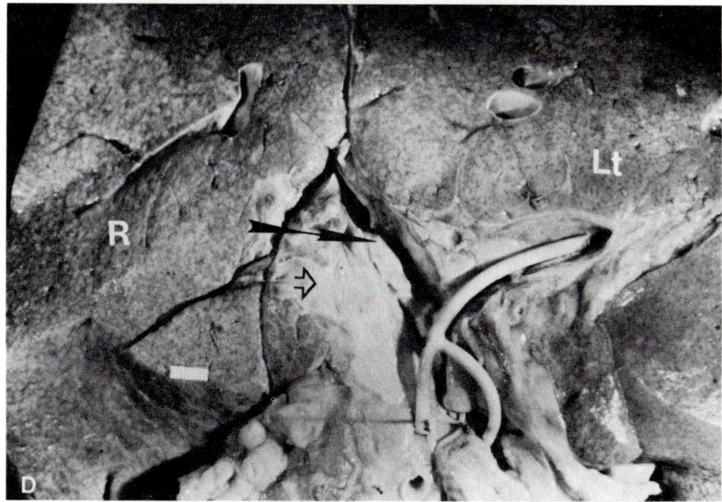

FIGURE 2.3. (c) The ERCP shows the localized obstruction of the right hepatic duct and the patent left ductal system, confirming the ultrasonic impression. (d) The obstructing cholangiocarcinoma (large arrow) accompanied by a proliferation of fibrotic tissue (arrowhead) was noted at the time of this patient's autopsy. A drainage catheter had been placed into the uninvolved left hepatic duct in an attempt to ensure continued patency. Right lobe liver = R; left lobe = Lt.

these proximal biliary tumors. Okuda[21] documented survival up to 3 years and 7 months.

Case History

A 70-year-old male underwent routine medical examination and the only abnormality was an isolated elevation of serum alkaline phosphatase. Ultrasound examination revealed dilatation of the right biliary ducts with a normal system on the left (Fig. 2.3a). Transhepatic percutaneous cholangiography confirmed the presence of dilated ducts, although only the right side was opacified (Fig. 2.3b). ERCP demonstrated non-filling of the right duct and a nondilated left duct (Fig. 2.3c). At surgery a small fibrotic tumor was found and the biliary system drained. After a rapid recovery and discharge from hospital, the patient was admitted in extremis and died. Postmortem examination showed a massive pulmonary embolus. The obstructing tumor is shown in Figure 2.3(d).

CURRENT APPLICATIONS OF ULTRASOUND IN THE DIAGNOSIS OF BILIARY TRACT TUMORS

Since tumors of the biliary tract present early with obstructive jaundice, the application of ultrasound for their diagnosis is essentially one of investigating the jaundiced patient. Many studies have reported the value of ultrasound for this application. The ultrasonic criterion of biliary duct obstruction is dilatation of the ducts proximal to that occlusion. In a review in the New England Journal of Medicine, Bismuth and Malt,[8] concluded that ultrasound "was the most sensitive noninvasive method to discriminate between obstructive jaundice and other forms of the disease." The largest series available to date is of 275 patients from this institution, in which jaundice due to extrahepatic obstruction was differentiated from that due to hepatocellular disease with an accuracy of 96%. The ability to detect obstruction at an early stage has now resulted in the possibility of diagnosing biliary obstruction by early tumors even before the onset of jaundice.[35]

Despite this sensitivity to the presence of extrahepatic obstruction, it is difficult to localize the anatomic site of obstruction and detect its cause by ultrasound alone. In our series, the precise anatomic site and cause of obstruction were delineated in only 55 percent of patients. The remaining 45 percent with obstruction are not diagnostic errors; we are aware of the limitations of ultrasound, and patients can be evaluated further by other diagnostic procedures, such as ERCP.

In our study of 275 jaundiced patients, 11 had carcinoma of the common bile duct. Dilated ducts were seen in all patients, correctly indicating the presence of extrahepatic biliary obstruction, but the tumor was not visualized in any patient.

Other authors have reported similar experiences. Koeningsberg[36] reviewed 32 patients with obstructive jaundice; only 2 had cholangiocarcinomas. Ultrasound indicated biliary dilatation and the anatomic level, but one was considered to be a pancreatic tumor. Chu, Cosgrove, and McCready located the site of the obstruction precisely in only 60 percent of their patients with obstruction.[37] Of 8 patients with biliary duct tumors, 2 showed identifiable masses, while 6 other tumors were inferred because of biliary dilatation.

Neiman and Mintzer[38] successfully imaged the common bile duct in 65 percent of their 30 patients and were able to identify the anatomic level of the obstruction in 73 percent of those successfully visualized. Morris[39] identified 13 of 25 obstructive lesions.[27]

In a recent paper by Gold,[40] ultrasound was only 72 percent accurate in distinguishing the presence of a dilated biliary tract; the site of obstruction was defined in only 47 percent and the etiology predicted in 37 percent. In contrast, transhepatic cholangiography was 100 percent accurate in all applications. However, the limited success at recognizing dilated ducts compared with all other reports must raise some doubts about the adequacy of their ultrasound experience.

Expectations for Earlier Diagnosis

Since the anatomic site of biliary tract tumors is so important to the surgeon, the radiologist must make every effort to predict this preoperatively by currently available diagnostic procedures, including ultrasound, CT, transhepatic cholangiography (THC), or ERCP. For ultrasound alone, this may prove to be difficult or impossible. Even when the site of obstruction is found, the etiology may not be determined, since the appearance of metastatic disease, pancreatic or bile duct tumors, may be identical. Where a mass is visualized, its histology can be determined by percutaneous skinny needle biopsy under ultrasonic or computerized tomographic guidance. So many tumors of the gallbladder and bile ducts present with obstructive jaundice, that a biliary bypass procedure is necessary and allows open biopsy. However, the spread of percutaneous biliary bypass procedures may preclude the need for open surgery in patients with extensive tumors and in those with evidence of distant spread.

In conclusion, ultrasound remains a valuable tool in the initial evaluation of patients suspected of having bile duct tumors and has the following advantages:

1. Ultrasound is the most sensitive technique to detect obstructive biliary dilatation, and allows simultaneous search of the liver and adjacent viscera for metastatic lesions, at times disclosing totally unsuspected pathology. To document the spread of tumor, CT is also valuable, especially when ultrasound is hampered by air in overlying gut.

2. When early distal lesions of the bile ducts have caused only dilatation of the extrahepatic ducts, transhepatic cholangiography may be unsuccessful, since the small caliber of the intrahepatic bile ducts make them difficult to cannulate.[41, 42] Repeated failure to opacify intrahepatic bile ducts may be falsely reassuring. Ultrasound, however, can be used as an accurate means to

document the caliber of the extrahepatic bile ducts, thereby prompting earlier diagnosis of obstructing lesions.

3. For patients with elevated serum alkaline phosphatase, ultrasound localizes unilateral biliary dilatation. Such patients are especially benefited by earlier diagnosis, although these Klatskin tumors do appear to have a better prognosis than tumors arising in other anatomic sites.

As clinical confidence in ultrasound techniques grows and our experience expands, more patients with biliary tract tumors should be discovered at a resectable stage. Ultrasound is presently one of the more hopeful devices for the earlier diagnosis of these tumors.

Acknowledgments

The author gratefully acknowledges the able editorial advice and technical assistance of Robin Charney, Janina Frankel, Bari Prince, and Vivian Carter in the preparation of this manuscript.

References

1. Fraumeni JF: Cancer of the pancreas and biliary tree: Epidemiological considerations. Cancer Res 35:3437–3446, 1975.
2. Adson MA: Carcinoma of the gallbladder. Surg Clin N Am 53:12-3-1215, 1973.
3. Robbins SL: The Liver and Biliary Tract. Pathologic Basis of Disease, Philadelphia, WB Saunders Co, 1974, p. 1050.
4. Krain L: Gallbladder and extrahepatic bile duct carcinoma—analysis of 1808 cases. Geriatrics 12:111–117, 1972.
5. Wenckert A, Robertson B: The natural course of gallstone disease. Gastroenterology 50: 376–381, 1966.
6. Spiro HM: Tumors. In: Clinical Gastroenterology. Toronto, The MacMillan Co, 1970, p 777.
7. Piehler JM, Crichlow RC: Primary carcinoma of the gallbladder. Surg Gynecol Obstet 147:929–942, 1978.
8. Bismuth H, Malt RA: Current concepts in cancer—carcinoma of the biliary tree. N Engl J Med 301:704–706, 1979.
9. Berk RN, Armbruster TG, Saltzstein SL: Carcinoma in the porcelain gallbladder. Radiology 106:29–31, 1973.
10. Olken SM, Bledsoe R, Newmark H: The ultrasonic diagnosis of primary carcinoma of the gallbladder. Radiology 129:481–482, 1978.
11. Phillips G, Goodman J, Robinson K, et al: Ultrasonic evaluation of carcinoma of the gallbladder. Proceedings of the Annual Meeting of the American Institute of Ultrasound in Medicine, August, 1979, Montreal, Canada, Paper 347.
12. Yeh H: Ultrasonography and computed tomography of carcinoma of the gallbladder. Radiology 133:167–173, 1979.
13. Mindell HJ, Ring BA: Gallbladder wall thickening: Ultrasonic findings. Radiology 133: 699–701, 1979.
14. Marchal G, Crolla D, Baert AL, et al: Gallbladder visualized by gray scale cholecystosonography. J Clin Ultrasound 6:177–179, 1978.

15. Crade M, Taylor KJW, Rosenfield AT, et al: Ultrasonic imaging of pericholecystic inflammation. J Am Med Assoc (in press).
16. Bergman AB, Neiman HL, Kraut B: Ultrasonic evaluation of pericholecystitic abscess. Am J Roentgenol 133:201–203, 1979.
17. Kane RA: Ultrasonographic diagnosis of gangrenous cholecystitis and empyema of the gallbladder. Radiology 134:191–194, 1980.
18. Handler SJ: Ultrasound of gallbladder wall thickening and its relation to cholecystitis. Am J Roentgenol 132:581–585, 1979.
19. Crade M, Taylor KJW, Rosenfield AT, et al: The varied ultrasonic character of gallbladder tumor. JAMA 241:2195–2196, 1979.
20. Patton RB, Horn RC Jr: Primary liver carcinoma. Autopsy study of 60 cases. Cancer 17: 757–768, 1961.
21. Okuda K, Kubo Y, Okazaki N, et al: Clinical aspects of intrahepatic bile duct carcinoma including hilar carcinoma. A study of 57 autopsy proven cases. Cancer 39:232–246, 1977.
22. Neibling HA, Dockerty MB, Waugh JM: Carcinoma of the extrahepatic bile ducts. Review of the literature and report of six cases. Surgery 41:416, 1957.
23. Andersson A, Bergdahl L, Van der Linden W: Malignant tumors of the extrahepatic bile ducts. Surgery 81:198–202, 1977.
24. Ross AP, Braasch JW, Warren KW: Carcinoma of the proximal bile ducts. Surg Gynecol Obstet 136:923–928, 1973.
25. Braasch JW: Carcinoma of the bile ducts. Surg Clin N Am 53:1217–1227, 1973.
26. Kagawa Y, Kashihara S, Kuramoto S, et al: Carcinoma in a congenitally dilated biliary tract: Report of a case and review of the literature. Gastroenterology 74:1286–1294, 1978.
27. Akwari OE, Van Heerden JA, Foulk WT, Baggenstoss AH: Cancer of the bile ducts associated with ulcerative colitis. Ann Surg 181:303–309, 1975.
28. Lord Smith Marlow: Obstructions of the bile duct. Br J Surg 66:69–79, 1979.
29. Spiro HM: Tumors. In: Clinical Gastroenterology. Toronto, MacMillan Co, 1970, p 779.
30. McDermott WV, Peinert RA: Carcinoma in the supra-ampullary portion of the bile ducts. Surg Gynecol Obstet 149:681–686, 1979.
31. Longmire WB Jr, McArthur MS, Bastounis EA, Hiatt J: Carcinoma of extrahepatic biliary tract. Ann Surg 178:333–345, 1973.
32. Tsunekawa H, Suga S, Miyata K, Shimaji T: A case of carcinoma of the common bile ducts, diagnosed at the non-icteric stage of disease. Gastroenterol Jap 12:490–494, 1974.
33. Cahow CE: Intrahepatic cholangiojejunostomy: A simplified approach. Am J Surg 137: 443–447, 1979.
34. Klatskin G: Adenocarcinoma of the hepatic duct at its bifurcation within the porta hepatis. An unusual tumor with distinctive clinical and pathological features. Am J Med 38: 241–256, 1965.
35. Taylor KJW, Rosenfield AT, Spiro HM: Diagnostic accuracy of gray scale ultrasonography for the jaundiced patient—A report of 275 cases. Arch Intern Med 139:60–63, 1979.
36. Koeningsberg M, Wiener JN, Walzer A: The accuracy of sonography in the differential diagnosis of obstructive jaundice: A comparison with cholangiography. Radiology 133: 157–165, 1979.
37. Chu JMG, Cosgrove DO, McCready VR: Ultrasonic tomography of the liver: Non invasive method of choice for differential diagnosis of jaundice. Aust N Z J Med 8:615–619, 1978.
38. Neiman HL, Mintler RA: Accuracy of biliary ultrasound: Comparison with cholangiography. Am J Roentgenol 129:979–982, 1977.
39. Morris A, Fawcitt RA, Wood R, et al: Computed tomography, ultrasound and cholestatic jaundice. Gut 19:685–688, 1978.

40. Gold RP, Casarella WJ, Stern G, Seaman WB: Transhepatic cholangiography: The radiological method of choice in suspected obstructive jaundice. Radiology 133:39–44, 1979.
41. Levine E, Maklad NF, Wright CH, Lee KR: Computed tomographic and ultrasonic appearance of primary carcinoma of the bile duct. Gastrointestinal Radiol 4:147–151, 1979.
42. Jacques PF, Mauro MA, Scatliff JH: The failed transhepatic cholangiogram. Radiology 134:33–35, 1980.

3 Pancreas

DAVID P. WEINSTEIN
BARBARA J. WEINSTEIN

The incidence of pancreatic cancer has tripled in the United States in the last 40 years. It is now the fourth most common cause of death from cancer. The 5-year survival is one of the lowest, being less than 1 percent, with 97 percent of the patients dying within 1 year. Despite recent advances in diagnosis, no improvement in survival has been achieved. Ultrasound provides a safe, noninvasive means to evaluate the pancreas for the presence of tumor, and information regarding nonresectability is often obtained. In view of the alarming increase in incidence and the bleak outlook in this disease, it is important that the ultrasonographic manifestations of pancreatic cancer be learned in order to achieve rapid and accurate diagnoses, thereby minimizing expense and suffering.

Several excellent reviews of pancreatic cancer have been published recently, covering epidemiology, incidence, clinical features, laboratory diagnosis, and treatment.[1-4] The ultrasound diagnosis of pancreatic disease has recently been presented in this series by Sample and Sarti, and by Simeone and Simonds.[5,6] The authors recommend reviewing this information as background material for this chapter, which will cover the application of ultrasound to the diagnosis of pancreatic cancer.

ADENOCARCINOMA

Adenocarcinoma is the most common variety of pancreatic cancer, representing 95 percent of cases. The pertinent clinical and pathologic features of this disease are listed in Table 3.1. The ultrasonic features of adenocarcinoma are listed in Tables 3.2 and 3.3.

The ultrasonic texture of adenocarcinoma is less echogenic than normal pancreas, allowing clear differentiation of tumor from adjacent pancreatic tissue.[5,7] This textural difference allows tumor detection within a gland that is entirely normal in size (Fig. 3.1). Unfortunately, the abnormal texture of adenocarcinoma is not specific. As will be discussed below, other tumors and chronic pancreatitis may have an identical echo pattern.

TABLE 3.1. Clinical and pathologic features of pancreatic malignancies.

Clinical and pathologic features	Adenocarcinoma	Islet cell carcinoma	Cystadenocarcinoma
Incidence	Common	Rare	Rare
Prognosis	Poor	Good	Good
Age predilection	60 average, incidence increases with age	None	49 average, less in elderly
Sex predilection	Males by 2:1	None	Females by 6:1
Presentation	Pain, weight loss, jaundice	Endocrine hypersecretion 75% or mass 25%	Mass, pain
Size	Large unless early jaundice	Small (unless nonfunctioning)	Large
Usual site in gland	Head	Head	Tail, body
Usual gross pathology	Solid, nodular, homogeneous	Solid with cystic zones	Cystic with solid zones
Calcifications	Very rare	No	Common
Differential diagnosis	Chronic pancreatitis, other periampullary tumor	Cystadenocarcinoma, adenocarcinoma	Pseudocyst, islet cell carcinoma

TABLE 3.2. Ultrasonic features of pancreatic masses.

Ultrasound finding	**Adenocarcinoma (other periampullary tumors)**	**Islet cell carcinoma**	**Cystadenocarcinoma**	**Chronic pancreatitis with a focal mass**
Texture (compared to normal pancreas)	Predominantly low level echoes	Predominantly low level echoes; possible cystic zones	Predominantly cystic with septations	Variable; may be same as adenocarcinoma
Attenuation (compared to normal pancreas)	Same	Same in solid areas decreased in cystic zones	Decreased	Same, except associated pseudocyst
Shape	Lobulated	Well circumscribed	Lobulated	Irregular, may be lobulated
Calcifications	None	None	Yes	Yes

TABLE 3.3 Associated ultrasound findings in adenocarcinoma.

Pancreatic duct dilatation
Biliary tract dilatation
Liver metastases
Nodal metastases
Portal venous system involvement
Superior mesenteric artery displacement
Ascites

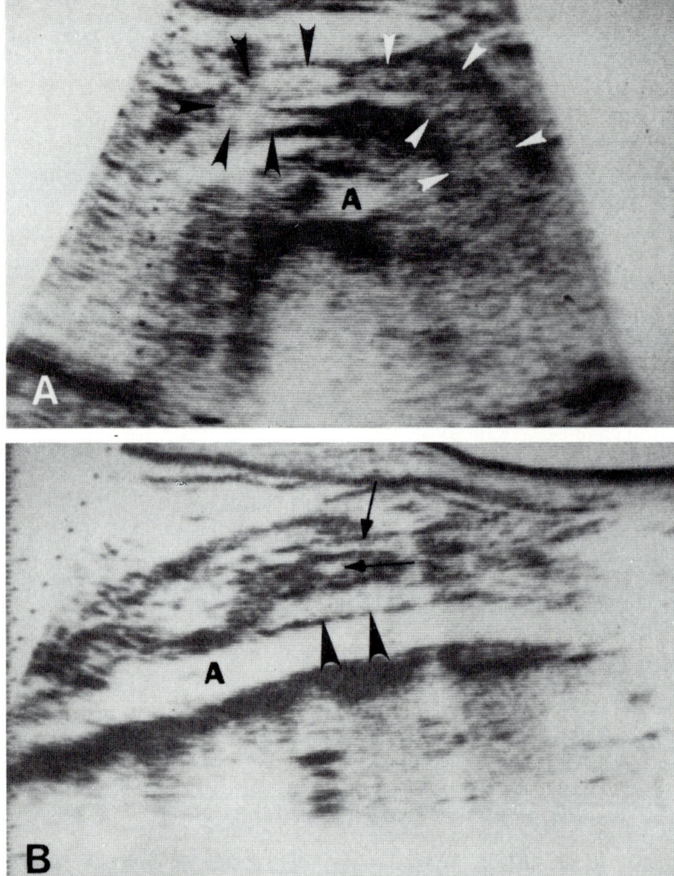

FIGURE 3.1. Adenocarcinoma of pancreas. (a) Oblique scan of pancreas. The tumor (black arrowheads) is seen as distinctly different echo texture from normal pancreas (white arrowheads). Note lack of enlargement or distortion of pancreas. A = aorta. (b) Midline longitudinal scan. Arrowheads point to enlarged paraaortic nodes, indicating metastatic spread. The mesenteric vessels (arrows) are displaced anteriorly by the nodal mass. (Weinstein, DP, Wolfman, NT, Weinstein, BJ: Ultrasonic characteristics of pancreatic tumors. Gastrointest Radiol 4:245–251, 1979.)

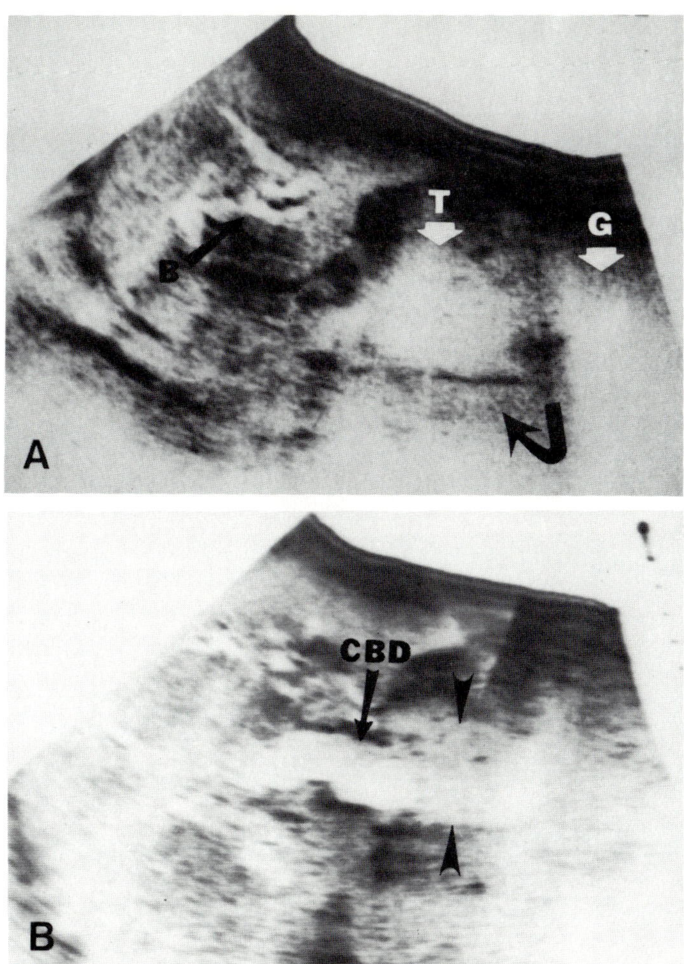

FIGURE 3.2. Adenocarcinoma of pancreatic head. (a) Longitudinal scan best demonstrates tumor (T) with typical low level acoustic pattern. Adjacent gas artefact (G) has similar acoustic pattern. Differentiation is made by visualization of structures behind tumor (arrow). B = dilated intrahepatic bile ducts. (b) 45° oblique scan shows dilated common bile duct (CBD). Tumor (arrowheads) is seen obstructing the duct.

Most adenocarcinomas are similar to other solid structures in their attenuation of sound energy.[7] The absence of relatively increased sound transmission prevents misinterpreting a tumor as a cystic lesion, even in those troublesome masses nearly devoid of internal echoes. Strangely, it is often difficult to differentiate an adenocarcinoma from the low-level reverberation pattern produced by adjacent gas collections, when only the texture itself is considered. A tumor will transmit sound energy, and structures beyond the area of interest can be recognized, a finding that is absent with a gas collection (Fig. 3.2). It is possible to overlook a fairly large adenocarcinoma by

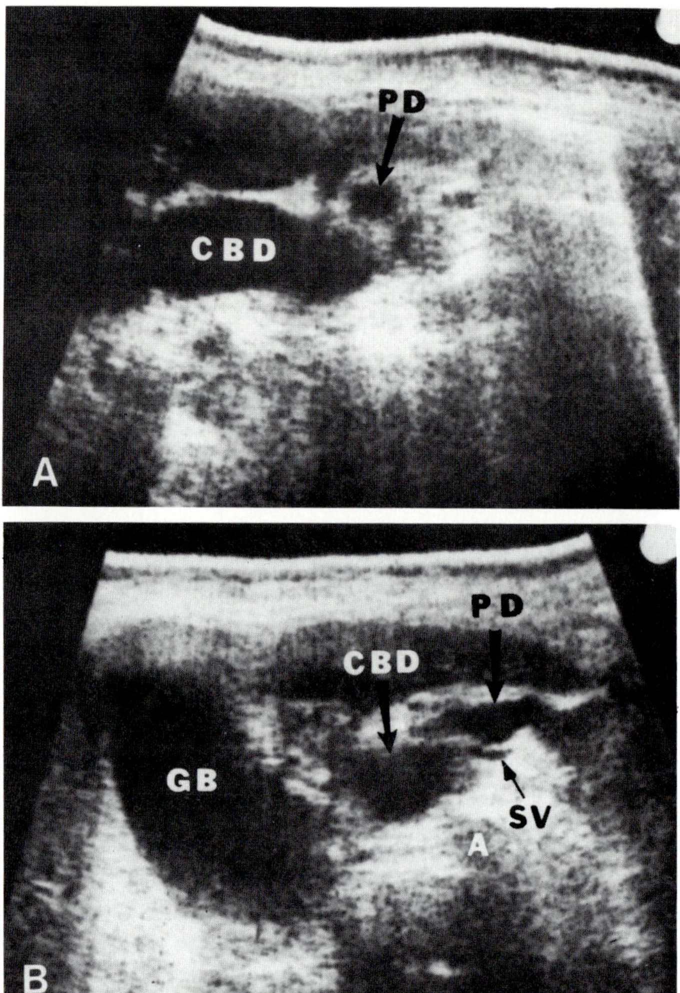

FIGURE 3.3. Adenocarcinoma of pancreatic head. (a) 45° oblique scan demonstrating dilatation of common bile duct (CBD) and pancreatic duct (PD). (b) Transverse scan showing marked dilatation of gallbladder (GB), common bile duct (CBD), and pancreatic duct (PD). Note relative increased sound transmission behind common duct. SV = splenic vein.

not realizing that a low-level echo pattern is a solid mass transmitting sound. To avoid this error the presence of through transmission must be deliberately sought.

Most pancreatic tumors are focal, lobulated enlargements of the gland. Due to biologic variations of gland morphology, size alone is a poor diagnostic criterion.[5, 8] The shape of the entire gland must be considered in evaluating a region of the pancreas for enlargement. The abnormal echo texture and bor-

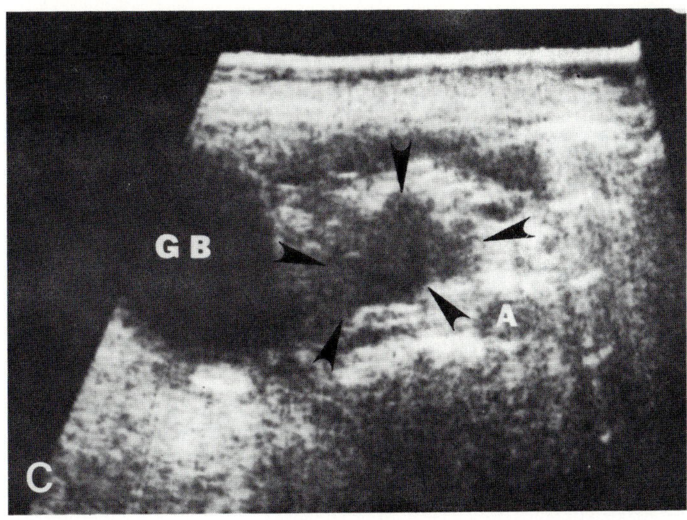

FIGURE 3.3. (c) Transverse scan at lower level showing lobulated tumor in pancreatic head (arrowheads). Note normal sound transmission behind tumor. GB = gallbladder; A = aorta.

der irregularities of tumors make it unnecessary to rely on size alone in ultrasound diagnosis.

Two-thirds of adenocarcinomas arise in the pancreatic head. Both the normal and the enlarged pancreatic head are better demonstrated in longitudinal scans (Fig. 3.2). Transverse and oblique scans of the pancreas usually underestimate the size of a pancreatic head mass. Since most adenocarcinomas involve the head, there is a high incidence of obstructive jaundice and biliary dilatation (Figs. 3.2 and 3.3). Biliary obstruction can also be caused by nodal metastases at the liver hilum. Biliary dilatation should be looked for in the nonjaundiced patient as well, since this finding precedes hyperbilirubinemia in developing obstruction.[9]

An obstructing tumor may produce dilatation of the pancreatic duct,[7] (Fig. 3.3) which may explain the high frequency of pancreatitis in adenocarcinoma of the pancreas. The practical significance of pancreatic duct dilatation is that it alerts the examiner to the possible presence of a mass in the periampullary region. It also facilitates surgical reconstruction after resection.[10]

Survival in adenocarcinoma of the pancreatic head is usually the result of early discovery due to obstructive jaundice. Adenocarcinomas of the body and tail have no potential early warning signs and almost invariably present late. Survival from an adenocarcinoma in these locations is exceedingly rare.

The ultrasound features of body and tail adenocarcinomas are similar to those of tumors of the head. These tumors usually present as hypoechoic, lobulated focal enlargements of the gland. Pancreatic body masses are best seen on transverse or oblique scans, as is true of the normal pancreatic body (Fig. 3.4). This scanning plane also allows visualization of the splenic vein.

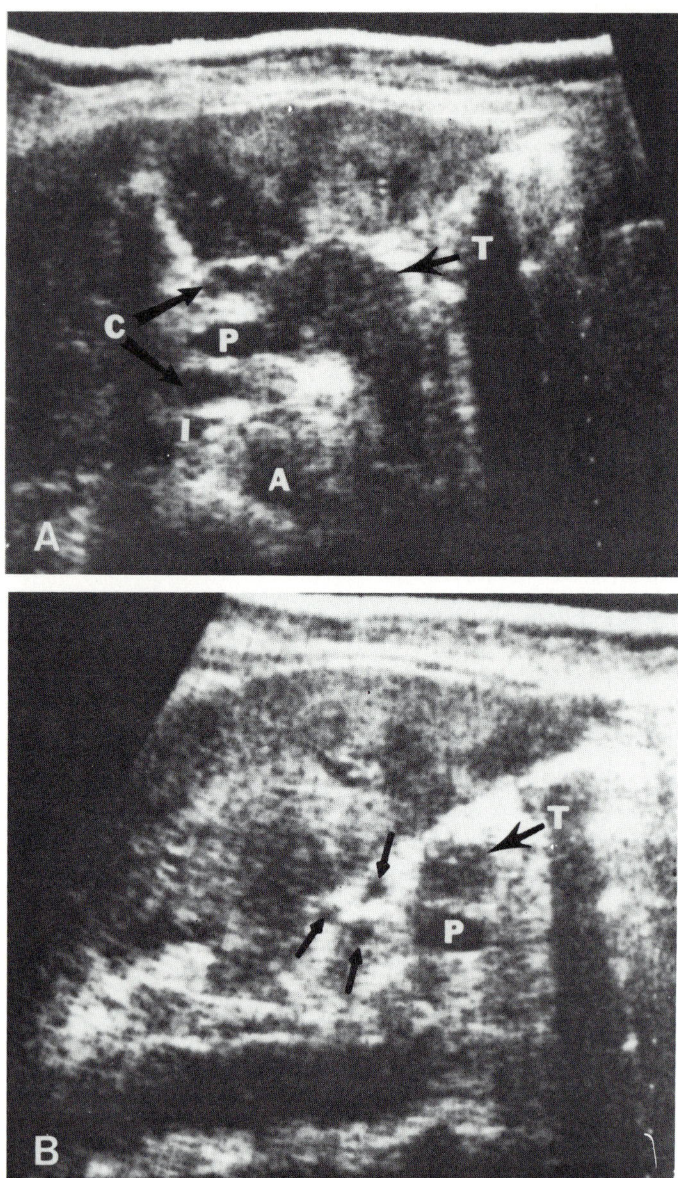

FIGURE 3.4. Adenocarcinoma of pancreatic body. (a) Transverse scan showing tumor mass (T) in pancreatic body as well as numerous liver metastases. Splenic vein is blocked and collateral veins (C) can be seen. P = portal vein; I = inferior vena cava; A = aorta. (b) Longitudinal scan showing right edge of tumor (T) above portal vein (P). Three vascular structures (arrows) are seen cephalad to pancreas, 1 being the hepatic artery and 2 the collateral veins. Note numerous liver metastases.

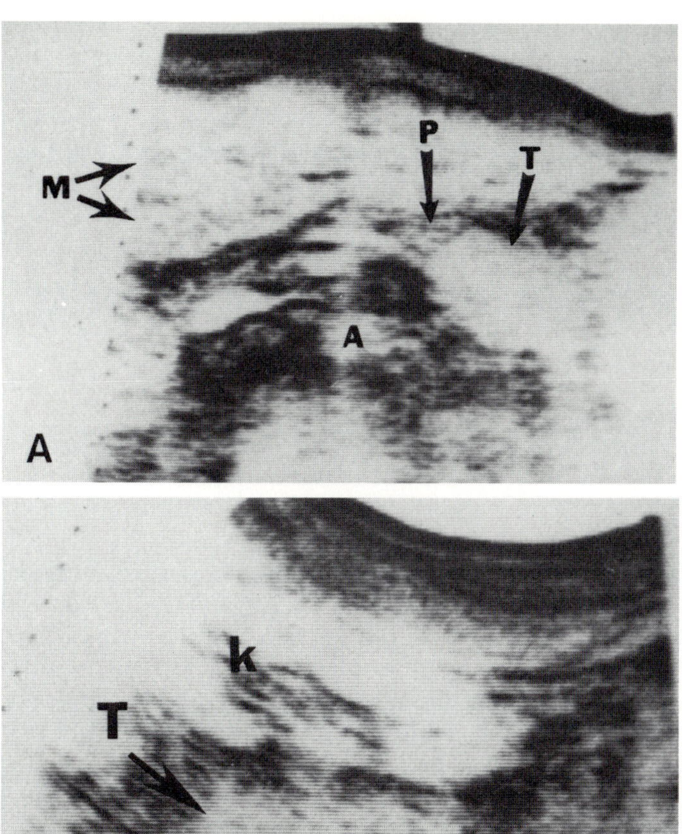

FIGURE 3.5. Adenocarcinoma of pancreatic tail. (a) Transverse scan demonstrating tumor (T) in tail. Normal pancreatic tissue (P) is seen adjacent to mass. Numerous metastases (M) are shown in the liver. A = aorta. (b) Prone longitudinal scan demonstrating tumor (T) anterior to kidney (K).

The inability to visualize the entire splenic vein is frequent in body adenocarcinomas, indicating obstruction. In this situation collateral veins may occasionally be demonstrated.

Pancreatic tail masses are the most difficult to demonstrate by ultrasound. Examination with the patient prone often aids in the identification of a tail mass[11] (Fig. 3.5). As in all left upper-quadrant sonograms, right lateral decubitus scans can be quite helpful.

The various associated ultrasound findings in adenocarcinoma (Table 3.3) are doubly significant. If one of these findings is detected during ultrasonography, a pancreatic adenocarcinoma should carefully be sought. Secondly, these findings may well indicate nonresectability and alter the future course of treatment.

Liver metastases are usually small and multiple[1] (Figs. 3.4 and 3.5). Nodal masses are also frequent, occurring in the liver hilum, mesentery, and para-aortic region[1] (Fig. 3.1). Large nodal masses may be mistaken for lymphoma, if the pancreatic primary is overlooked.

In addition to splenic vein involvement, pancreatic adenocarcinoma may affect the superior mesenteric vessels and the portal vein by displacement or obstruction. The superior mesenteric vessels are frequently displaced posteriorly by pancreatic masses, as opposed to anteriorly by lymphomas.[8] Nodal metastases from a pancreatic adenocarcinoma or a tumor of the uncinate process can also produce anterior displacement, limiting the reliability of this sign (Fig. 3.1).

Compression of the inferior vena cava has been described in adenocarcinoma of the head.[12] This sign is also limited since the normal pancreatic head can produce a similar appearance.

A finding indicating nonresectability of an adenocarcinoma does not eliminate the need for histologic diagnosis, since a treatable rare tumor or lymphoma must not be overlooked.

A percutaneous needle aspiration biopsy under ultrasonic guidance is simple to perform and may obviate the need for diagnostic laparotomy.[13] Even in the presence of obstructive jaundice, a laparotomy can be omitted by a percutaneous aspiration biopsy and a percutaneous transhepatic catheterization to relieve the obstruction.[14] The reduction in cost and suffering made possible by this combined approach is the most significant accomplishment of ultrasound in this disease to date.

Since adenocarcinoma can be recognized prior to gland enlargement, there is hope that early diagnosis is possible with ultrasound. The barrier to early diagnosis is the inability to suspect the presence of disease until symptoms occur, at which time the disease is nearly always incurable. The limitation is clearly demonstrated in Figure 3.1, where the presence of nodal metastases indicates advanced disease even though the primary tumor is apparently confined to the pancreas. If an inexpensive, reliable screening test is developed, patients could be examined by ultrasound before symptoms develop, providing the ultimate challenge to this modality in the diagnosis of adenocarcinoma.

ISLET CELL CARCINOMA

Islet cell carcinoma is a rare tumor that has gained great attention due to the various endocrine hypersecretory disorders associated with it. Ten percent of islet cell tumors are malignant and 25 percent of these are nonfunctioning.[15] The clinical and pathologic features are listed in Table 3.1. Table 3.2 lists the ultrasound features of islet cell carcinoma. However, only limited experience has been acquired in this entity.

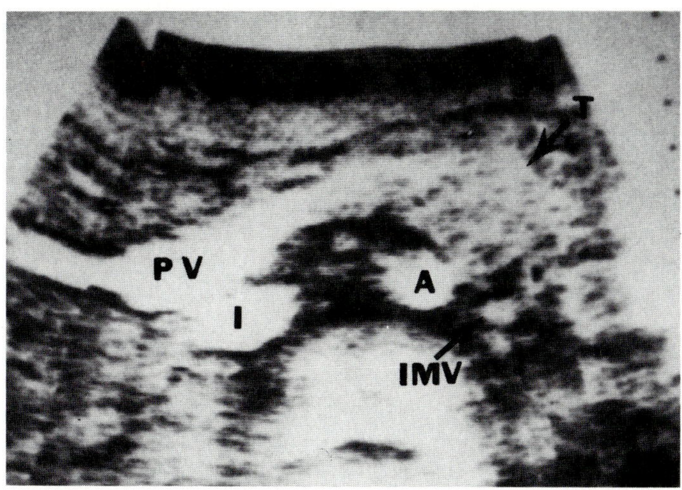

FIGURE 3.6. Islet cell carcinoma. Transverse scan demonstrating tumor (T) in pancreatic body. Splenic vein is obstructed. Prominent inferior mesenteric vein (IMV) suggests collateralization. PV = portal vein; I = inferior vena cava; A = aorta.

A large nonfunctioning islet cell carcinoma is shown in Figure 3.6. This tumor was solid, with a texture similar to an adenocarcinoma. Islet cell tumors may contain cystic areas, and resemble a cystadenocarcinoma.[16] The mass shown in Figure 3.6 also produced splenic vein obstruction. The important consideration in these rare tumors is their better prognosis than adenocarcinoma, even when metastatic at discovery.

CYSTADENOCARCINOMA OF THE PANCREAS

Pancreatic cystadenocarcinoma is the malignant counterpart of the mucinous cystadenoma. There are no gross pathologic differences between benign and malignant mucinous cystadenomas. All mucinous cystadenomas are treated like malignancies, due to their actual or potential malignant behavior.[17] The features of pancreatic cystadenocarcinoma are listed in Tables 3.1 and 3.2. There is a second variety of cystadenoma of the pancreas, which is truly benign, the glycogen rich cystadenoma.[18] This variety of tumor contains microscopic cysts producing a solid ultrasonic texture, and probably accounts for the reports of cystadenomas misinterpreted as adenocarcinoma.[8]

Cystadenocarcinoma may be suspected because unlike adenocarcinoma it occurs more commonly in the pancreatic tail and body in females and in younger patients. Additionally, the ultrasonic appearance of cystadenocarcinoma is predominantly cystic with decreased attenuation, which is unlike adenocarcinoma[19] (Fig. 3.7). As is the case in islet cell carcinoma, cystadenocarcinoma has a much better prognosis than adenocarcinoma. Aggressive therapy is warranted in these two rare tumors in an attempt for cure.

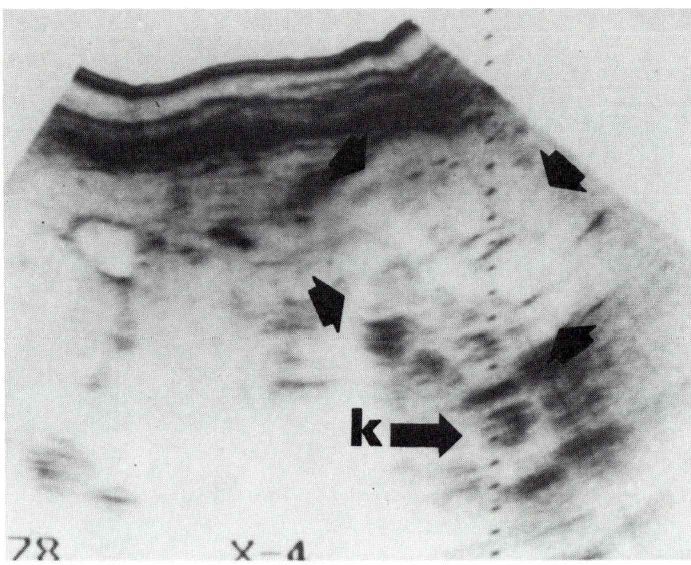

FIGURE 3.7. Cystadenocarcinoma. Transverse scan showing large tumor (arrows) of pancreatic tail containing multiple cystic areas. K = kidney. (Courtesy of Neil T. Wolfman, MD)

NONPANCREATIC PERIAMPULLARY TUMORS

Tumors arising from the duodenum, extrahepatic bile duct, or ampulla of Vater have a clinical presentation similar to that of adenocarcinoma of the pancreatic head. Prognosis with these tumors is better than for pancreatic adenocarcinoma, and more aggressive therapy is indicated. The ultrasonic appearance of the ampullary carcinoma shown in Figure 3.8 is identical to that of adenocarcinoma. Both pancreatic duct and biliary duct obstruction are produced by ampullary carcinoma. Differentiation between these periampullary tumors and pancreatic adenocarcinoma cannot be made by ultrasound alone.[8] An upper gastrointestinal series and endoscopy may be helpful in this differential.

OTHER TUMORS

The pancreas is the second most common site of intraabdominal lymphoma.[20] The internal echo texture of lymphoma is usually similar to that of adenocarcinoma; however, most lymphomas are less attenuating and relatively increased sound transmission is common. Lymphomas also tend to be large masses, with associated lumpy masses seen in nodal areas. The superior mesenteric vessels are often displaced anteriorly by lymphoma, as

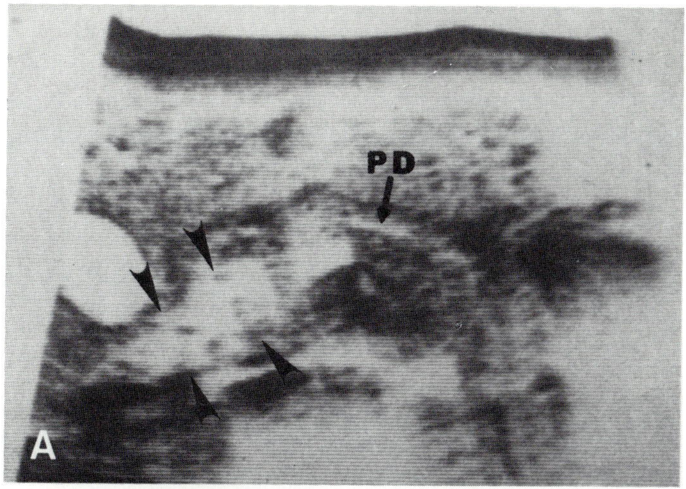

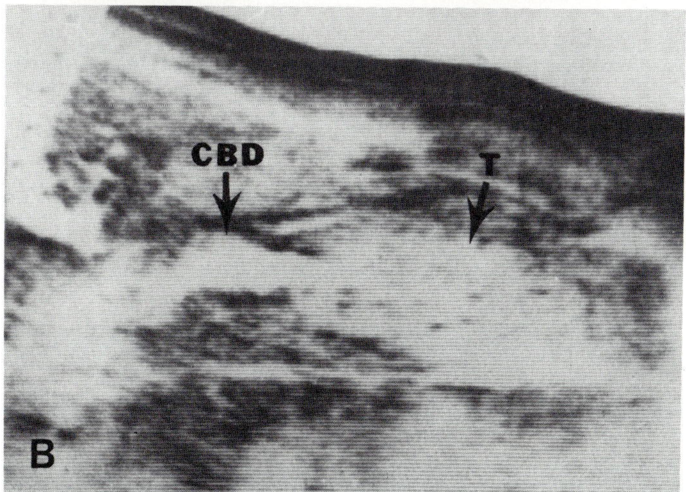

FIGURE 3.8. Ampullary carcinoma. (a) Transverse scan showing tumor (arrowheads) involving pancreatic head. Pancreatic duct (PD) is obstructed by the tumor. (b) Longitudinal scan showing full length of tumor (T). Common bile duct (CBD) is obstructed by the tumor.

compared to adenocarcinoma (Fig. 3.9). Other findings, such as pleural effusion and splenomegaly, can be clues to the diagnosis of lymphoma.[8]

Carcinoma of the stomach or colon occasionally may have an appearance similar to a pancreatic tumor (Fig. 3.10). Routine barium examinations will provide the diagnosis in these cases.

Retroperitoneal sarcomas can involve the pancreatic area. Further experience is needed to determine if these tumors can be differentiated from adenocarcinomas by ultrasound.

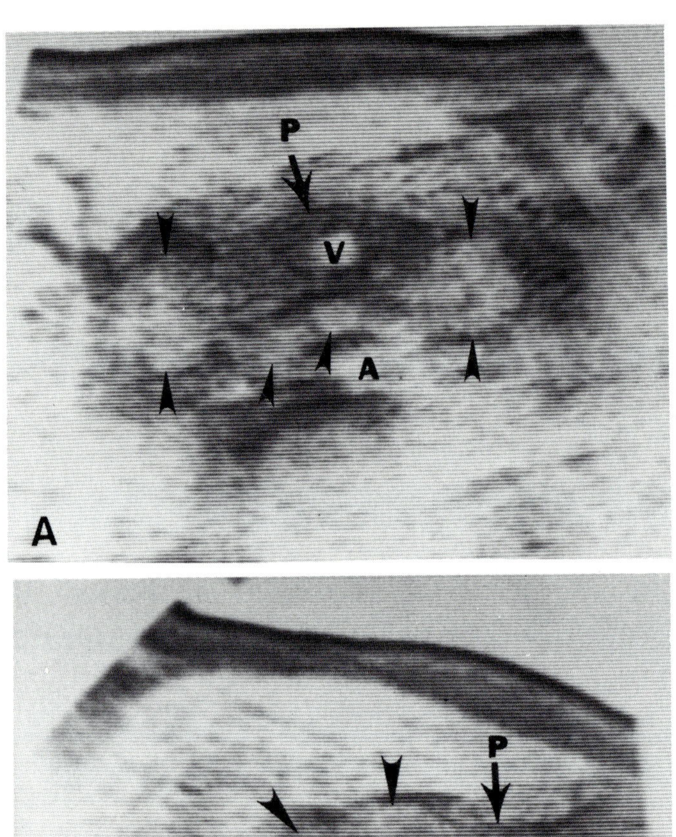

FIGURE 3.9. Lymphoma. (a) Transverse scan showing two masses (between arrowheads) involving pancreas (P) and two para-aortic nodal masses (arrowheads). V = superior mesenteric vein; A = aorta. (b) Longitudinal scan showing multiple celiac and paraaortic nodal masses (arrowheads). P = pancreas; V = superior mesenteric vein.

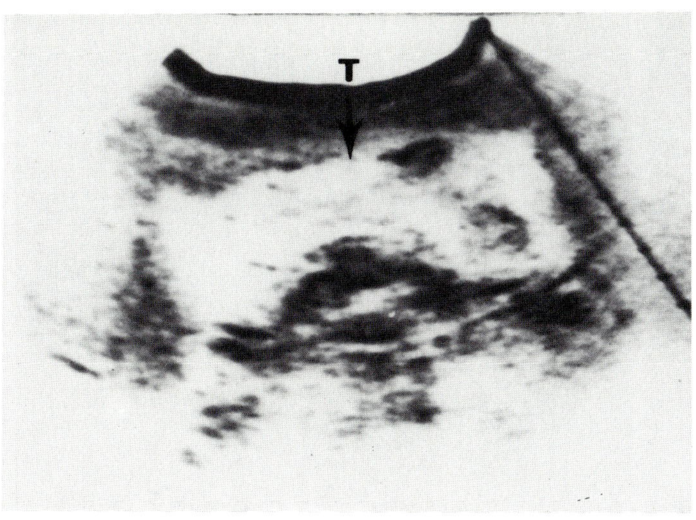

FIGURE 3.10. Gastric carcinoma. Transverse scan demonstrating large tumor (T). Pancreas is obscured by the tumor, which arises from stomach.

FOCAL MASSES IN CHRONIC PANCREATITIS

A focal mass due to chronic pancreatitis can present with an ultrasound appearance similar to that of an adenocarcinoma. The ultrasonic features of focal masses due to chronic pancreatitis are listed in Table 3.2. Although the echo texture of chronic pancreatitis is variable, a texture identical to that of adenocarcinoma can occur. The shape of the mass may be more irregular than an adenocarcinoma, or quite similar.[8]

Associated ultrasound findings overlap between adenocarcinoma and chronic pancreatitis. Pancreatic duct dilatation and biliary dilatation can occur in both disorders as well as in obstruction of the portal venous system. Certain ultrasound findings help to differentiate chronic pancreatitis from tumor. Calcifications within a mass highly favor chronic pancreatitis since calcification in an adenocarcinoma is rare (Fig. 3.11). The presence of metastases in the liver or nodes obviously indicates malignancy.

In addition to the ultrasound findings, valuable clues in the patient's clinical history will usually suggest benign or malignant disease. The differential diagnosis may be impossible without a biopsy or even surgery. The difficulty that both the surgeon and pathologist have in this differential diagnosis should be remembered, and the inability to separate these entities by ultrasound must be expected on occasion.

ACCURACY

A concise discussion of the accuracy and limitations of ultrasound evaluation of the pancreas can be found in a recent article by Sample and Sarti.[5] The ac-

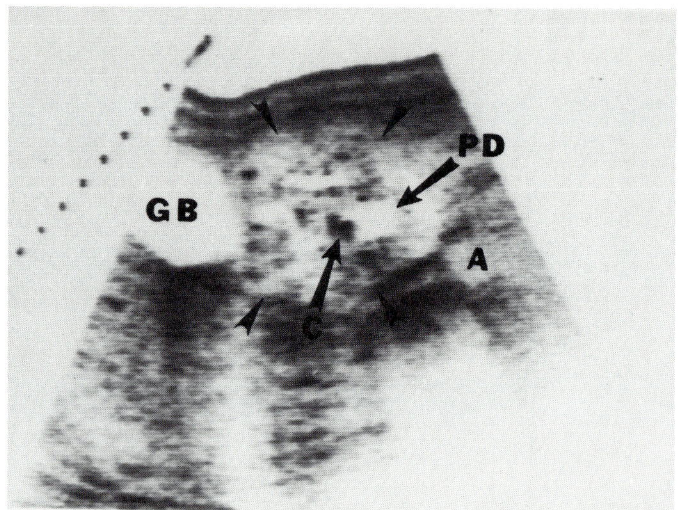

FIGURE 3.11. Chronic pancreatitis. Transverse scan demonstrating focal enlargement of pancreatic head (arrowheads), pancreatic duct dilatation (PD), and calcification (C). Calcification favors chronic pancreatitis rather than tumor. GB = gallbladder; A = aorta.

curacy of ultrasound in pancreatic disease is approximately 85 percent with a specificity of 90 percent, indicating that few false positives occur. The most limiting factor is gas-produced obscuration of the pancreas, resulting in a 15 percent unsatisfactory examination rate. Ultrasound is a reliable means of evaluation for pancreatic cancer, and less costly than the other reliable noninvasive technique, computed tomography. Ultrasound is therefore the logical method to employ primarily in suspected pancreatic cancer.[5] Further evaluation by computed tomography and other modalities should be obtained when necessary.

CONCLUSION

Ultrasound is a safe and reliable means for the evaluation of pancreatic cancer. Tumors can be recognized by their abnormal echo texture and significant information obtained about biliary obstruction, vascular involvement, and metastatic spread. Most cancers of the pancreas are adenocarcinomas; however, the rarer tumors may be suspected by clinicopathologic and ultrasonographic analysis. Focal masses in chronic pancreatitis present a difficult differential diagnosis. Exploratory surgery can be avoided by using an ultrasound guided biopsy. Survival in pancreatic cancer has not been improved to date; however, a saving in hospitalization time, cost, and suffering has been achieved.

References

1. del Regato JA, Spjut HJ: In: Cancer: Diagnosis, Treatment and Prognosis. St Louis, CV Mosby, 1977, pp 572–584.
2. Malagelada JR: Pancreatic Cancer. An overview of epidemiology, clinical presentation and diagnosis. Mayo Clin Proc 54:459–467, 1979.
3. Howard JM, Jordan GL Jr: Cancer of the pancreas. Curr Prob Cancer 2:5–52, 1977.
4. Hermann RE, Cooperman AM: Current concepts in cancer: Cancer of the Pancreas. N Eng J Med 301:482–485, 1979.
5. Sample WF, Sarti DA: Diagnosis of pancreatic disease by ultrasound and computed tomography. In: Clinics in Diagnostic Ultrasound 1, Diagnostic Ultrasound in Gastrointestinal Disease, 1979, pp 85–101.
6. Simeone JF, Simonds BD: Normal anatomy of the pancreas by computed tomography and diagnostic ultrasound. In: Clinics in Diagnostic Ultrasound 1, Diagnostic Ultrasound in Gastrointestinal Disease, 1979, pp 73–84.
7. Weinstein DP, Wolfman NT, Weinstein BJ: Ultrasonic characteristics of pancreatic tumors. Gastrointest Radiol 4:245–251, 1979.
8. Weill FS: In Ultrasonography of Digestive Diseases. St Louis, CV Mosby, 1978.
9. Weinstein BJ, Weinstein DP: Biliary tract dilatation in the non-jaundiced patient. Am J Roentgenol 134:899–906, 1980.
10. Braasch JW, Gray BN: Technique of radical pancreatoduodenectomy with consideration of hepatic arterial relationships. Surg Clin N Am 56:631–647, 1976.
11. Goldstein HM, Katragadda CS: Prone view ultrasonography for pancreatic tail neoplasms. Am J Roentgenol 131:231–234, 1978.
12. Wall WJ, Templeton AW: The ultrasonic demonstration of inferior vena caval compression: A guide to pancreatic head enlargement with emphasis on neoplasm. Rad 123: 165–167, 1977.
13. Holm HH, Als O, Gammelgaard J: Percutaneous aspiration and biopsy procedures under ultrasound visualization. In: Clinics in Diagnostic Ultrasound 1, Diagnostic Ultrasound in Gastrointestinal Disease, 1979, pp 137–149.
14. Ring EJ, Husted JW, Oleaga JA, Freiman DB: Multihole catheter for maintaining long-term percutaneous antegrade biliary drainage. Rad 132:752–754, 1979.
15. Khandekar JD: Islet cell tumors of the pancreas: Clinico-biochemical correlations. Ann Clin Lab Sci 9:212–218, 1979.
16. Gold J, Rosenfield AT, Sostman D, et al: Nonfunctioning islet cell tumors of the pancreas: Radiographic and ultrasonographic appearances in two cases. Am J Roentgenol 131: 715–717, 1978.
17. Compagno J, Oertel JE: Mucinous cystic neoplasms of the pancreas with over and latent malignancy. (Cystadenocarcinoma and Cystadenoma.) A clinicopathologic study of 41 cases. Am J Clin Pathol 69:573–580, 1978.
18. Compagno J, Oertel JE: Microcystic adenomas of the pancreas (glycogen-rich cystadenomas). A clinicopathologic study of 34 cases. Am J Clin Pathol 69:289–298, 1978.
19. Freeny PC, Weinstein CJ, Taft DA, Allen FH: Cystic neoplasms of the pancreas: New angiographic and ultrasonographic findings. Am J Roentgenol 131:795–802, 1978.
20. Gorelick FS, Spiro HM: The gastroenterologist's view of the indications and efficacy of ultrasound examination. In: Clinics in Diagnostic Ultrasound 1, Diagnostic Ultrasound in Gastrointestinal Disease, 1979, pp 1–21.

4 Lymphoma

BARBARA A. CARROLL

Malignant lymphomas generally arise within the lymph nodes or thymus. They are classified into two separate groups: Hodgkin disease and non-Hodgkin lymphoma. Approximately 40 percent of newly diagnosed lymphomas consist of Hodgkin disease; the remainder represent non-Hodgkin lymphomas. Non-Hodgkin lymphomas are further subdivided into nodular and diffuse histopathologies. There are predictable differences in abdominal distribution of disease in these three different groups of lymphomas. Effective therapeutic management, using radiotherapy and chemotherapy, in patients with malignant lymphoma requires both accurate histologic classification and reliable definition of the anatomic regions of involvement.[1]

While lymphangiography has proved particularly accurate in the diagnosis of paraaortic and paracaval adenopathy, it fails to detect disease at numerous other abdominal sites, including mesenteric, perisplenic and perihepatic nodes, and extranodal sites, including the spleen and liver.[1-3] Ultrasound can detect retroperitoneal disease and provides additional information, not detectable by lymphangiography, with respect to the extent of abdominal lymphoma involvement.

PARAAORTIC LYMPH NODES

Paraaortic nodes are involved with lymphoma in approximately 25 percent of newly diagnosed patients with Hodgkin disease and in 40 percent of patients with non-Hodgkin lymphoma.[2,4] Over 12 percent of patients with Hodgkin disease, who have a normal lymphangiogram, may have positive celiac, perisplenic or mesenteric nodes.[4] In non-Hodgkin nodular lymphoma, more than 40 percent of patients with normal lymphangiograms had involvement of mesenteric nodes, while 76 percent of patients with abnormal lymphangiograms demonstrated coexistent mesenteric disease.[4] Ultrasound detects retroperitoneal nodal lymphoma with an 80 to 90 percent level of accuracy.[5,6] This degree of accuracy compares favorably with those reported for other imaging modalities, including computed tomography (CT) body scanning,

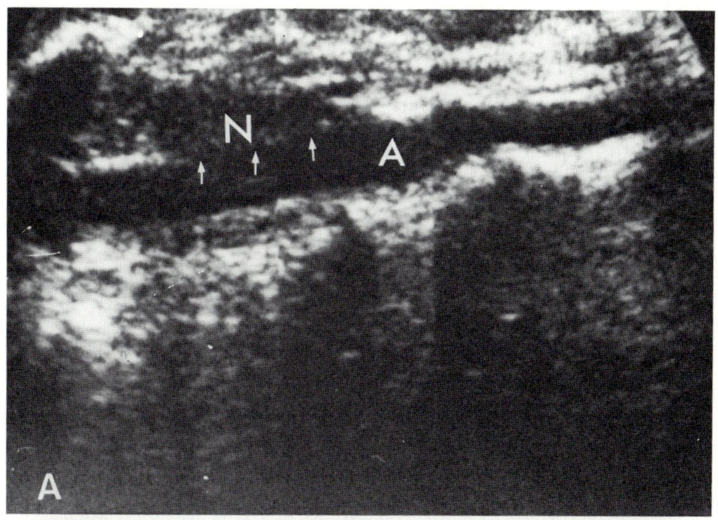

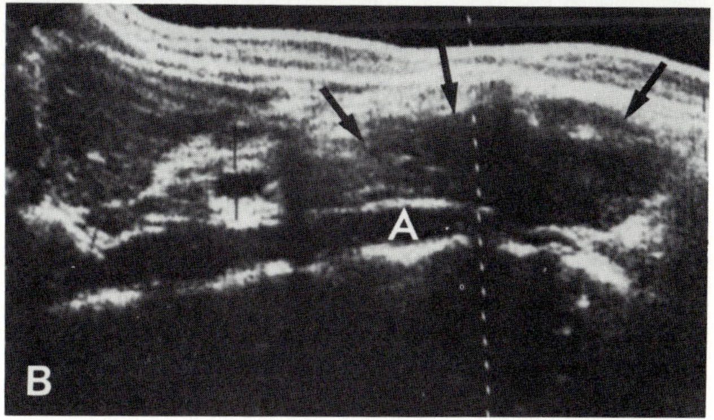

FIGURE 4.1. (a) A sagittal sonogram performed 1 cm to the left of midline demonstrates ''silhouetting'' of the anterior margin (arrows) of the abdominal aorta (A) by a mass of paraaortic lymph nodes (N). (b) A sagittal supine sonogram performed 1 cm to the left of midline demonstrates a large periumbilical mass of mesenteric nodes (arrows) which do not create ''silhouetting'' of the anterior margin of the abdominal aorta (A); dotted line-level of umbilicus.

lymphangiography, and gallium 67 citrate scanning.[5-8] Brascho et al. reported 98 percent accuracy in the sonographic estimation of nodal size in retroperitoneal nodes greater than 2 cm in diameter.[5] Both Brascho and Rochester et al. reported sonographic accuracy in the detection of retroperitoneal lymphadenophy comparable to that of lymphangiography.[5, 6] In addition to the detection of nodal pathology in areas demonstrated on lymphangiograms, sonography demonstrates adenopathy in the celiac, perisplenic, mesenteric, and perihepatic nodes in a manner similar to that reported for CT body scanning.[9, 10] While bowel gas may obscure retroperitoneal structures and a large amount of retroperitoneal fat degrades sonographic resolution, the relatively

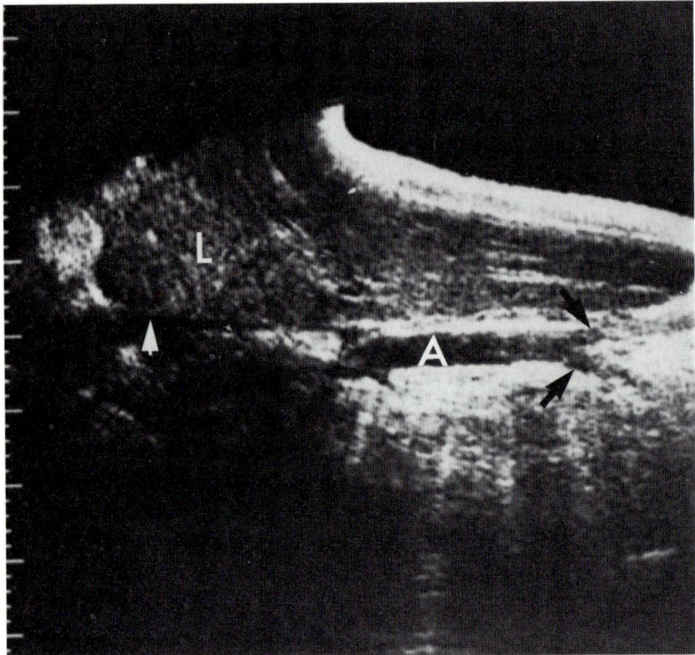

FIGURE 4.2. A right decubitus, (coronal) longitudinal projection sonogram showing the abdominal aorta (A) and its bifurcation (arrows). Liver (L); proximal vena cava (arrowhead).

high degree of accuracy with which abdominal disease is detected in these areas, as well as other nodal and extranodal abdominal regions, suggests a useful role for ultrasound in initial patient staging, especially in non-Hodgkin lymphomas with extensive abdominal disease in areas not visualized by lymphangiography. Approximately 10 percent of normal-sized lymph nodes can be expected to contain disease foci, which would likely only be detected by lymphangiography.[2, 10] However, ultrasound could be used to screen for retroperitoneal disease to detect individuals who required lymphangiography, based on clinical parameters.

The sonographic appearance of paraaortic nodes involved by malignant lymphoma has been described as low echo or anechoic enlargement of lymph nodes.[11] While these sonographic appearances constitute the most typical appearance of lymphomatous nodal involvement, the findings are nonspecific. Occasionally, anechoic nodal masses may resemble cystic structures. The distinction between anechoic solid nodal masses and cysts may be difficult due to the proximity of the anechoic retroperitoneal nodes to the spine, which makes the evaluation of posterior acoustic transmission or refractory shadowing problematic. Nodal enlargement secondary to other neoplasms or inflammatory processes, such as retroperitoneal fibrosis, may be indistin-

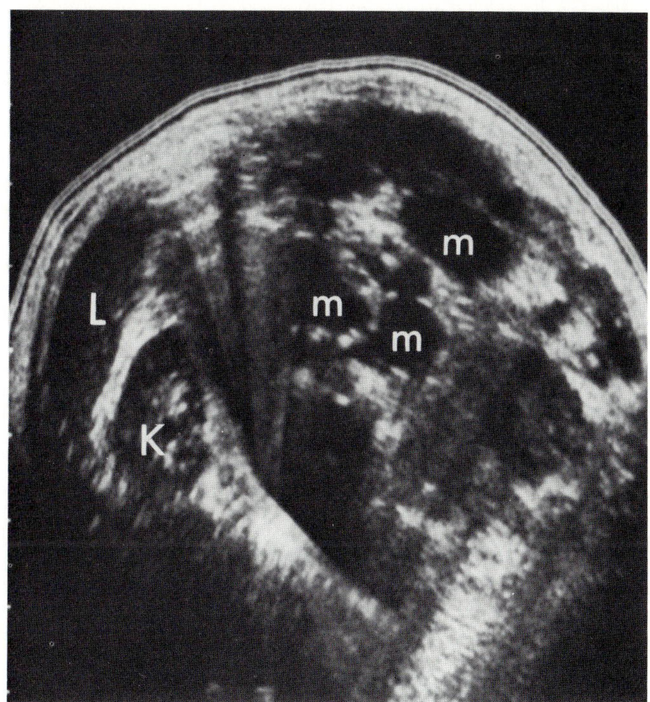

FIGURE 4.3. A transverse supine sonogram at the umbilical level demonstrates multiple "cystic" masses of abnormal enlarged mesenteric lymph nodes (m) involved by lymphoma. K = right kidney; L = liver.

guishable from lymphomatous lymphadenopathy.[12] Conversely, atypical, more echogenic inhomogeneous nodal masses may occur in lymphoma. Paraaortic or paracaval nodes frequently obscure the sharp anterior vascular border, providing a "sonographic silhouette" that may help distinguish paraaortic nodes from adjacent mesenteric nodes (Fig. 4.1a and b). Decubitus viewing facilitates sonographic imaging of the retroperitoneal area down to the aortic bifurcation (Fig. 4.2).

While no detectable correlation has been observed between the sonographic appearance of abnormal paraaortic nodes and the histology of the lymphoma, the largest paraaortic nodal masses demonstrated have usually been in non-Hodgkin lymphoma. Additional work is required to correlate the intrinsic sonographic features of abdominal nodes and the histopathology they contain.

OTHER ABDOMINAL NODAL SITES

Mesenteric nodal involvement in non-Hodgkin lymphoma is important to document as it may exclude a staging laparotomy or result in altered radia-

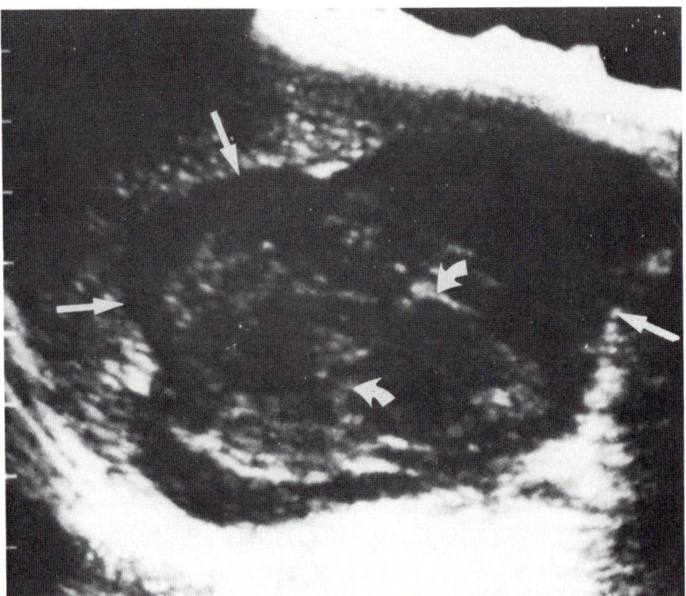

FIGURE 4.4. A sagittal supine sonogram obtained 8 cm to the right of midline demonstrates a large, heterogeneous infrahepatic mass of nodes (arrows). Central areas of increased echogenicity representing necrosis (curved arrows).

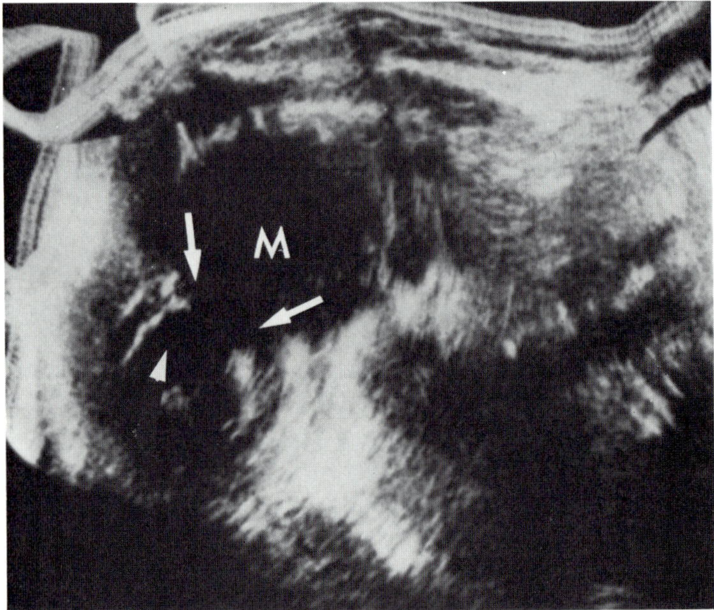

FIGURE 4.5. A transverse supine sonogram at the umbilical level demonstrates a mass of lymphomatous nodes in the right renal hilar area (M) invading the medial aspect of the kidney (arrows) producing hydronephrosis (arrowhead).

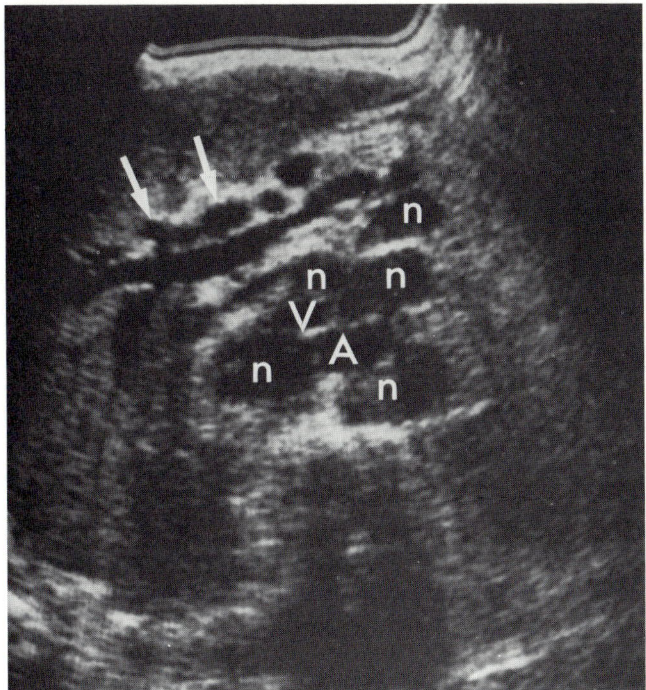

FIGURE 4.6. A transverse sonogram 5 cm inferior to the xiphoid process demonstrates multiple enlarged nodes in the porta hepatis (n) and resultant biliary obstruction (arrows). A-aorta; V-inferior vena cava.

tion therapy ports.[3] While less than 4 percent of newly diagnosed Hodgkin patients will demonstrate mesenteric disease, more than 50 percent of non-Hodgkin patients will have mesenteric nodal involvement.[4] Of particular importance, 40 percent of nodular nonHodgkin lymphomas present with mesenteric nodal involvement in the presence of a normal lymphangiogram.[4] Ultrasound frequently detects such mesenteric masses secondary to lymphomatous involvement. The appearance of mesenteric nodes can resemble that of retroperitoneal nodes; however they do not usually demonstrate a "silhouette sign" with respect to obscuration of the anterior margin of the abdominal great vessels. Mesenteric masses may also appear as multiple cystic or septated masses that may resemble fluid-filled bowel loops (Fig. 4.3). While bowel gas may obscure small mesenteric masses, and it is unlikely that normal sized mesenteric nodes can be sonographically visualized, ultrasound examination should be able to demonstrate most masses greater than 4 cm in diameter.

Perihepatic nodes, celiac axis nodes, splenic-hilar and renal-hilar nodes may also be demonstrated sonographically and manifest a spectrum of appearances similar to that of retroperitoneal adenopathy. While most are hypoechoic to anechoic, inhomogenous areas of increased echogencity can be found in areas of focal necrosis within large nodes (Fig. 4.4). Lymphomatous retroperitoneal nodes can encase or invade adjacent organs and produce significant organ displacement (Fig. 4.5). While portal nodes can produce biliary obstruction (Fig. 4.6) 11 of 13 recently evaluated cases presenting with significant portal adenopathy showed no evidence of biliary obstruction.[13] Of interest is the fact that periportal adenopathy was found in 13 of 24 cases with documented lymphoma involvement of the liver.

SPLEEN

Splenic involvement may be the only site of abdominal disease in a significant number of patients with newly diagnosed Hodgkin disease.[7] However, clinicopathologic correlations have demonstrated that while an enlarged spleen in a patient with non-Hodgkin lymphoma usually indicates lymphomatous involvement, one-third of Hodgkin patients with splenomegaly will not have splenic disease. Conversely, approximately one-third of normal-sized spleens will be involved by lymphoma in both Hodgkin and non-Hodgkin patients.[4] In such instances, non-Hodgkin patients usually evidence other sites of abdominal involvement.

Sonographic critera for the detection of splenomegaly have been difficult to establish. Splenic extension below the left costal margin on supine scans and anterior to the anterior margin of the vertebral bodies or midaxillary line have been used as critera for splenic enlargement, as has an anterior-posterior diameter greater than half that of the abdomen.[6, 13] However, detection of splenomegaly by any critera correlates poorly with lymphomotous involvement.[6, 7, 13] Some authors have reported a correlation between splenic enlargement with decreased splenic echogenicity and lymphomatous involvement.[14] However, neither splenomegaly nor splenic echogenicity correlated with disease involvement in the experience of those at our institution.[7, 13] Rochester et al. reported an equally discouraging correlation between splenic appearance and involvement by lymphoma.[6] The sonographic demonstration of a focal anechoic splenic defect in a patient with lymphoma, resembling an abscess, has been reported.[15] Focal splenic defects have been correlated with a high incidence of lymphomatous involvement, using CT body scanning.[2, 10] However, focal splenic masses may also occur in cases of splenic infarction and hemorrhage.[13]

While splenomegaly and splenic echogenicity correlated poorly with disease involvement, splenomegaly associated with splenic hilar adenopathy or focal hepatic defects correlated more closely with splenic involvement by lymphoma.[13] The left coronal or lateral decubitus views facilitated viewing of the splenic hilum (Fig. 4.7). All cases in which sonographic hepatic abnormalities were demonstrated also showed concomitant splenic involvement.[13]

EXTRANODAL LYMPHOMA

Hepatic lymphomatous involvement is present at initial diagnosis in approximately 5 percent of patients with Hodgkin disease and 15 percent of non-

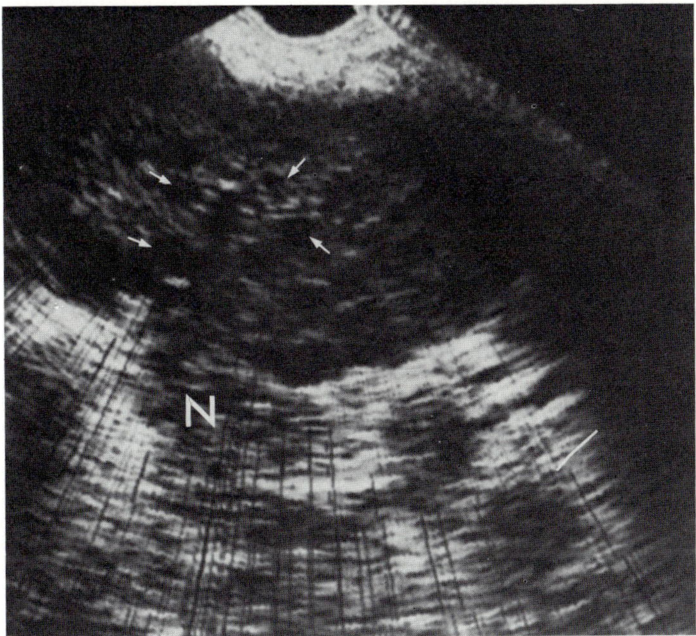

FIGURE 4.7. Left decubitus longitudinal sonogram (coronal) shows an enlarged spleen containing multiple hypoechoic masses (arrows) and associated splenic hilar adenopathy (N).

Hodgkin lymphomas. This involvement is usually microscopic and beyond the limits of resolution of ultrasound or CT body scan.[4,7] However, focal hepatic deposits of 5 mm in diameter can be sonographically detected in cases of lymphomatous involvement[13] (Fig. 4.8). Advanced hepatic lymphomatous involvement may have a variety of sonographic appearances. The most common manifestations include multiple hypoechoic or anechoic focal parenchymal defects. While these anechoic lesions may resemble cystic structures, they rarely demonstrate enhanced posterior acoustic transmission or peripheral refractory shadowing.[13] Occasionally, more echogenic inhomogenous focal lesions indistinguishable from other neoplastic metastatic lesions will be found. Hepatic abscesses, metastases from sarcomas or melanomas, focal areas of cholangitis, radiation fibrosis, and extensive hemosiderosis have presented with findings sonographically indistinguishable from hepatic lymphoma.[13] Earlier sonographic manifestations of hepatic lymphoma include diffuse hepatic parenchymal inhomogeneity with focal lesions smaller than 5 mm in diameter associated with decreased parenchymal echogenicity and hepatomegaly. In cases presenting with focal hepatic defects, concomitant retroperitoneal nodal disease is frequently present, as is portal or perihepatic nodal disease. Direct invasion of hepatic parenchyma from contiguous perihepatic nodes occurs more frequently in non-Hodgkin lymphomas.

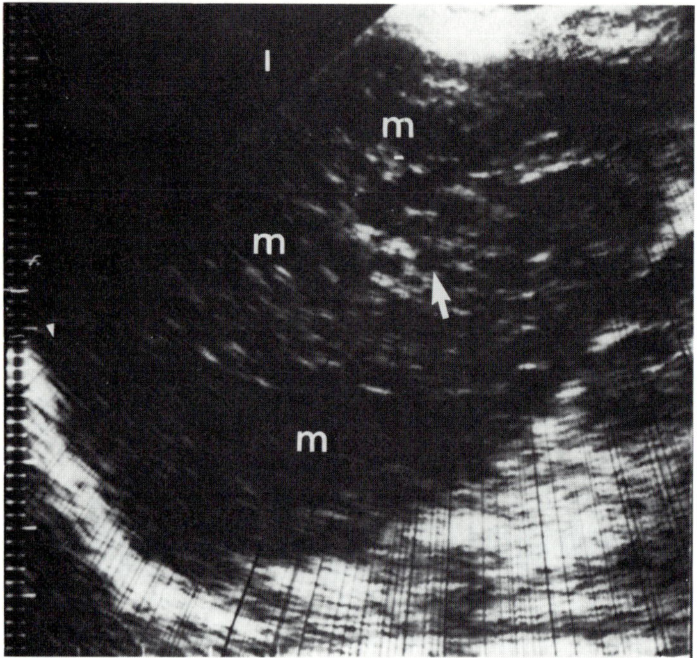

FIGURE 4.8. A sagittal supine sonogram obtained through the right lobe of liver demonstrates multiple anechoic masses of varied sizes (m). Some focal deposits are as small as 5 mm in diameter (arrow).

Less than 3% of all non-Hodgkin lymphomas present with renal involvement, mainly Burkitt lymphoma or diffuse hystiocytic lymphomas.[16] Common sonographic manifestations of renal lymphoma include focal hypoechoic or anechoic lesions.[16, 17] While some anechoic lesions may demonstrate enhanced posterior sound transmission and refractory shadowing similar to renal cysts, the margins of such lesions are usually poorly defined and suggest a different etiology.[13] Focal renal masses may be only slightly less echogenic than adjacent renal parenchyma and may resemble a variety of primary or metastatic neoplasms.[13, 17] Additional findings include diffusely enlarged kidneys without focal masses or obstruction (Fig. 4.9a and b), and direct invasion of the kidney from adjacent nodal masses. As in cases of focal hepatic abnormalities or enlarged nodal masses, there is no definite correlation between the sonographic appearance of renal masses and the lymphomatous histologic subtype. The lateral decubitus view facilitates detection of renal hilar nodes, which, like splenic hilar or retroperitoneal nodes, may be more echogenic than splenic or renal parenchymal involvement, probably reflecting an admixture of fat and/or collagen within abnormal lymphomatous nodes (Fig. 4.10).

Fifteen percent of non-Hodgkin lymphomas may present with gastrointes-

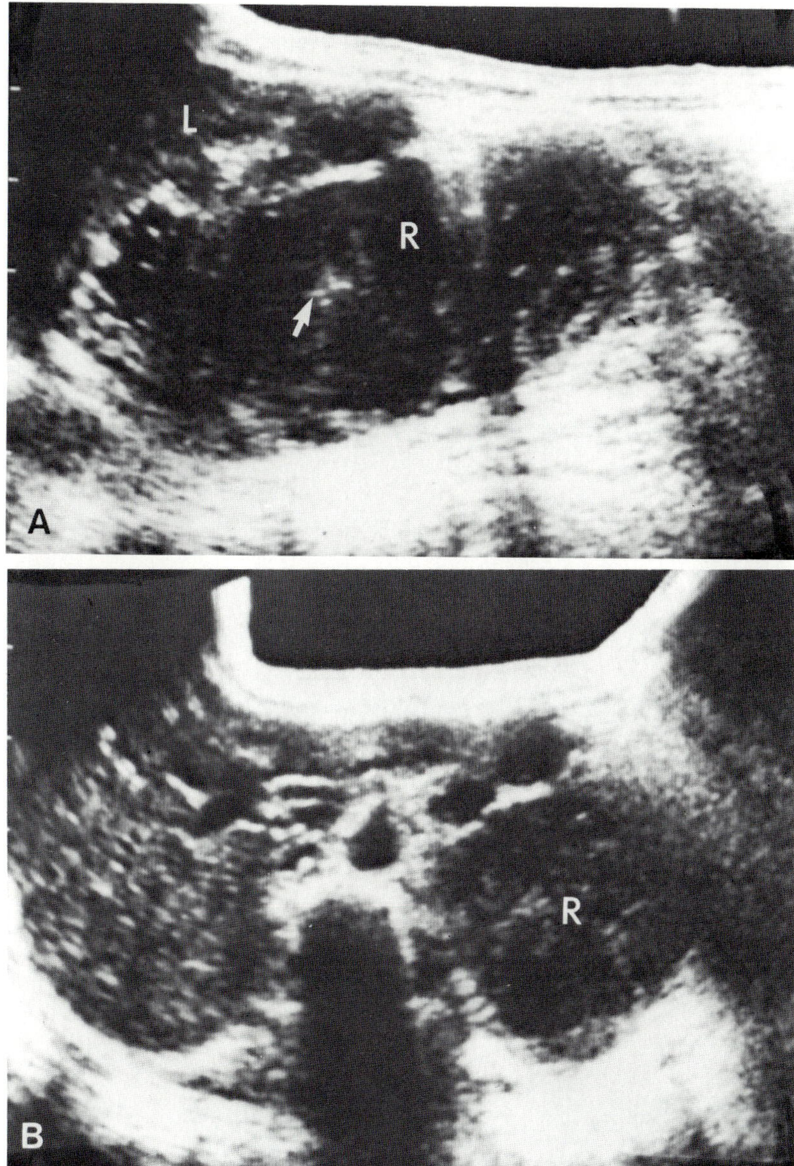

FIGURE 4.9. (a) A sagittal supine sonogram through the left upper quadrant reveals a reniform mass in the region of the left kidney (R) with only a suggestion of central calyceal echoes (arrow). L = left lobe of liver. (b) A transverse supine sonogram obtained in the same patient demonstrating the abnormally enlarged left kidney infiltrated by lymphoma (R).

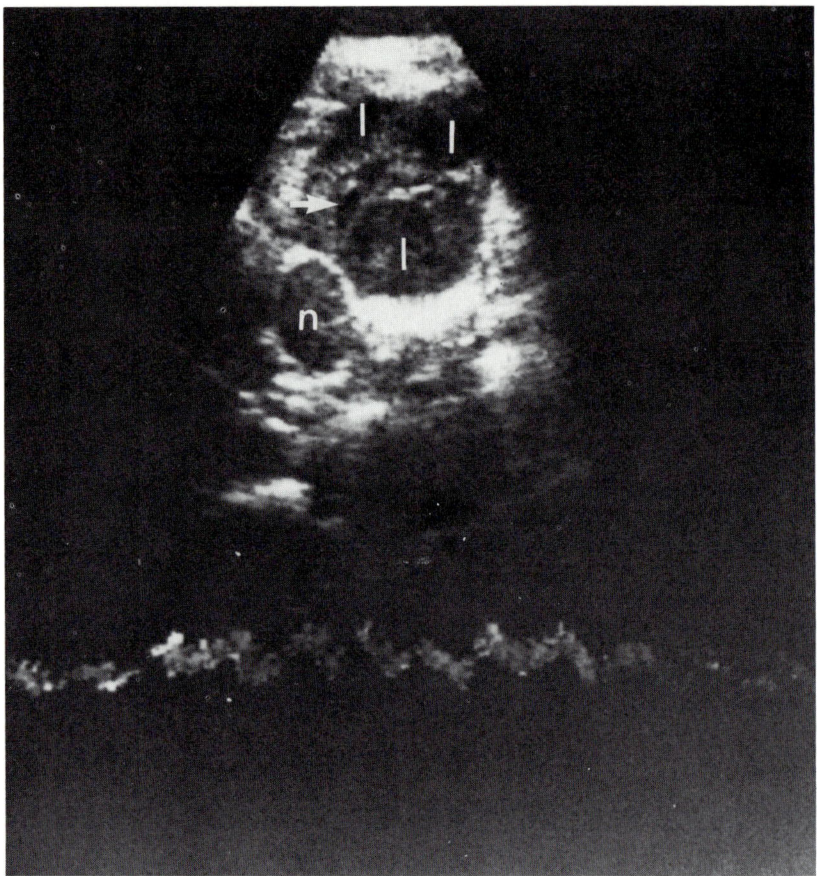

FIGURE 4.10. Left transverse decubitus scan through the left kidney demonstrates multiple focal intrarenal lymphomatous deposits (1), mild hydronephrosis in a distorted collecting system (arrow) and renal hilar nodes (n).

tinal involvement, usually symptomatic in nature.[4] Sonographic features of gastrointestinal lymphoma include a relatively hypoechoic mass with a central sonodensity (Fig. 4.11).[18] The demonstration of such a mass suggests a gastrointestinal lesion. However, such findings are not specific for lymphomatous involvement, as gastric carcinoma or gastric wall edema may have a similar appearance. Intrinsic gastrointestinal disease may be difficult to distinguish sonographically from contiguous celiac, retrogastric, or peripancreatic nodes, which frequently coexist. Real-time viewing of the gastric fundus through a fluid path facilitates the identification of the gastric etiology of the lesion. While sonographic examinations will not replace barium studies, they may prove useful in directing attention to abnormal areas on subsequent x-ray exams of the gastrointestinal tract.

Approximately 10 percent of the non-Hodgkin patients present with pan-

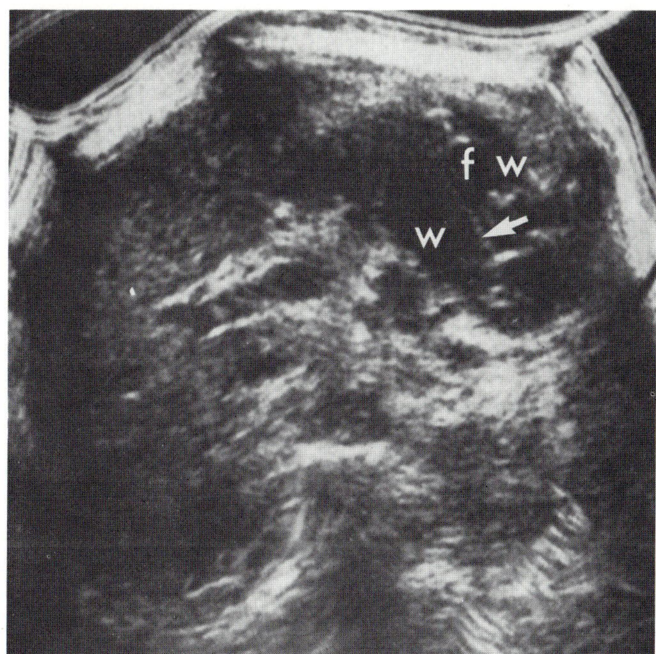

FIGURE 4.11. A transverse supine sonogram at 4 cm inferior to the xiphoid shows hypoechoic thickening of the gastric wall (w) and a central sonodense line representing the mucosal surface (arrow). The lumen of the stomach is fluid-filled (f).

creatic disease.[4] Sonographic features of pancreatic involvement include replacement of portions of pancreatic tissue by focal hypoechoic or anechoic masses (Fig. 4.12). Peripancreatic adenopathy, which commonly coexists, is usually sonographically indistinguishable from intrinsic pancreatic disease and may occur in the presence of a normal lymphangiogram.[13] Sonographic features of pancreatic involvement by lymphoma may be simulated by atypical pseudocysts, abscesses of the pancreas, or less commonly pancreatic carcinoma.

Lymphomatous thyroid masses appear similar to extranodal lymphomatous metastases at other sites. Hypoechoic, poorly marginated masses, which may be indistinguishable from other primary or secondary thyroid neoplasms, can be detected using high frequency (greater than 5 MHz) transducers. Lymphomatous metastases to the pleura, chest wall, breast, and ovaries usually manifest an appearance similar to that previously described for the involvement of other extranodal sites. Muscular involvement by lymphoma may be detected in a variety of sites. Sonographic findings include diffuse enlargement of the muscle without well-defined focal masses, or focal anechoic, featureless soft tissue masses resembling hematomas or abscesses (Fig. 4.13). The sonographic features demonstrated by extranodal lymphomatous

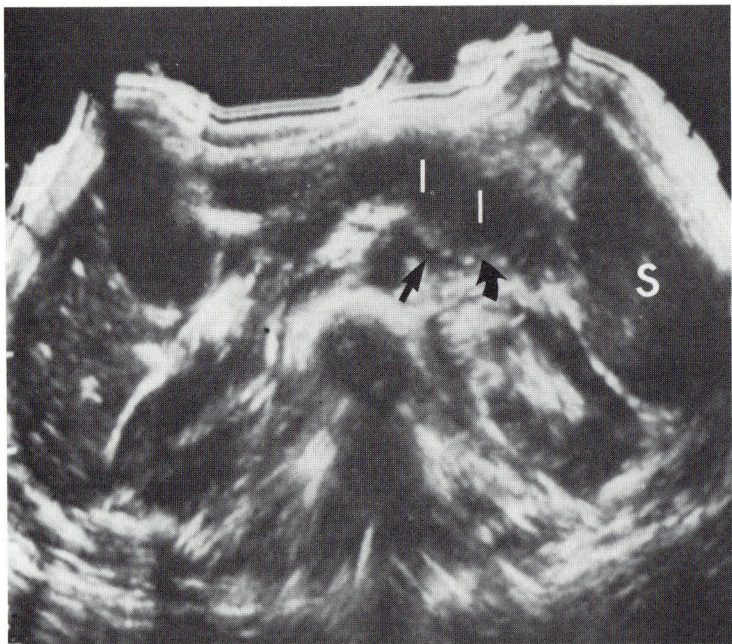

FIGURE 4.12. A transverse supine sonogram at 3 cm inferior to the xiphoid reveals hypoechoic, focal replacement of normal pancreatic tissue in the tail and body of the pancreas by lymphoma (1). A small amount of normal pancreatic tissue is observed (curved arrow) as is a portion of the splenic vein (arrow). Splenomegaly is also present (S).

metastases are not specific for the histologic subtype of lymphoma; however non-Hodgkin lymphomas have been detected more frequently in extranodal sites.

ULTRASOUND AND OTHER IMAGING MODALITIES IN THE DETECTION OF ABDOMINAL LYMPHOMA

The sonographic accuracy for the detection of retroperitoneal lymphadenopathy has been well described.[5-7] Computed tomography, which images similar abdominal anatomy, has been reported to be 90 percent accurate in the detection of paraaortic adenopathy.[3, 9, 10] Retroperitoneal fat, which degrades sonographic resolution, facilitates CT evaluation of the retroperitoneum. Bowel gas provides an additional source of diagnostic inaccuracy in the sonographic evaluation of the retroperitoneum. However, because ultrasound is an accurate imaging procedure that can be done rapidly, does not involve exposure to ionizing radiation or contrast media, and is relatively inexpensive, it should provide valuable diagnostic screening information, particular-

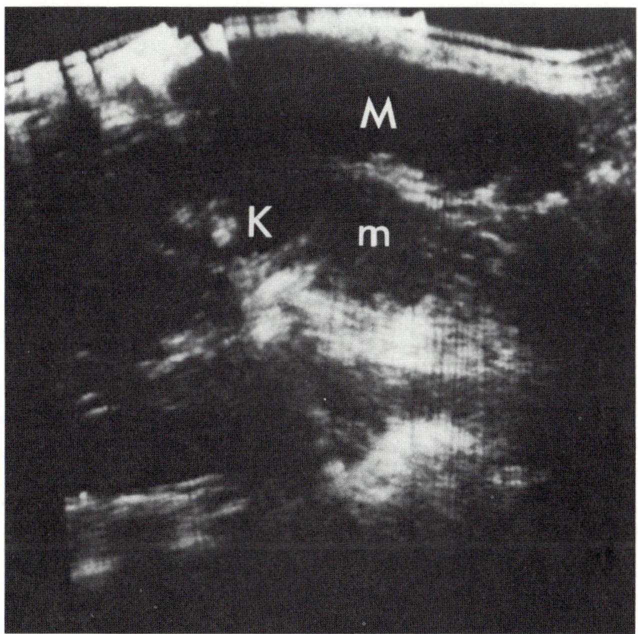

FIGURE 4.13. A sagittal prone scan 6 cm left of midline demonstrates a large, featureless anechoic mass involving the superficial paraspinous muscles (M). m = iliopsoas muscle; K = left kidney.

ly in the staging of non-Hodgkin patients, as well as in the surveillance of Hodgkin and non-Hodgkin patients.

One preliminary prospective study reports that lymphangiography is more accurate than ultrasound or CT in assessing opacified abdominal nodes.[7] (Table 4.1). Other authors report that sonography and gallium 67 citrate scanning is as accurate as lymphangiography in detecting abdominal nodal involvement.[5, 6, 8] Still others found gallium 67 citrate scanning a rather disappointing imaging modality, which detected less than 50 percent of abdominal disease.[19] A recent paper maintains that an abnormal CT scan may eliminate the need for lympangiography; these authors suggest CT scanning, performed at 2 cm intervals, provides a reliable means of excluding abdominal disease.[9] While the detection of abnormally enlarged nodes suggests lymphomatous involvement, a false positive diagnosis can result due to hyperplastic reactive changes within nodes. As many as 10 percent of normal sized nodes may be involved with lymphoma at the time of presentation.

A careful prospective study comparing CT, ultrasound, and lymphangiography is necessary to better define the accuracies of these modalities and their appropriate roles in the staging and surveillance of malignant lymphomas. It is possible that the demonstration of significant nodal disease by ultrasound or CT body scanning may obviate the need for lymphangiography

TABLE 4.1. Paraaortic/paracaval adenopathy—staging.[a]

LAG	+	−
+	16	1
−	1	34

CT	+	−
+	14	6
−	2	30

US	+	−
+	4	0
−	2	11

	LAG	*CT*	*US*
Sensitivity	16/17 = 94%	14/16 = 88%	4/6 = 67%
Specificity	34/35 = 97%	30/36 = 83%	11/11 = 100%
Accuracy			
Overall	50/52 = 96%	44/52 = 85%	15/17 = 88%
+ Report	16/17 = 94%	14/20 = 70%	4/4 = 100%
− Report	34/35 = 97%	30/32 = 94%	11/13 = 85%

[a]Fifty-two cases, 38 with Hodgkin and 14 with non-Hodgkin lymphoma lymph node pathology. (From Castellino RA, Noon M, Carroll BA, et al: Lymphography, computed tomography and ultrasound in staging Hodgkin's disease and non-Hodgkin's lymphoma. Proceedings of the Seventh International Congress of Lymphology. Florence, Italy, October 28–November 1, 1979.) Abbreviations: LAG = lymphangiography; CT = computed tomography; US = ultrasound.

in most cases. However, because lymphangiography accurately detects disease in normal size nodes, is easy to use for surveillance imaging, and is useful for directing surgical node samplings, CT and ultrasound must be evaluated very carefully before they replace lymphangiography in the diagnostic imaging workup of lymphoma.

References

1. Deforges JF, Rutherford CJ, Piro A: Hodgkins disease. N Engl J Med 301:1212–1222, 1979.
2. Harell GS, Breiman RS, Glatstein EJ, Marshall WH, Castellino RA: Computed tomography of the abdomen in the malignant lymphomas. Rad Clin N Am 15:391–400, 1977.
3. Alcorn FS, Mategrano VC, Petasnick JP, et al.: Contributions of computed tomography in the staging and management of malignant lymphomas. Radiology 125:717–723, 1977.
4. Goffinet DR, Warnke R, Dunnick WR, Castellino R, Glatstein E, Nelsen TS, Dorfman RF, Rosenberg SA, Kaplan HS: Clinical and surgical laparotomy—evaluation of patients with non-Hodgkin's lymphomas. Cancer treat Rep 61:981–992, 1977.
5. Brascho DL, Durant JR, Green LE: The accuracy of retroperitoneal ultrasonography in hodgkin's disease and non-Hodgkin's lymphoma. Radiology 125:485–487, 1977.
6. Rochester D, Bowie JD, Kunzmann A, Lester E: Ultrasound in the staging of lymphoma. Radiology 124:483–487, 1977.
7. Castellino RA, Noon M, Carroll BA, Hoppe RT, Young SW, Blank N, Marglin SI, Harell GS: Lymphography, computed tomography and ultrasound in staging Hodgkin's disease and non-Hodgkin's lymphoma. Proceedings of the Seventh International Congress of Lymphology. Florence, Italy, October 28–November 1, 1979.
8. Rudders RA, McCaffrey JA, Kahn PC: The relative roles of gallium-67-citrate scanning and lymphangiography in the current management of malignant lymphoma. Cancer 40: 1439–1443, 1977.

9. Lee JKT, Stanley RJ, Sagel SS, et al.: Accuracy of computed tomography in detecting intraabdominal and pelvic adenopathy in lymphoma. Am J Radiol 131: 311–315, 1978.
10. Breiman RS, Castellino RA, Harell GS: CT-pathologic correlations in Hodgkin's disease and non-Hodgkin's lymphoma. Radiology 126: 159–166, 1978.
11. Filly RA, Marglin S, Castellino RA: The ultrasonographic spectrum of abdominal and pelvic Hodgkin's disease and non-Hodgkin's lymphoma. Cancer 38: 2143–2148, 1946.
12. Sanders RC, Duffy T, McLoughlin MG, Walsh PC: Sonography in the diagnosis of retroperitoneal fibrosis. J Urol 118: 1977.
13. Carroll BA, Tal NH: The ultrasonic appearance of extranodal abdominal lymphoma. Radiology, in press.
14. Taylor KJW, Milan J: Differential diagnosis of chronic splenomegaly by gray-scale ultrasonography: clinical observation and digital A-scan analysis. Br J Radiol 49: 519–525, 1976.
15. Cunningham JJ: Ultrasonic findings in isolated lymphoma of the spleen simulating splenic abscess. J Clin Ultrasound 6: 412–414, 1973.
16. Shawker TH, Dunnick NR, Head GL, Magrath IT: Ultrasound evaluation of American Burkett's lymphoma. J Clin Ultrasound 7:279–283 August, 1979.
17. Kaude, JV, Lacy GD: Ultrasonography in Renal Lymphoma. J Clin Ultrasound 6: 321–323, 1978.
18. Salem S, Hiltz CW: Ultrasonographic appearance of gastric lymphosarcoma. J Clin Ultrasound 429–430, December, 1978.
19. Horn NL, Ray GR, Kriss JP: Gallium-67 citrate scanning in Hodgkin's disease and non-Hodgkin's lymphoma. Cancer 37: 250–257, 1976.

5 Kidneys

ROGER C. SANDERS

Ultrasonic criteria for the distinction between a renal neoplasm and a renal cyst have been available for several years. Most series document an accuracy, in making this distinction, of about 95 percent.[1-4] Little or no trouble occurs in the distinction between normal renal parenchyma, a simple cyst, and a neoplasm that has numerous internal echoes within it, but echogenicity greater than the surrounding renal parenchyma within a renal neoplasm is unusual.[5] Occasional inaccuracies occur when attempts to distinguish between a cyst and a mass, which contains essentially no internal echoes (a solid homogeneous mass), are made. Such solid masses may mistakenly be called cysts, and rarely, cysts that contain atypical fluid are called solid masses. Increased transonicity is almost always seen in cysts but is also often seen in neoplasms. Comparison with a known cystic structure, such as the gallbladder, helps. Providing that it lies at the same depth, a similar echo-free appearance and degree of through transmission will be seen (see Fig 5.1 and 5.2). The distinction between cystic and solid can be accentuated if a transducer of higher frequency is used and can be checked by the use of A-mode, which may be a little more sensitive in the detection of subtle echoes within a mass. One should ensure that a transducer of the correct focal length is used. The walls of renal cysts are generally smooth, although lobulation may occur, whereas those of renal neoplasms are almost always irregular. An irregularity in the wall of a cyst may be due to septum. If such septa are clearly present, this is good evidence that the mass is filled with fluid. A thin echo-free area distal to the lateral walls of a cyst is commonly seen and represents a refraction artifact. This "lateral shades" sign is helpful in the diagnosis of a cyst.[6] A few internal echoes may be seen within cysts in the dependent area, although this is unusual. Such echoes may be due to debris or to an artifact presumed to be related to the beam partially transecting fluid. Echoes occur within the center of almost all renal neoplasms and are often, although sparse, bright reflectors.[5]

A good deal of progress has been made in correlating various sonographic patterns within neoplasms with the type of neoplasm. Hypernephroma

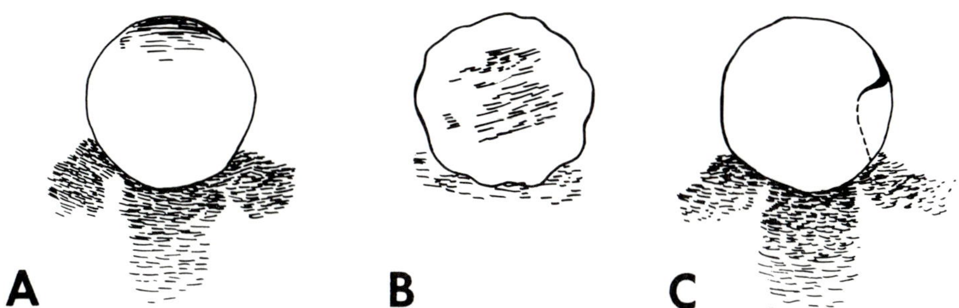

FIGURE 5.1. Diagram of the typical appearances of a cyst. Note in (a) acoustic enhancement through the mass. (b) Appearance of a homogeneous mass; a few internal echoes, practically no through transmission, and a slightly irregular wall. (c) Septum mimicking a mass arising from the wall of the cyst.

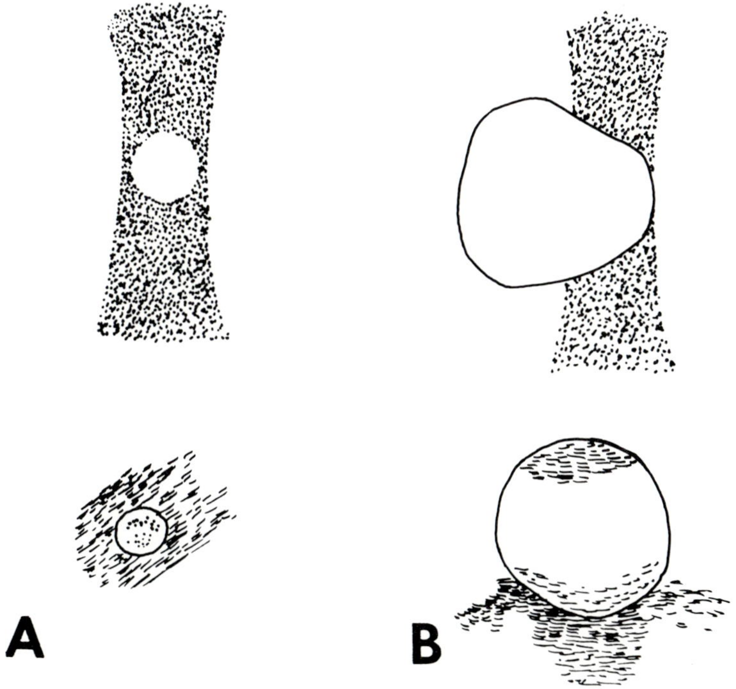

FIGURE 5.2. A cyst can appear to have internal echoes if it is included incompletely within the beam along with some adjacent tissue (a). (b) Typical artifacts within a cyst, which may wrongly suggest the presence of neoplasm. Reverberations in the anterior aspect of cysts cause parallel echogenic lines to the anterior wall of the cyst. These help to identify this as a fluid-filled structure. Artifactual echoes are also seen in the posterior aspect of the cyst thought to be due to partial volume effect when the beam transects the wall and the cyst at the same time.

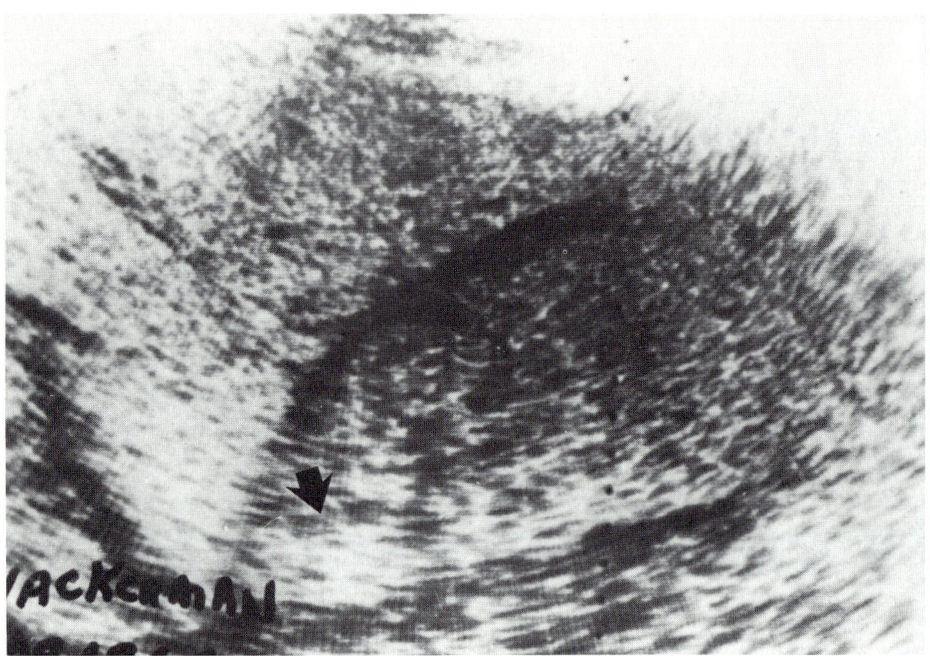

FIGURE 5.3. This kidney is almost completely involved with an echogenic hypernephroma. Only the upper pole is spared (arrow).

(otherwise known as von Grawitz or renal cell carcinoma), the most common type of renal neoplasm, vary in echogenicity. Some are highly echogenic (Fig. 5.3), others contain essentially no internal echoes. Coleman et al. have shown that echopenic hypernephroma (Figs. 5.4 and 5.5) that contain fewer echoes than the adjacent renal parenchyma are the most common variety.[5] Correlation with the variants of hypernephroma, such as papillary carcinoma or oncocytoma, which carry a more favorable prognosis, has not yet been sufficient to determine if a typical sonographic pattern exists, though the suggestion has been made that they will be solid homogeneous masses.[32] A moderate correlation between the echogenicity of a hypernephroma and the degree of vascularity was alleged[7] on the basis of bistable studies, but this did not prove reliable when gray scale comparisons were performed.[5] However, avascular masses, which might angiographically be either cyst or neoplasm, commonly contain internal echoes.[8]

In my experience the smallest neoplasms that can be detected by ultrasound are about 1 cm in size. Cysts are easier to discriminate from adjacent renal parenchyma than neoplasms, since there is such a marked difference in acoustic impedance; cysts as small as 2 to 3 mm in size can be seen if they lie in the appropriate focal zone. Since ultrasound is a tomographic technique, it does not represent a good screening method for the detection of hypernephroma. Neoplasms in locations that are relatively inaccessible, e.g., the left

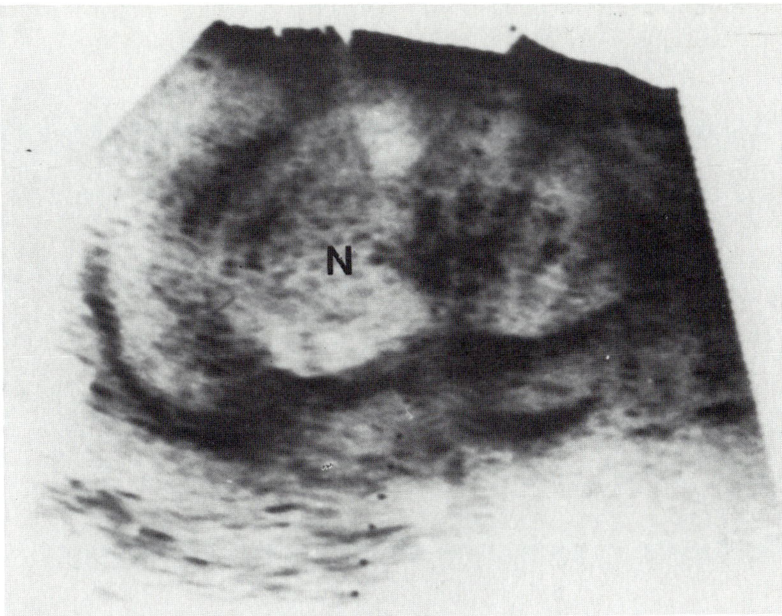

FIGURE 5.4. A large relatively echo-free hypernephroma at the upper pole of the kidney (N) shows some areas of echogenicity (decubitus view).

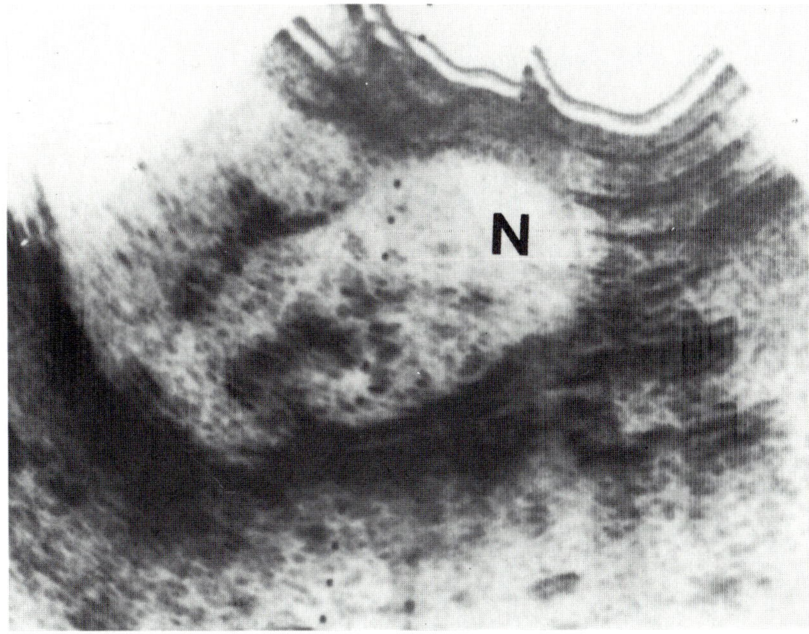

FIGURE 5.5. Essentially echo-free mass at lower pole of the kidney (N), which proved to be a hypernephroma.

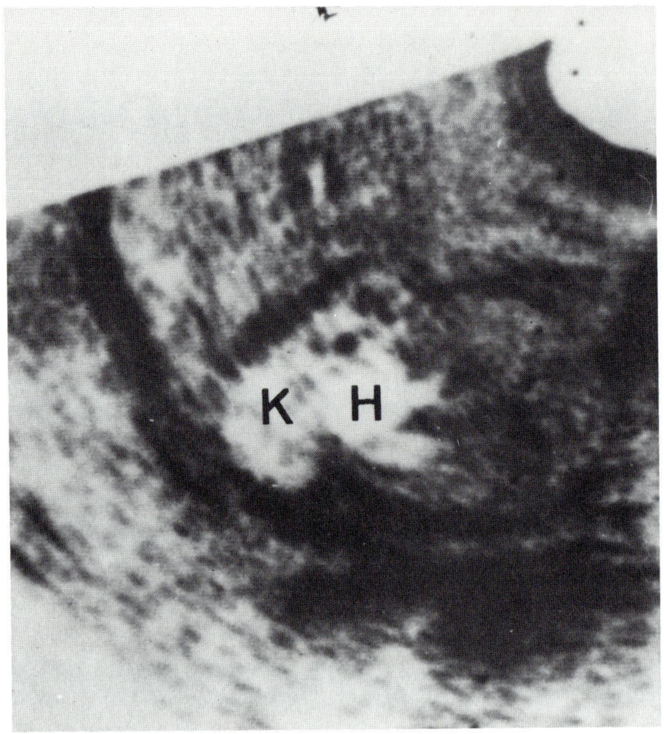

FIGURE 5.6. Longitudinal section of a Wilms tumor involving the lower pole of the right kidney. There is a small amount of hydronephrosis (H) superior to the Wilms tumor and a rim of renal parenchyma (K) remains.

upper pole, can be missed. Ultrasound is better used as a follow-up to an excretion urogram (EVU): it is essential that the EVU be available at the time the sonogram is performed so that smaller lesions can be located when a written description leaves one uncertain as to exactly where they lie. However, some exophytic lesions arising from the lateral aspect of the kidney and invisible on the EVU, can be seen sonographically. It may therefore be worthwhile to perform a sonogram in a patient who has a negative EVU but in whom the clinical suspicion of renal neoplasm is high.

Wilms' tumors, the most common tumors in childhood, have an acoustic pattern slightly less varied than that of hypernephroma. Most such tumors do contain internal echoes (Fig. 5.6), and a significant subsegment have sonolucent areas within, which represent areas of necrosis (Fig. 5.7).[9] These echo-free areas usually represent liquified material. The amount of sonolucent material may reach quite sizable amounts, so that rarely the neoplasm may appear largely cystic at sonography. On occasion, a fluid-fluid level may be seen within such a sonolucent area and is thought to represent bleeding into an area of necrosis. When a Wilms' tumor evolves into a rhabdomyoma, the acoustic pattern, in two cases, has resembled that of a fibroid.

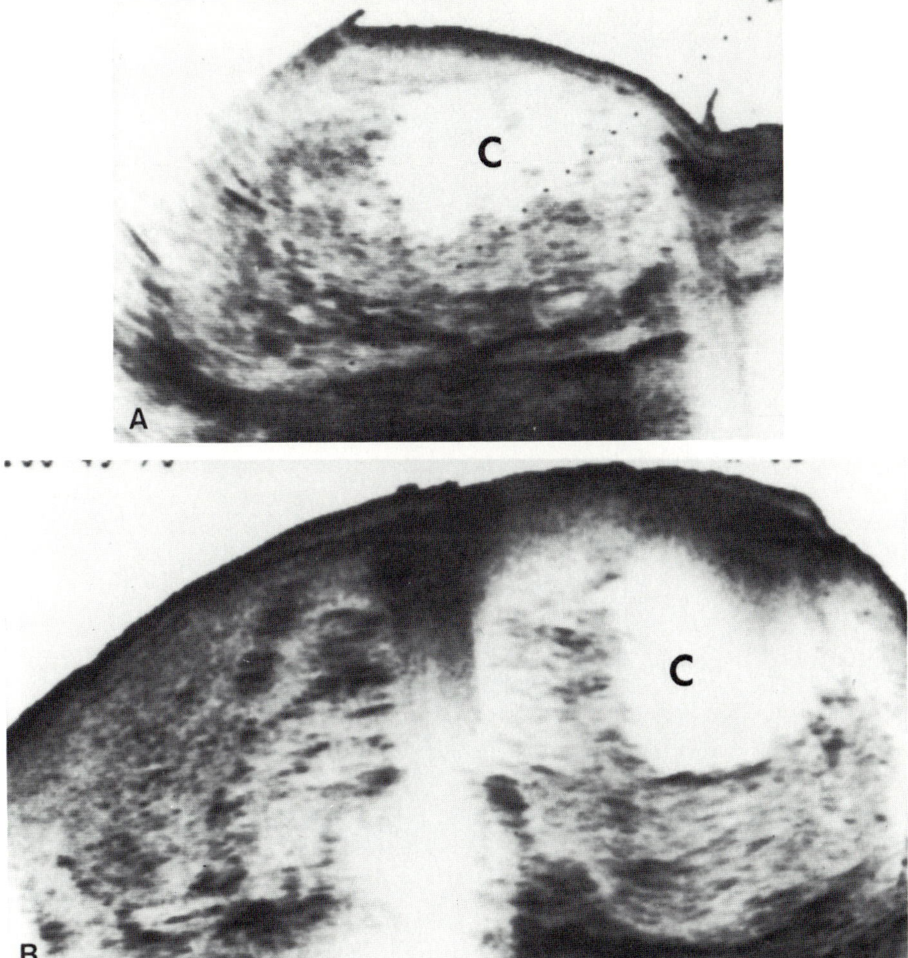

FIGURE 5.7. (a) Longitudinal section through a large Wilms tumor arising from the anterior aspect of the kidney, which has a necrotic component (C). (b) Transverse section of the same patient.

Benign mesoblastic nephroma is generally considered to be a separate entity distinct from Wilms' tumor. Experience with these rare tumors is limited,[10, 11] but a review of four cases at the AFIP showed two to be highly echogenic (Fig. 5.8) and a third to contain cysts.[12] The pattern appears to be as variable as that of hypernephroma.

Transitional cell carcinomas have a typical ultrasonic appearance, containing only low-level echoes.[13] Unfortunately, the appearances are easily confused with blood clot or sloughed papilla. These tumors occur in the central part of the kidney and separate the "sinus" echoes (Fig. 5.9). Although on the EVU they can be confused with uric acid calculi, stones, whatever their com-

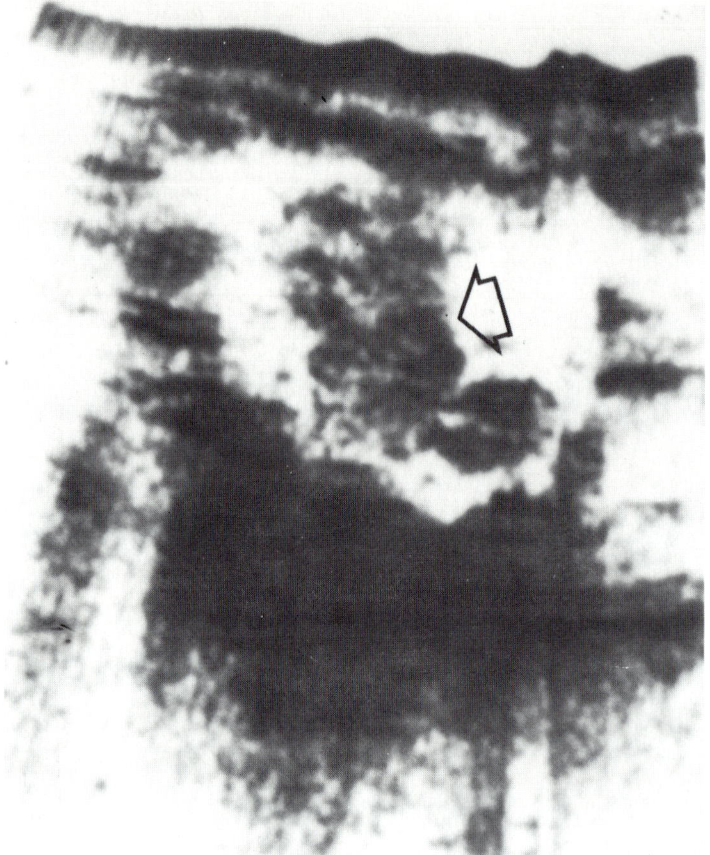

FIGURE 5.8. Longitudinal section. This neonate has a mesoblastic nephroma. This tumor contains a large echogenic component (arrow) (Courtesy of St. Judes Hospital, Fullerton, California.)

position, provided they are of sufficient size, cause distinctive acoustic shadowing. Serial studies should allow distinction of tumor from clot, since the latter will change in shape and acoustic character over the course of time.

Benign neoplasms of the kidney are not common, but one benign mass that can be specifically diagnosed by more modern imaging modalities does occur with some frequency. An angiomyolipoma (otherwise known as renal hamartoma) is a benign neoplasm composed of a mixture of muscle and fat. This neoplasm is reported to produce a highly echogenic pattern in the kidney whenever it is seen (Fig. 5.10).[14-16] The echogenicity is a tip-off that a computerized axial tomogram should be performed; the fat within the mass will have a pathognomonic low density number. Angiomyolipomas as small as 1.5 cm have been diagnosed with this technique.[17] It has been suggested that any renal tumor that contains fat will have a similar sonographic appearance. A myolipoma was also echogenic.[18]

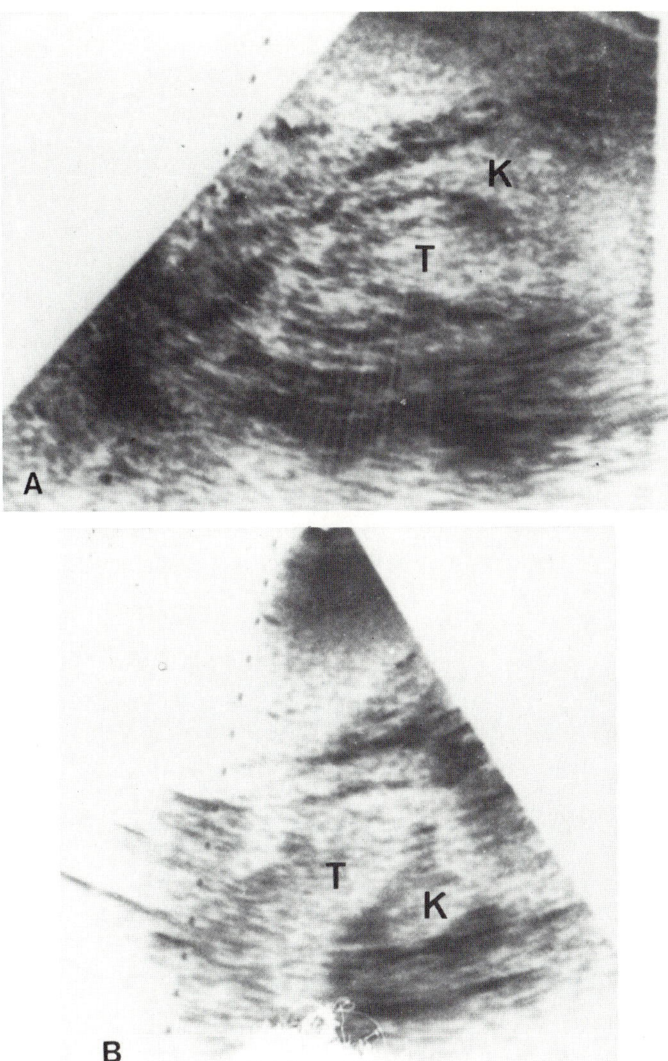

FIGURE 5.9. (a) Longitudinal section through the left kidney. The sinus echoes are separated by a large transitional cell tumor (T). It has almost the same echogenicity as the rest of the renal parenchyma (K). (b) A transverse section shows that the tumor is proceeding down the pelvis into the ureter.

Lymphomas also have a fairly characteristic appearance. In the kidney, lymphomatous lesions are generally echo-free, although histiocytic lymphoma may have an echogenic pattern. Distribution of lymphomatous deposits is variable. In some instances there is a localized deposit of lymphoma that causes a mass, distorting the usual sonographic anatomy (Fig. 5.11); in others there are multiple, smaller, echo-free deposits causing a generalized renal enlargement without major distortion of renal outline or of sinus

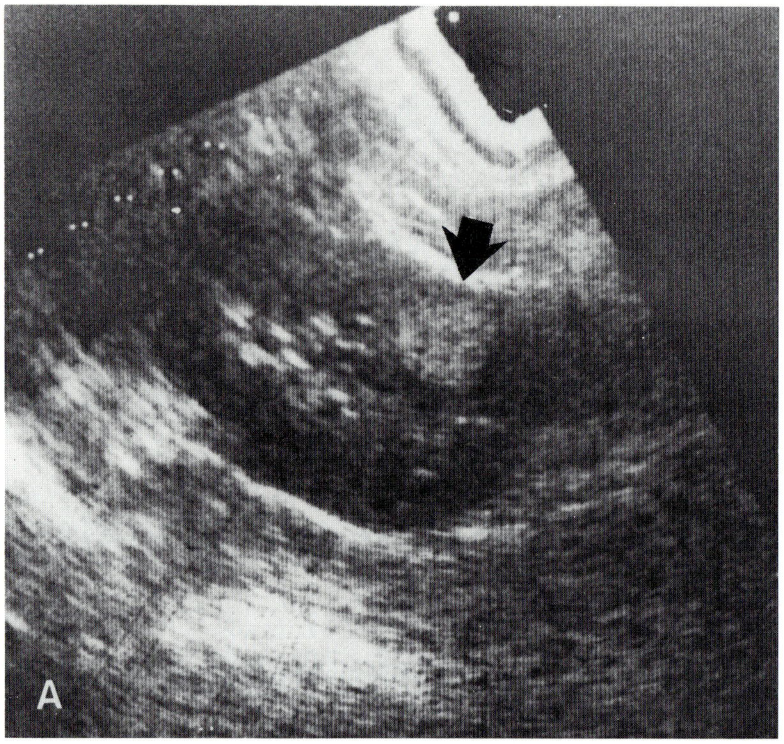

FIGURE 5.10. (a) Longitudinal section. An echogenic mass can be seen within the renal parenchyma (arrow).

echoes (Fig. 5.12). The echo-free areas may be mistaken for unduly obvious renal pyramids.[19] Leukemic deposits can give a similar picture.[20] Figure 5.13 summarizes diagrammatically some of the typical ultrasonic appearances of neoplasms.

Experience with metastatic lesions of the kidney is limited, although these are common at autopsy. When seen, metastases have often been hypoechogenic (Fig. 5.14), which is somewhat surprising in view of their variable origin and the varied pattern of metastases in other organs, such as the liver.

At least 99 percent of the cysts seen on sonography and computerized tomography are benign lesions of no clinical significance, unless they are causing secondary compression of a calyx or infundibulum, or are responsible for abdominal pain. How does one distinguish the small minority that are neoplastic from the benign? Seven neoplasms within cysts have been seen at Johns Hopkins. In those cases in which a good quality sonogram was available, a localized echogenic area within the cyst could be seen (Fig. 5.15). In many instances, such an echogenic focus in a cyst proves to be of no significance when the patient is subsequently punctured, for it represents a lobulation or septum. However, the presence of echoes does appear to be a moder-

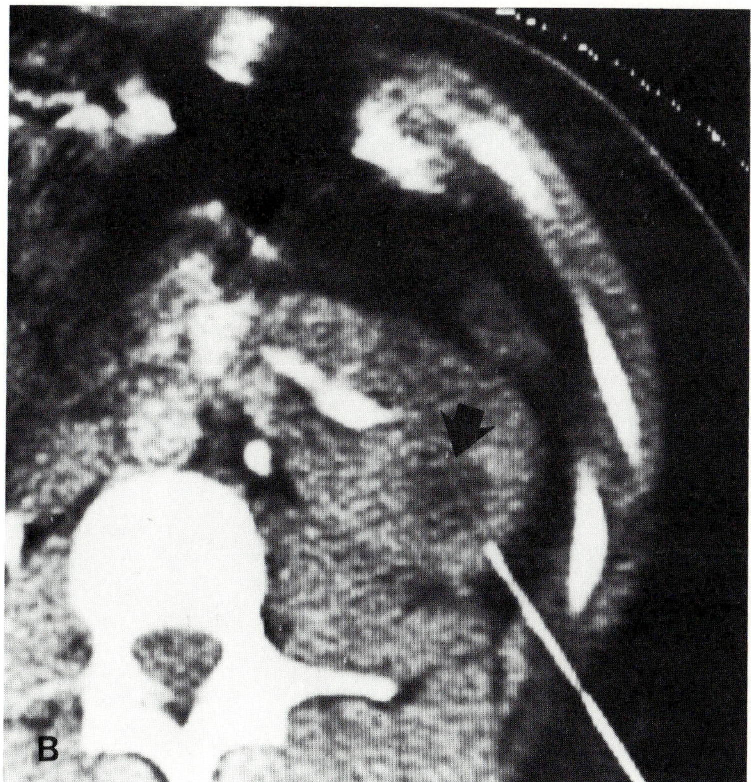

FIGURE 5.10. (b) Percutaneous biopsy of this mass under CT control was performed. The CT image shows a zone of decreased density (arrow) corresponding to the echogenic mass. The white line represents a needle which was inserted into the mass. The lesion proved to be an angiomyolipoma. (Courtesy of E. Lipsit, MD, George Washington Hospital, Washington, DC)

ately useful criteria when trying to decide whether or not to puncture a cyst. Other helpful criteria appear to be an abnormal CT number on the computed tomogram, or symptoms and signs suggestive of neoplasia.

A variant of a cyst, which may or may not have malignant potential, is a benign multilocular cyst. This condition, often seen in middle-aged women, has a characteristic sonographic appearance (Fig. 5.16). Although the cyst appears empty at angiography and nephrotomography, it contains numerous irregular thick septa that are readily seen both on sonography and CT.

Two benign conditions that give rise to lesions that may be mistaken for a neoplasm are hematoma and abscess. These entities may contain internal echoes. Both can mimic the ultrasonic appearances of a neoplasm but are generally recognizable on the basis of their history.

The detection of a renal neoplasm, thought to be malignant, within the kid-

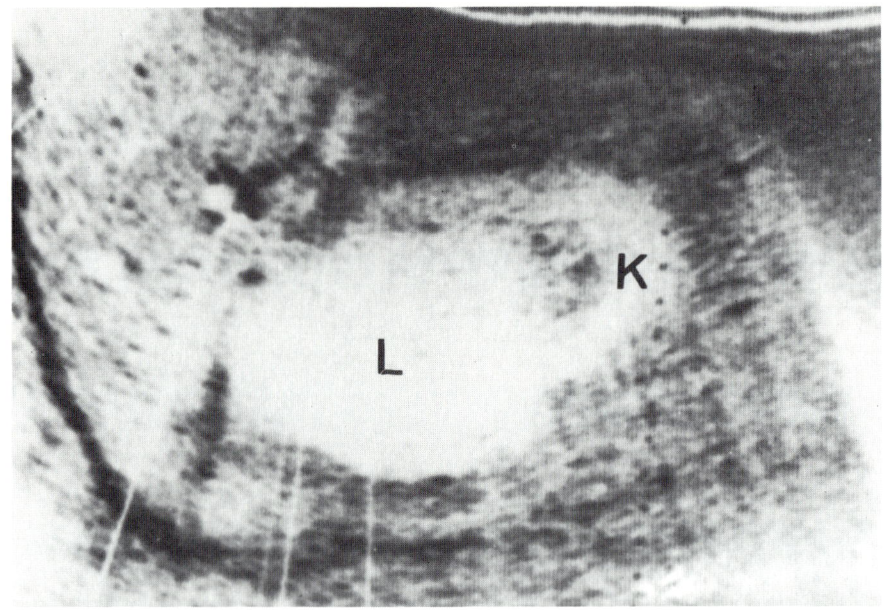

FIGURE 5.11. Longitudinal section. Large lymphomatous deposit (L) in the upper pole of the kidney (K).

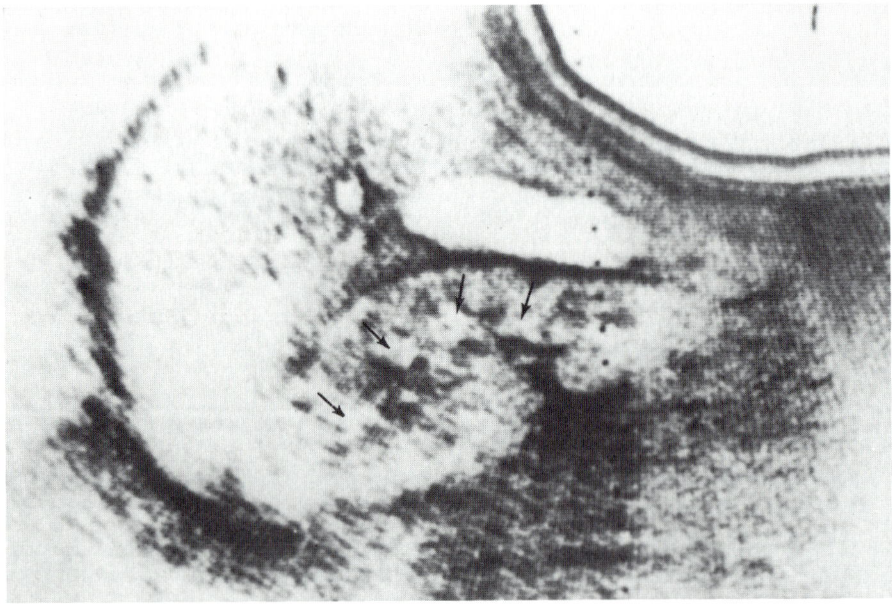

FIGURE 5.12. Numerous small deposits of lymphoma (arrows) are scattered throughout the kidney. A subsequent sonogram performed 6 month's later showed complete disappearance of these areas and return to normal size of the enlarged kidney.

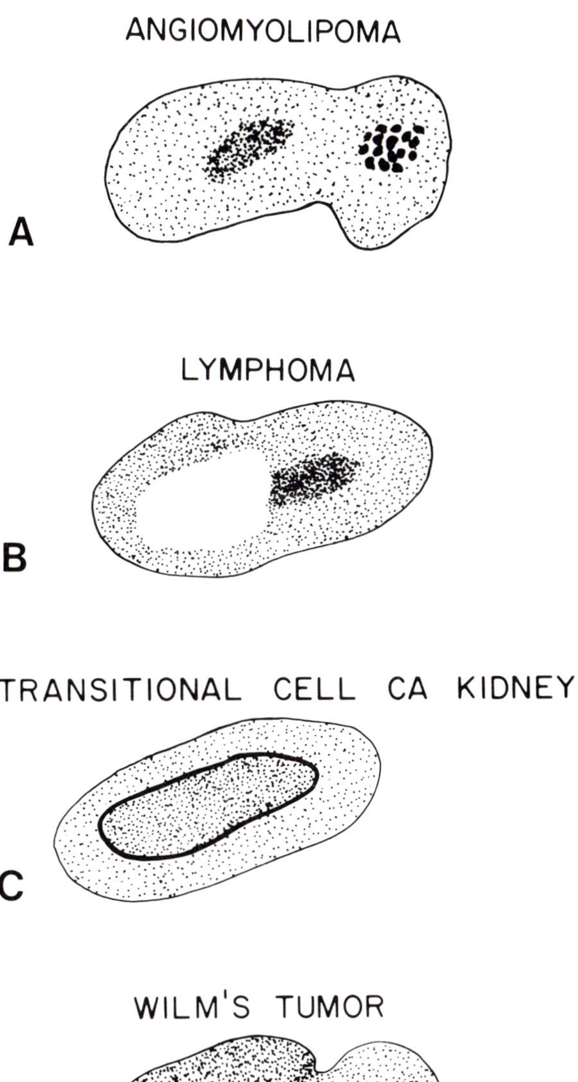

FIGURE 5.13. Diagram showing the typical appearance of some renal neoplasms. (a) The echogenic area at the lower pole represents an angiomyolipoma. (b) Echo-free mass suggestive of lymphoma. (c) The renal sinus echoes are split by the presence of a tumor due to transitional cell cancer. (d) Within the Wilms tumor one can see numerous sonolucent areas which represent areas of necrosis; in one there is a fluid-fluid level which represents blood within an area of necrosis.

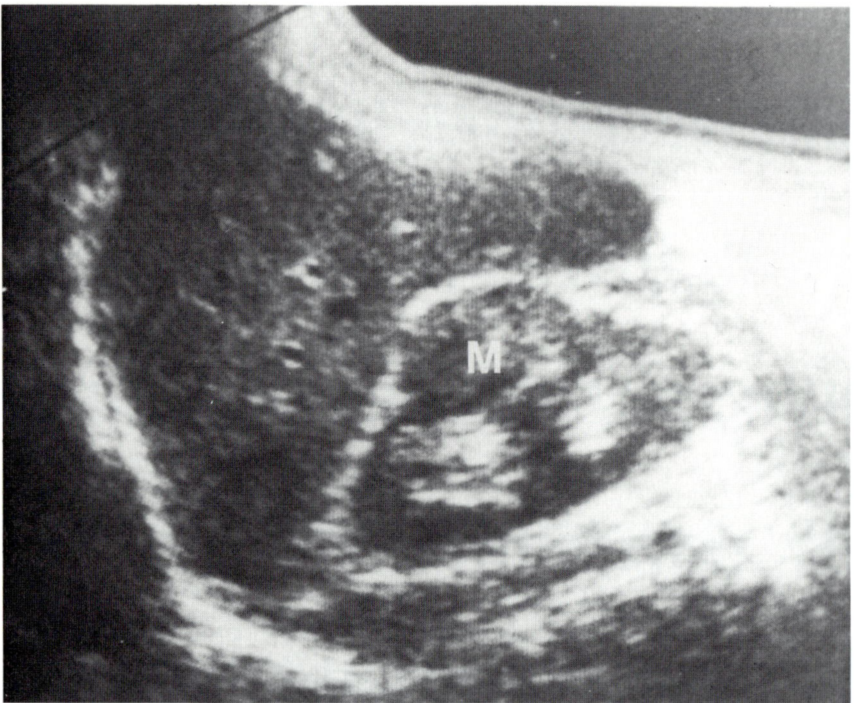

FIGURE 5.14. Longitudinal section. A metastatic lesion (M) can be seen distorting the anterior aspect of the kidney. It contains about the same number of echoes as the renal parenchyma.

ney signals the need for a number of ancillary ultrasonic views.[21, 22] It is important to define whether or not the neoplasm has penetrated the capsule of the kidney, for this interferes with operability. Although the fascial planes around the kidney are not as well delineated by sonography as by CT, it is usually possible to visualize penetration of the capsule, for the contour of the kidney will be irregular and the usually well-defined linear margin around the normal kidney, which represents the capsule, will be lost. Disruption of this capsule by a neoplasm is usually evident, but several sites around the kidney, notably the left upper pole, are inaccessible or difficult to demonstrate, due to overlying ribs. In some hypernephroma (and indeed in other renal neoplasms) a confusing picture can be seen if the neoplasm has caused secondary hydronephrosis (Fig. 5.5). A cystic lesion will be seen superior to the neoplasm.

A common site for hypernephroma invasion is along the renal vein;[23] renal vein invasion may be difficult to detect sonographically, but involvement of the inferior vena cava is a simple problem[24] (Fig. 5.17) as long as gas does not obscure the area. An echogenic mass within the caval lumen will be seen.

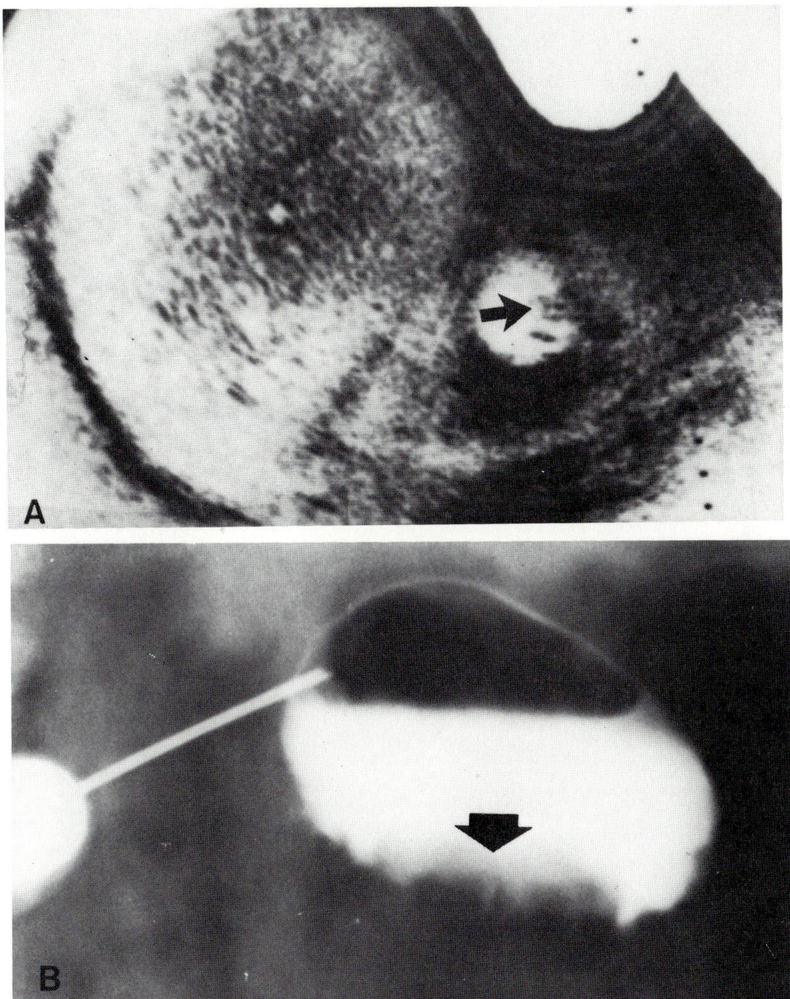

FIGURE 5.15. (a) Cystic lesion in the anterior aspect of the right kidney. There are a number of internal echoes within this cyst (arrows). (b) Because of a suspicion of a neoplasm, a puncture was performed. It showed a neoplasm involving the inferior aspect of the cyst (arrow), which proved to be a hypernephroma.

Sonography cannot distinguish venous tumor invasion from clot but it can differentiate the confusing washout appearance in the area of the renal vein on the cavogram from a true lesion.

Although most metastic lesions from hypernephroma occur in the lungs or bones, a small proportion metastasize early to the liver. Therefore, whenever a possible hypernephroma is discovered, the liver should be exhaustively surveyed to rule out metastases. Commonly found at surgery, though often

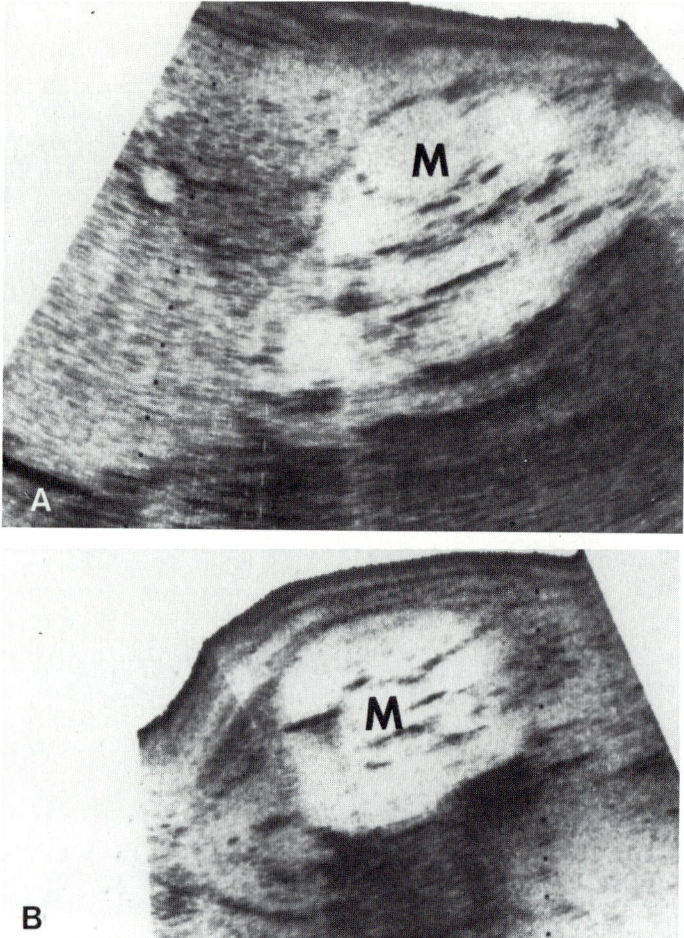

FIGURE 5.16. (a) Longitudinal section through a large multiloculated cystic mass (M) arising from the anterior aspect of the kidney. This was a multilocular cyst. (b) Transverse section of this same mass showing that it is bascially round in shape with numerous septum within.

too small to be detected by sonography, are paraaortic nodes. Hence, it is important to examine the paraaortic area in detail, particularly the area around the left renal hilum.[25] Although most nodal spread from hypernephromas takes place into adjacent nodes, the lymphatic spread from the kidney is not clearly mapped and examples have been seen in which nodal spread has occurred down to the level of the aortic bifurcation (Fig. 5.18). The hepatopathy that accompanies hypernephroma has no associated sonographic signs, apart from splenomegaly. Splenomegaly is also occasionally seen when the splenic vein has been directly involved by the renal neoplasm.

On more than one occasion, it has been unclear whether a mass in the kidney

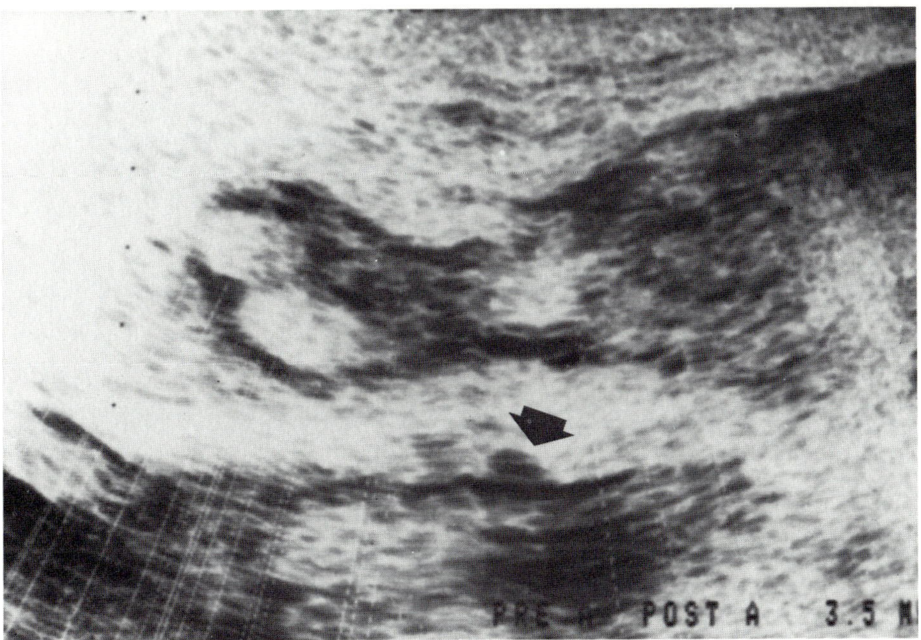

FIGURE 5.17. Longitudinal section through the inferior vena cava in a patient with a known hypernephroma. Proven neoplastic invasion of the inferior vena cava can be seen (arrow).

represents the primary lesion with metastatic lesions in the liver or whether another primary neoplasm is responsible for masses in the liver and kidney. Percutaneous puncture of the renal mass via a 22- or 23-guage needle is a simple procedure that has successfully clarified such confusing situations. In two instances there were two neoplasms—a hypernephroma and another primary.

A particularly difficult situation arises when a hypernephroma is calcified. The presence of calcification around or within a mass makes sonographic evaluation difficult. One may mistake the acoustic shadowing for an area of gas in adjacent bowel, when it is really a calcified mass. A cyst with a calcified rim may be indistinguishable from a hypernephroma.

Invasion of the kidney by neoplasms that arise in structures near the kidney is a sonographic problem. It is hard to distinguish whether the neoplasm is renal or adrenal in origin when invasion has occurred, and no interface is present (Fig. 5.19). The sonographic pattern of neuroblastoma is generally more varied than that of a Wilms tumor with high-level echoes. Areas of necrosis are more common in Wilms tumors than in neuroblastoma. Retroperitoneal sarcomas also develop necrotic areas, which appear as sonolucent spaces. Such necrotic centers are presumed to be a consequence of rapid sarcomatous growth.

The sonographic appearance of a column of Bertini is not particularly dis-

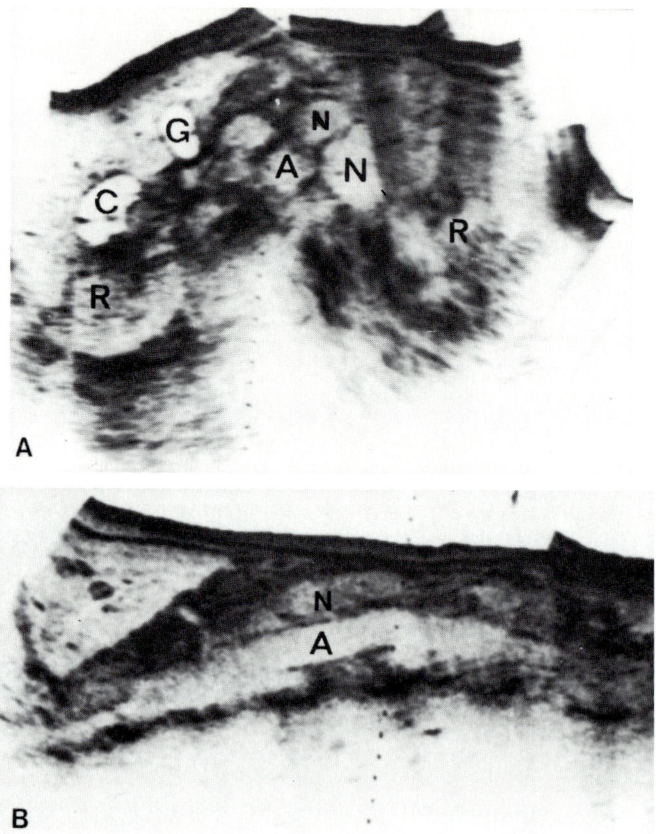

FIGURE 5.18. (a) Transverse section of the upper abdomen of a patient with a left hypernephroma. Several large nodes can be seen (N) surrounding the aorta (A). Gallbladder = G. At the anterior aspect of the right kidney there is a cyst (C) that contains a septum. R = kidneys. (b) Longitudinal section shows nodes (N) surrounding aorta (A).

tinct. An area of normal sonographic tissue invaginates into the renal sinus echoes (Fig. 5.20). A noninvasive method for distinguishing a column of Bertini from a neoplasm is a renal DMSA scan; the suspect area will take up isotope, if it is normal renal tissue.

Neoplasms can also be detected in the bladder. Several authors have attempted to assess the extent of neoplastic spread to see whether it has penetrated into or through the bladder wall.[26, 27] It has been suggested that a rigid wall or a reduced capacity indicates a grade B neoplasm with wall invasion and that a grade C neoplasm is indicated when a large pelvic mass or nodes are seen outside the bladder. Grade C neoplasms are certainly relatively easy to detect by ultrasound but experience with grade B neoplasms has not been very satisfactory. In my view, ultrasound, using a conventional static scanner, is not as accurate as computed tomography because it is hard to assess

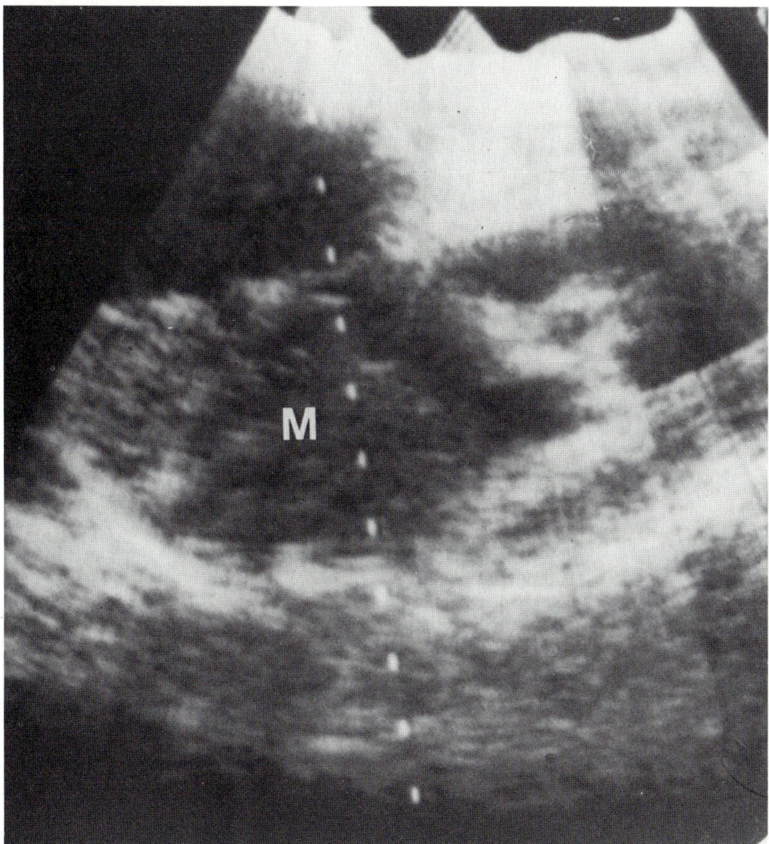

FIGURE 5.19. Longitudinal section through a small child, age 3, with a mass in the left upper quadrant. The mass (M) cannot be separated from the kidney. It proved to be neuroblastoma.

the extent of anteriorly placed neoplasms due to reverberation artifacts. Lesions on the lateral aspect of the wall of the bladder may be difficult to display because the beam is not at a satisfactory angle to show the degree of tissue penetration by the neoplasm. Wall rigidity is a difficult sign to assess; confusion can occur between clot and tumor. It is sometimes possible to see an echo-free area between a clot and the bladder wall, but this is not always present. It may well be that transrectal scanners will offer a better assessment of the degree of bladder wall invasion.

Most work using ultrasound in the assessment of prostatic neoplasia has been performed with transrectal scanners. Until the last year or so, experience with these scanners did not suggest that they would be used widely for the amount of clinical information obtained was limited and some neoplasms were missed. Recent work using transrectal scanners equipped with better gray scale has yielded impressive results.[28]

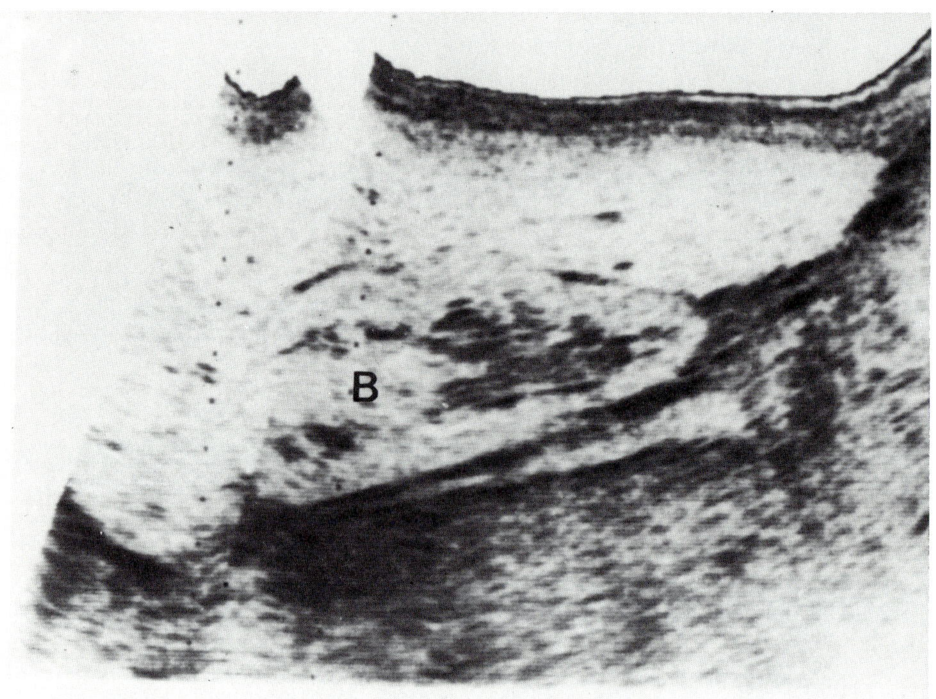

FIGURE 5.20. Longitudinal section through the left kidney and spleen. The sinus echoes are distorted by a mass (B) with the same acoustic texture as the remains of the kidney, which proved, on subsequent study, to be a column of Bertini.

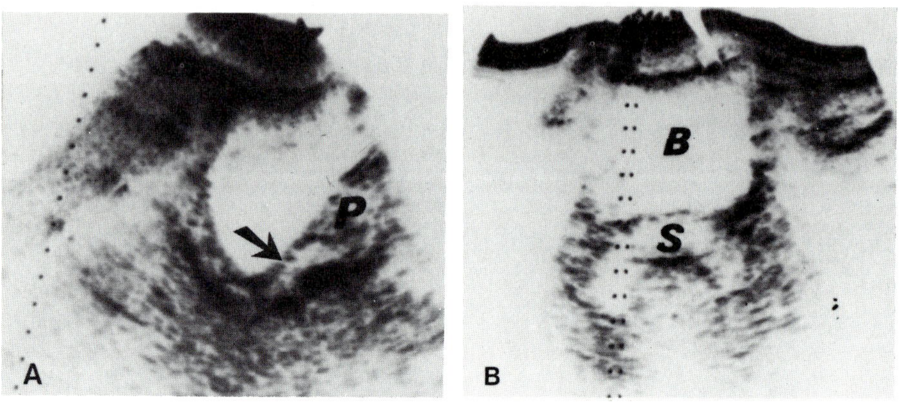

FIGURE 5.21. (a) Longitudinal section through normal prostate (P) and seminal vesicles (arrow). (b) Transverse section. B = bladder; S = seminal vesicle.

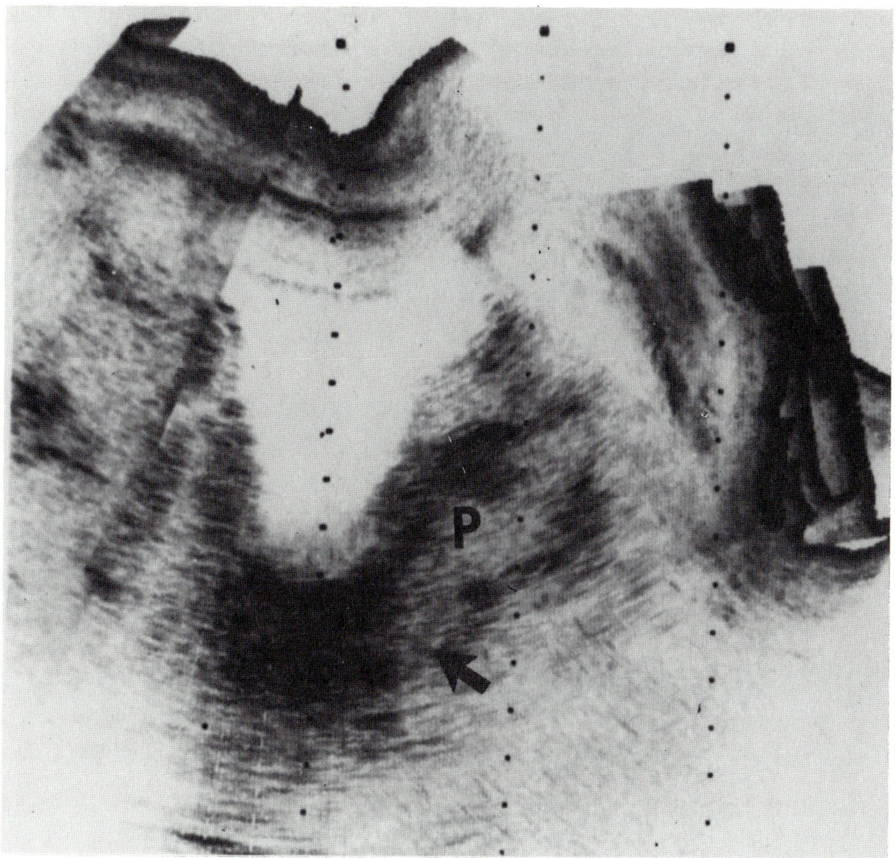

FIGURE 5.22. Longitudinal section. Both an abdominal and a perineal approach have been used. The prostate (P) is enlarged. There is a prostatic neoplasm invading the seminal vesicles (arrow).

It is possible to obtain valuable information about the prostate using a static scanner and scanning through the bladder[29, 30] (Fig. 5.21). One can visualize neoplastic invasion of the seminal vesicles and of the areas close to the bladder. Only part of the prostate can be seen on a routine anterior or posterior approach. An additional view can be obtained through the perineum but it is usually difficult to superimpose the perineal view on that obtained with a transabdominal approach (Fig. 5.22). A fairly accurate estimate of the volume of the prostate can be obtained using the anterior approach only.[31]

It is not clear from the literature whether prostatic neoplasms can be expected to be echogenic or echo free (Fig. 5.22). In all likelihood, the situation is similar to that with hepatic lesions—both types occur and the predominance of reports of echogenic lesions in the past is due to the ease with which they can be seen. B2 prostatic neoplasms (those confined to the capsule) are treated surgically, while the usual therapy for stage C and D prostatic carcinoma is irradiation. It seems unlikely that the critical distinction between a B2 and a C neoplasm can be obtained with a static scanner; for visualization of the lateral margin of the capsule is often difficult using an anterior approach. Nevertheless, a static scanner is helpful in evaluating the prostate in the management of prostatic neoplasms, for it can usefully define the extent of radiotherapy portals and show seminal vesicle invasion.

The ultrasonic assessment of renal neoplasms is no longer limited to a decision as to whether the mass is cystic or solid. The limits of neoplastic invasion can be defined for the surgeon. We are beginning to see the development of the ultrasonic characterization of renal tumors.

References

1. King DL: Renal ultrasonography. Radiology 105:633–640, 1972.
2. Romeiser RS, Walls WJ, Valk WL: B-scan ultrasound in the evaluation of renal mass lesions. J Urol 112:8–12, 1974.
3. Sherwood T: Renal masses and ultrasound. Br Med J 4:682–683, 1975.
4. Lingard DA, Lawson TL: Accuracy of ultrasound in predicting the nature of renal masses. J Urol 122:724–727, 1979.
5. Coleman BG, Arger PH, Mulhern CB, et al: Gray scale sonographic spectrum of hypernephromas. Accepted for publication in Radiology.
6. Bree RL, Silver TM: Differential diagnosis of hypoechoic and anechoic masses with gray scale sonography: New observations. J Clin Ultrasound 7:249–254, 1979.
7. Maklad NF, Chuang VP, Doust BD, et al: Ultrasonic characterization of solid renal lesions: Echographic, angiographic and pathologic correlation. Radiology 123:733–739, 1977.
8. Arger PH: The value of ultrasound in hypovascular hypernephromas. J Clin Ultrasound 4:5 371–373, 1976.
9. Gates GF, Miller JH, Stanley P: Necrosis of Wilm's tumors. J Urol, in press.
10. Gates GF: Atlas of Abdominal Ultrasonography in Children. New York, Churchill Livingstone, 1978.
11. Resnick M, Sanders R: Ultrasound in Urology. Baltimore, Williams and Wilkins, 1979.
12. Hartman D: Armed Forces Institute of Pathology, Washington, DC, personal communication, 1979.
13. Arger PH, Mulhern CB, Pollack HM, et al: Ultrasonic assessment of renal transitional cell carcinoma: Preliminary report. Am J Radiol 132:407–411, 1979.
14. Duffy P, Ryan J, Aldous W: Ultrasound demonstration of a 1.5 cm intrarenal angiomyolipoma. J Clin Ultrasound 5:2 111–112, 1976.
15. Lee TG, Henderson SC, Freeny PC, et al: Ultrasound findings of renal angiomyolipoma. J Clin Ultrasound 6:150–154, 1978.
16. Bush WH, Freeny PC, Orme BM: Angiomyolipoma. Urology 14:531–535, 1979.
17. Shawker TH, Horvath KL, Dunnick NR, Javadpour N: Renal angiomyolipoma: Diagnosis by combined ultrasound and computerized tomography. J Urol 121:675–676, 1979.
18. Scheible W, Ellenbogen PH, Leopold GR, Siao NT: Lipomatous tumors of the kidney and adrenal: Apparent echographic specificity. Radiology 129:153–156, 1978.
19. Kaude JV, Lacy GD: Ultrasonography in renal lymphoma. J Clin Ultrasound 6:295–382, 1978.

20. Goh TS, LeQuesne GW, Wong KY: Severe infiltration of the kidneys with ultrasonic abnormalities in acute lymphoblastic leukemia. Am J Dis Child 132:1204–1205, 1978.
21. McDonald DG: The complete echographic evaluation of solid renal masses. J Clin Ultrasound 6:377–456, 1978.
22. Green B, Goldstein HM, Weaver RM: Abdominal pansonography in the evaluation of renal cancer. Radiology 132:421–424, 1979.
23. Goncharenko V, Gerlock AJ, Kadir S, Turner B: Incidence and distribution of venous extension in 70 hypernephromas. Am J Roentgenol 133:263–265, 1979.
24. Goldstein HM, Green B, Weaver RM: Ultrasonic detection of renal tumor extension into the inferior vena cava. Am J Roentgenol 130:1083–1085, 1978.
25. Kratochwil A: Moglichkeiten and grenzen der ultraschalldiagnostik in der nachsorge urologischer tumorpatienten. Forschr Roentgenstr 122:95–99, 1975.
26. Edell SL, Pahira JJ: Ultrasound evaluation of bladder tumors. Paper presented at the Annual Meeting of the American Institute of Ultrasound in Medicine, Montreal, 1979.
27. McLaughlin IS, Morley P, Deane RF, et al: Ultrasound in the staging of bladder tumours. Br J Urol 47:51–56, 1975.
28. Harada K, Igari D, Tanahashi Y: Gray scale transrectal ultrasonography of the prostate. J Clin Ultrasound 7:45–49, 1979.
29. Sukov RJ, Scardino PT, Sample WF, et al: Computed tomography and transabdominal ultrasound in the evaluation of the prostate. J Comput Assist Tomogr 1:281–289, 1977.
30. Kihm RH, Flesh LH: Sonographic evaluation for prostatic carcinoma. Presented at the Annual Meeting of the American Institutes of Ultrasound in Medicine, Montreal 1979.
31. Henneberry M, Carter MF, Neiman HL: Estimation of prostatic size by suprapubic ultrasonography. J Urol 121:615–616, 1979.
32. Wills JS, Santos RM, Ashley PF: Renal papillary adenocarcinoma. Clin Radiol 30:53–57, 1979.

6 Retroperitoneum

HARVEY L. NEIMAN

The peritoneal cavity is a potential space that normally is empty except for a thin film of fluid. It is formed by the parietal and visceral peritoneum. These are serous membranes that line the abdominal wall and are reflected from the wall to cover various organs to a variable extent.[1]

The extraperitoneal portion of the abdomen is somewhat more difficult to define anatomically. This extraperitoneal space is bounded anteriorly by the posterior parietal peritoneum and posteriorly by the transversalis fascia. It extends from the diaphragm to the pelvic brim. Major organs and structures within it include: (1) the adrenal glands, kidneys, and ureters; (2) the descending, transverse, and ascending portions of the duodenum; (3) the pancreas; (4) abdominal vessels and major branches, adjacent lymph nodes; and (5) the ascending and descending colon. The space is C-shaped with the convexity pointing anteriorly in the midline.[2] Meyers[2] has pointed out that there are three well-defined extraperitoneal compartments, each with major fascial margins: (1) the anterior pararenal space, which extends from the posterior parietal peritoneum to the anterior renal fascia and includes the ascending and descending colon, the duodenal sweep, and the pancreas; (2) the perirenal space, which includes the kidney and its investing fat and the adrenal gland; and (3) the posterior pararenal space, which extends from the posterior renal fascia to the transversalis fascia. It consists of a thin layer of fat and contains no organs. The kidneys and pancreas will be discussed elsewhere. This chapter will confine itself to predominantly the adrenal gland and lymph nodes, as well as primary neoplasms of the retroperitoneum. The urinary bladder will also be discussed although it is not truly a retroperitoneal organ.

SCANNING TECHNIQUES

Demonstration of retroperitoneal pathology requires a great deal of interest and determination on the part of the ultrasound technologist. Abnormalities may be subtle and optimum technique is often necessary to achieve a high level of accuracy. The examination must be tailored to the clinical problem, with transverse and longitudinal supine scans serving as the initial basis of the procedure. Prone views, however, are often helpful, particularly for the adrenal glands and tail of the pancreas. We have found that supine oblique views are particularly useful, with excellent visualization being obtained even in a gaseous patient. The retrogastric area can frequently be visualized in this fashion when all other techniques have failed. Visualization of the pancreas, kidneys, prevertebral vessels, psoas muscles, and crura of the diaphragm should be noted to be certain that the entire extraperitoneal region is well studied.

In addition to visualization of a specific mass, the displacement of organs from their expected location should be noted. Particular attention should be paid to tissue-texture, as lymph node enlargement may be incorrectly evaluated with improper techniques.

Lymphadenopathy

Imaging of the lymph nodes by the most efficacious technique is an evolving topic. Ultrasound, computed tomography, and lymphangiography are currently of particular usefulness in lymph node imaging.[3-6] Each of these modalities has specific usefulness and qualities that recommend the technique, and yet each has disadvantages as well.

Lymphangiography has the unique advantage of displaying not only lymph node size, but internal nodal architecture as well. This allows for greater sensitivity, as metastases in normal sized lymph nodes can be detected and enlarged lymph nodes, secondary to hyperplasia, correctly diagnosed. Lymphangiography, however, has the disadvantage of requiring a minor surgical procedure as well as the inability to demonstrate lymph nodes in the upper paraaortic, mesenteric, splenic, and porta hepatis regions.

While the sensitivity of computed tomography and ultrasound may be less than that of lymphangiography, the ability to stage the extent of the abdominal disease may be greater. The sensitivity of ultrasound and CT is decreased by the fact that filling defects cannot be detected, making these techniques of less value in solid tumors, such as carcinomas of the cervix and prostate. Conversely, the noninvasive procedures may be falsely positive in the area of the left upper lumbar clump. Many slightly prominent nodes may normally be present in this area. Whether ultrasound or CT is utilized, is determined partially by the body habitus of the patient as well as the experience of the physician. The CT findings of lymph node enlargement are frequently more obvious than those of ultrasound. Although ultrasound can identify lymphadenopathy in the splenic hilum, porta hepatis, and retrocrural space, minimal enlargement may be subtle and difficult to accurately assess. In the pelvis, overlying small bowel loops may obscure detail, diminishing the sensitivity of the technique.

The particular usefulness of diagnostic ultrasound is in the area of therapy

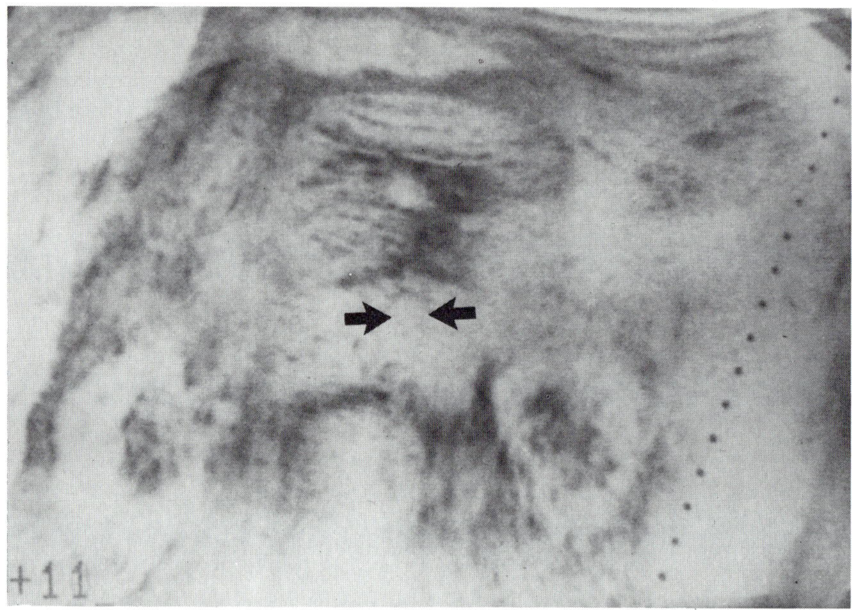

FIGURE 6.1. Transverse section of upper abdomen demonstrating a hypoechoic mantle "silhouetting" the abdominal aorta (arrow). Non-Hodgkin lymphoma.

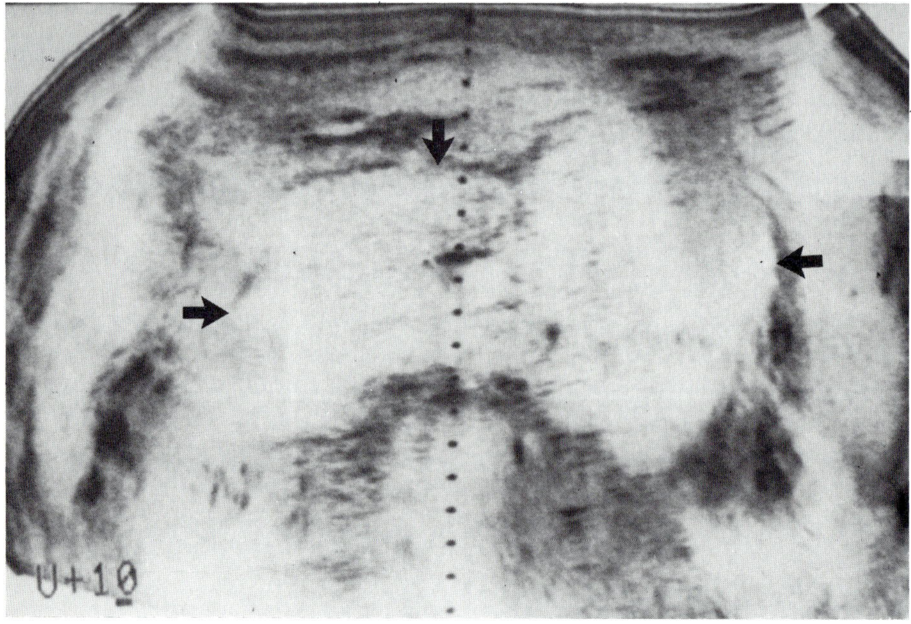

FIGURE 6.2. Hodgkin disease demonstrating a large volume of tumor which presents as a hypoechoic mass (arrows) displacing the abdominal aorta ventrally.

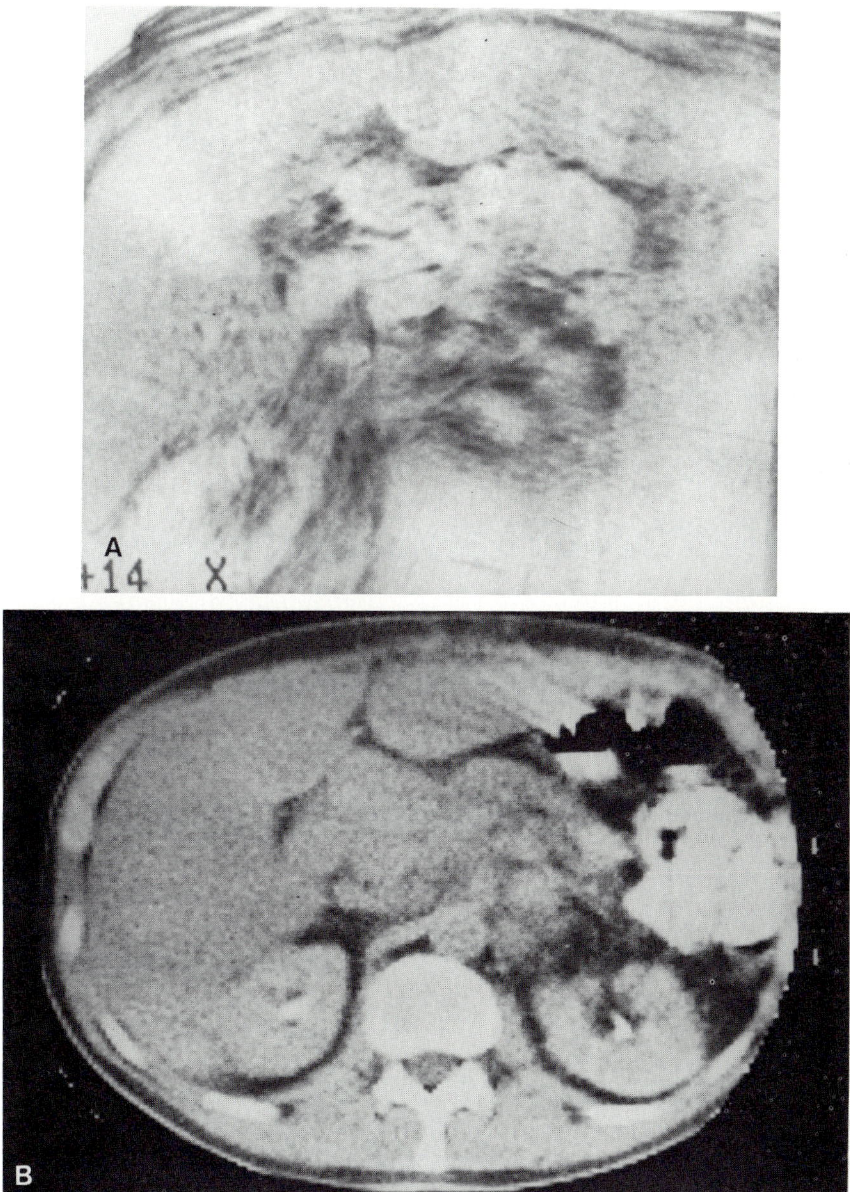

FIGURE 6.3. (a) Hodgkin disease demonstrating multiple discrete lymph node masses. (b) Computed tomographic section through same area demonstrating excellent correlation with the ultrasound findings.

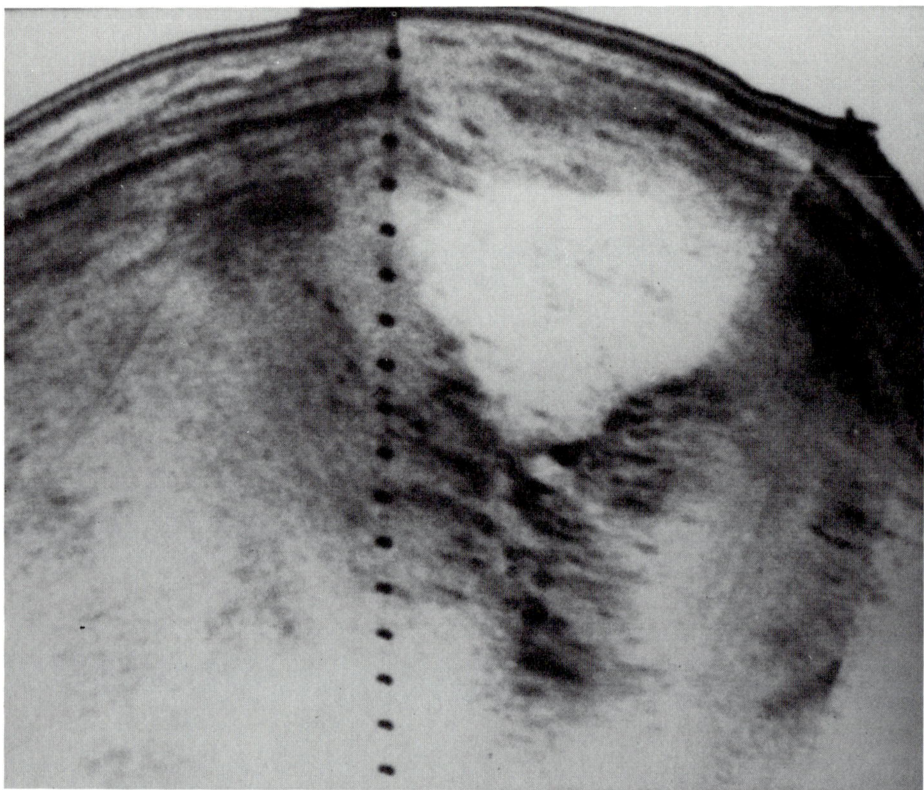

FIGURE 6.4. Large hypoechoic intraabdominal mass. While there is a large volume of bowel gas the mass remains clearly visualized. Skinny needle aspiration biopsy proven Hodgkin disease.

follow-up. Primary detection of neoplasms that cause lymph node enlargement is probably best carried out by lymphangiography and computed tomography. Ultrasound, however, is an excellent tool for following tumor volume changes once the initial disease process has been staged. Neoplasms that predominantly replace lymph nodes without increasing their size are best studied by lymphangiography.

Lymphadenopathy secondary to Hodgkin disease and non-Hodgkin lymphoma was initially described as demonstrating sonolucent masses. Particular attention was drawn to the fact that there was poor acoustic enhancement posterior to the mass, indicating its homogeneous solid nature. Frequently, this presents as a mantle shaped, midline, paraaortic mass. While lymphoma can present as an anechoic neoplasm, it has been our experience that with newer instrumentation, lymphadenopathy presents as a hypoechoic mass or masses (Figs. 6.1 and 6.2).

Not infrequently, the aorta and inferior vena cava may be obscured by the lymph node enlargement, demonstrating the "silhouette sign." In longitudi-

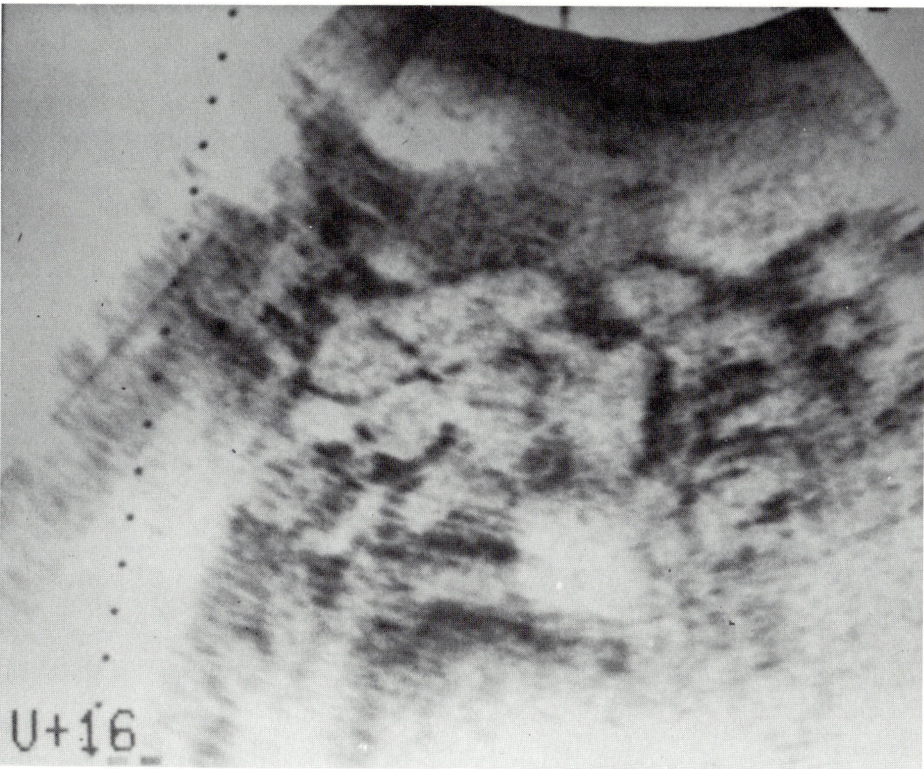

FIGURE 6.5. Colon carcinoma metastatic to the peripancreatic and porta hepatis lymph nodes. Note the discrete well-marginated hypoechoic masses.

nal section, the aorta may be seen to be displaced ventrally by enlarged lymph nodes and, in some cases, may appear to be "floating." With careful scanning technique, there is a slight tissue-textural difference (Fig. 6.1) between the surrounding volume of tumor and the encased great vessels. There is poor acoustic enhancement behind the lymph node mass. Care must be taken in assessing individual lymph node size (Fig. 6.3). While a normal node is ovoid and less than 2 cm in length, an occasional solitary single node may be as large as 3 cm in length.[8] Multiple abnormal nodes should therefore be the basis for diagnosis. Lymphoma can also cause large solitary abdominal masses (Fig. 6.4).

While Hodgkin disease and non-Hodgkin lymphoma frequently cause lymph node enlargement in addition to internal architectural distortion, other neoplasms more likely cause small filling defects within the node. These metastatic neoplasms often present a normal sonographic appearance of the retroperitoneum. In some solid tumors, however, such as malignant melanoma and some testicular tumors,[9] lymph node enlargement may be a

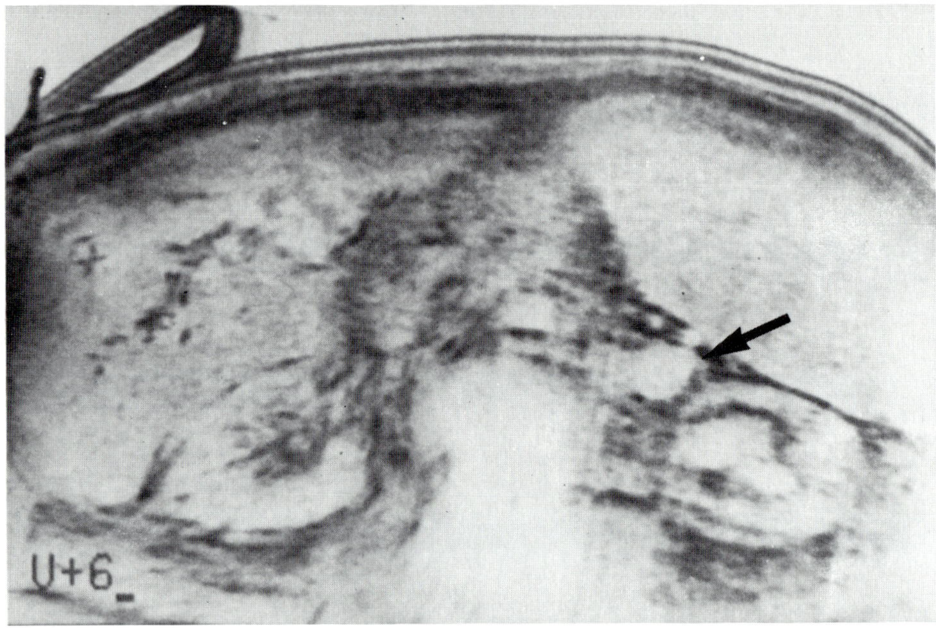

FIGURE 6.6. Dilatation of the left renal collecting system from metastatic testicular carcinoma. The left renal hilar lymph nodes are demonstrated (arrow).

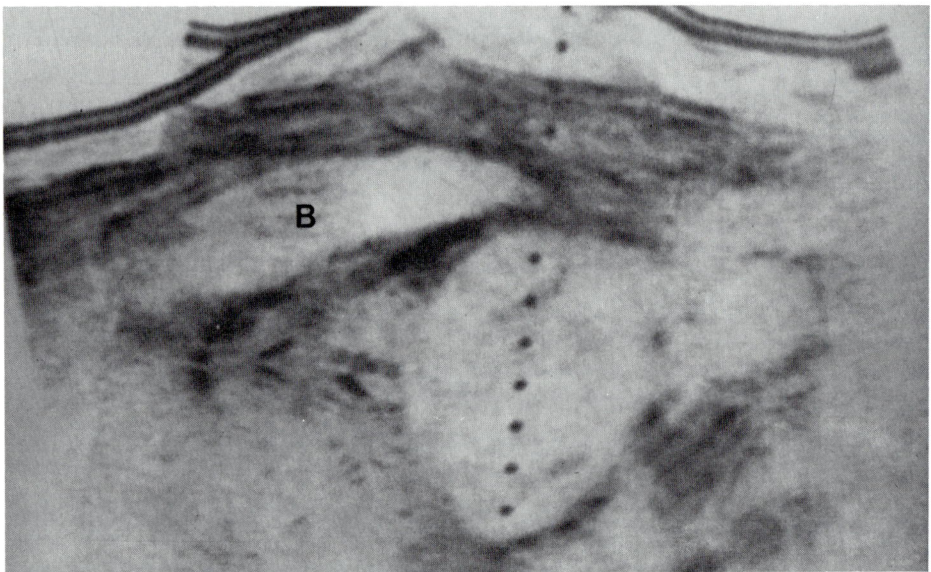

FIGURE 6.7. Multiple large lymph node masses from non-Hodgkin lymphoma is seen displacing the urinary bladder to the right and anterior. Bowel gas was not a problem in this case.

feature and noninvasive sectional imaging may aid in staging the disease process (Fig. 6.5). When they can be identified, metastatic neoplasms present as hypoechoic masses that may be well marginated, separate masses, or occasionally as a poorly defined mantle of tumor in the retroperitoneum. The tissue texture of these abnormal nodes is usually homogeneous but clearly different from adjacent organs.

Particular attention should be paid to the pelvis, renal fossae, porta hepatis, and splenic hilum, as well as to the retrocrural areas during scanning to completely evaluate the extent of disease (Figs. 6.6 and 6.7). Associated changes, such as hydronephrosis and ascites, can be detected by ultrasound as well as the occasional obstruction of the biliary tree by lymph node masses.

Primary retroperitoneal neoplasms are rare and are usually sarcomas.[10] Frequently, these neoplasms are large and present a variable ultrasonic appearance. The masses usually are obvious but may present as either a hypoechoic or echogenic lesion. Anechoic zones, representing areas of necrosis, may also be seen.

Adrenal Gland

Multiple imaging techniques also exist for visualization of the adrenal gland. These include iodocholesterol radionuclide scans, computed tomography, adrenal venography, and diagnostic ultrasound. The choice of technique depends on the clinical situation, body habitus, pregnancy, and so on. At Northwestern Memorial Hospital/Northwestern University, computed body tomography is the imaging procedure of choice for mass lesions. Ultrasound, however, has been effective in delineating adrenal masses, particularly in thin adults and when the lesions are large.[11, 12] Ultrasound can demonstrate adrenal enlargement from carcinoma, pheochromocytoma, metastases, and pseudocysts. The exact role of this procedure in patients with suspected adrenal adenoma and hyperplasia is less certain. Adrenal venography has the benefit of providing venous samples for biochemical analysis. The disadvantage, however, is the clearly obvious technical problem in carrying out the procedure by people not specifically trained in its performance.

Although computed tomography is utilized as the primary imaging technique, ultrasound is frequently necessary as an adjunctive method. Additionally, incidental adrenal abnormalities are often noted during ultrasound examination for renal masses, occult neoplasms, lymphadenopathy, and others.

Sample has described the optimum views for identification of the adrenal glands as well as the normal anatomy.[12] Coronal sections are also frequently of value in demonstrating the adrenal glands, particularly the left.[13] Additionally, right and left anterior oblique views, with the patient supine, are sometimes helpful. Optimum technique is essential to visualize the low echogenicity of the normal adrenal gland and to differentiate it from the surrounding fat and adjacent structures, such as the diaphragmatic crura.

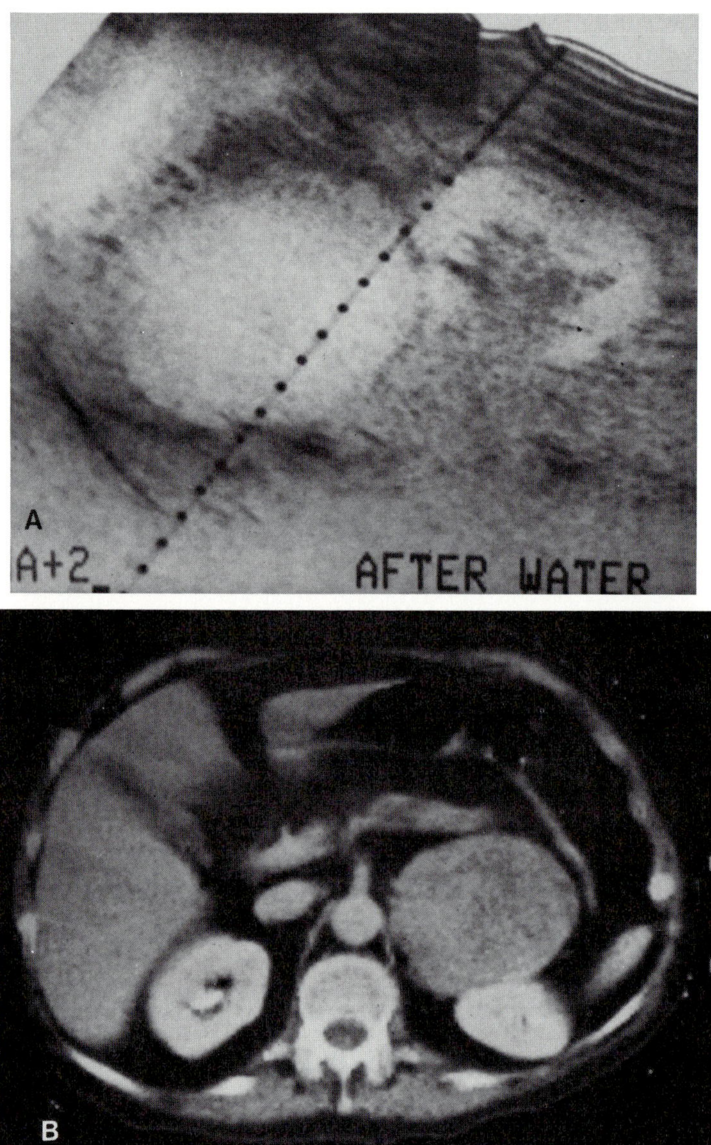

FIGURE 6.8. Large left adrenal pheochromocytoma well-demonstrated by ultrasound (a) and computed tomography (b). The lesion is well-marginated and hypoechoic on the ultrasound study. Although it is large, it was only well seen on the prone views.

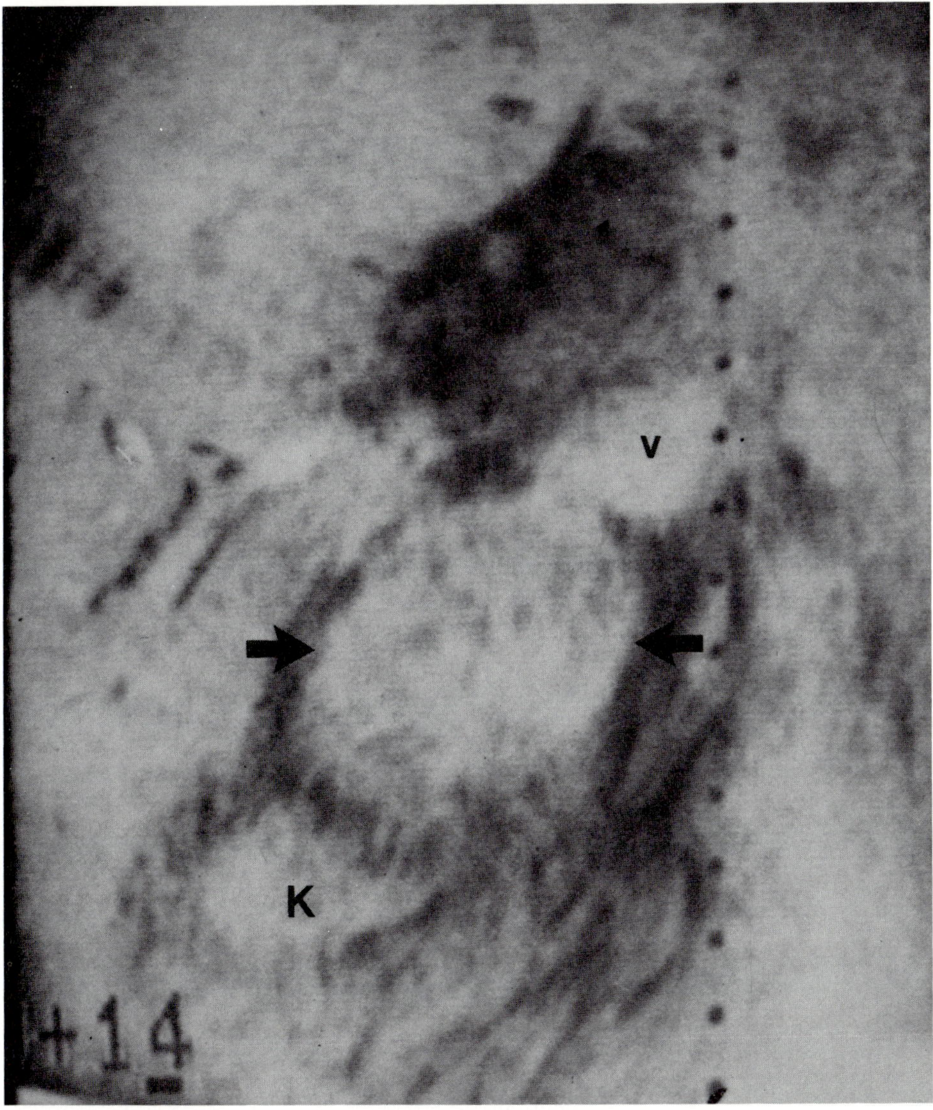

FIGURE 6.9. Right adrenal carcinoma (arrows) causing an impression on the kidney (K) and a slight posterior indentation on the inferior vena cava (V).

Primary carcinoma of the adrenal gland and metastatic disease cause enlargement with echo-architecture being that of a solid mass[15-18] (Fig. 6.8). Of course, any tumor may undergo necrosis and present as a complex ultrasonic pattern. Changes in the tissue-texture without enlargement are not a useful sign.[12] The adrenal gland being a retrocaval structure on the right, may cause a posterior indentation or ventral displacement of the inferior vena cava if a

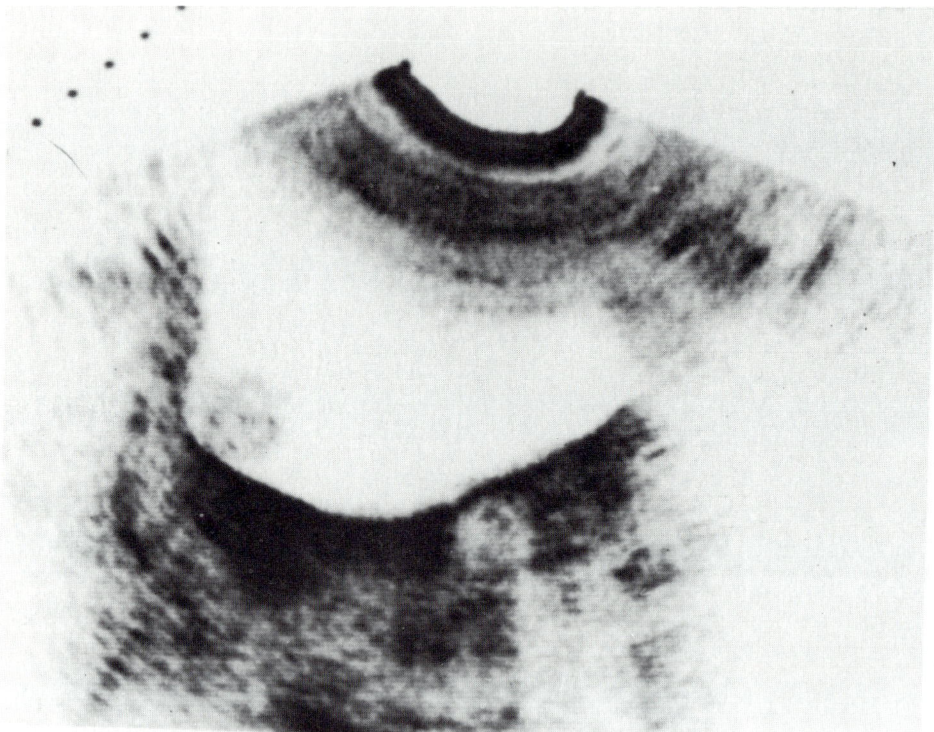

FIGURE 6.10. Polypoid hypoechoic mass from transitional cell carcinoma located on right side of the urinary bladder. (Courtesy of Terry Silver, MD, Ann Arbor, Michigan.)

mass is large enough (Fig. 6.9). This differentiates the mass from other abnormalities, such as a lesion of the head of the pancreas.

Adrenal pseudocysts can also occur in the adult patient and have a characteristic anechoic appearance. The lesion must be differentiated by its location from renal, pancreatic, and splenic cysts. Adrenal hemorrhage also may be noted with enlargement of the gland and a variable internal appearance, depending on the stage of the organization.

URINARY BLADDER

Diagnostic ultrasound can be of use in the detection and staging of vesical and perivesical neoplasms.[19, 20] There have been, however, few papers concerning the sensitivity of the technique. Neoplasms present as echogenic masses that arise from the bladder wall and protrude into the lumen (Fig. 6.10). Filled-bladder techniques are essential for noting the abnormality. Unlike calculi, a change in position does not affect the mass and acoustic shadowing is not present. The mass may be polypoid or pedunculated or,

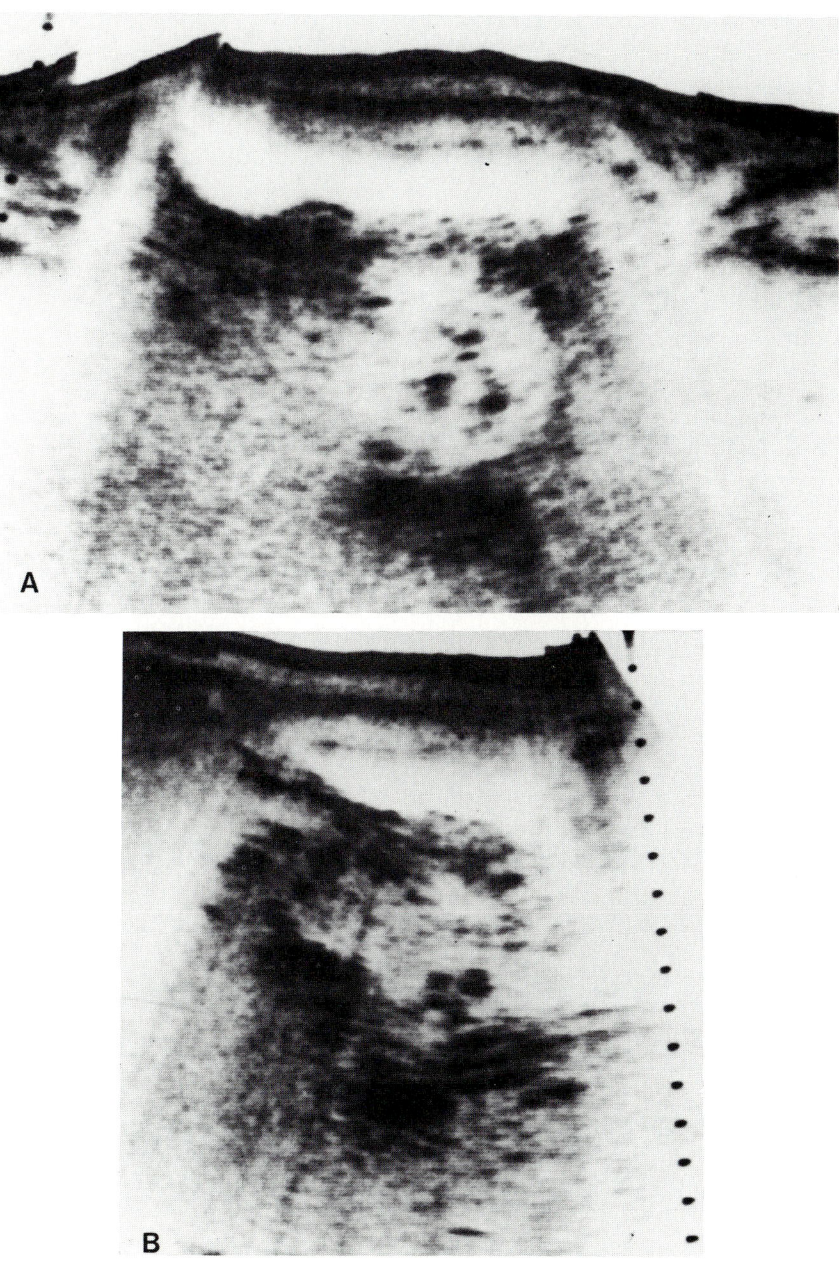

FIGURE 6.11. Transverse (a) and longitudinal (b) scans demonstrating prostatic carcinoma invading the urinary bladder.

more frequently, demonstrates a thickened segment of wall, often with low-level echogenicity. When larger, the mass may be irregular in its luminal border.

Gynecologic neoplasms have been well described. Prostatic carcinoma can also be detected. Enlargement of the prostate can be quantitatively assessed.[21] Additionally, an area of carcinoma can be suggested. The use of ultrasound to stage prostatic carcinoma has received less attention, but appears promising (Fig. 6.11).

References

1. Gardner E: Anatomy, ed. Gardner E, Gray DJ, O'Rahilly R: Philadelphia, WB Saunders, 1963, p 476–477.
2. Meyers MA: Dynamic Radiology of the Abdomen. New York, Springer-Verlag, 1976, p 115–119.
3. Brascho DJ, Durant JR, Green LE: The accuracy of retroperitoneal ultrasonography and Hodgkin's disease and non-Hodgkin's lymphoma. Radiology 125:485–487, 1977.
4. Davidson JK, Moorley P, Hurley GD, et al.: Adrenal venography and ultrasound in the investigation of the adrenal gland: An analysis of 58 cases. Br J Radiol 48:435–450, 1975.
5. Filly RA, Marglin S, Castellino RA: The ultrasonographic spectrum of abdominal and pelvic Hodgkin's disease and non-Hodgkin's lymphoma. Cancer 38:2143–2148, 1976.
6. Lecky JW, Wolfman NT, Modic CW: Current concepts of adrenal angiography. Radiol Clin N Am 14:309–352, 1976.
7. Rochester D, Bowie JD, Kunzmann A: Ultrasound in the staging of lymphoma. Radiology 124:483–487, 1977.
8. Jackson BT: The Lymphatics, ed. Kinmonth JB. London, Arnold, 1972, p 44–56.
9. Tyrell CJ, Cosgrovedo McReady VR, et al: The role of ultrasound in the assessment of abdominal metastases testicular tumors. Clin Radiol 28:475–481, 1977.
10. Bree RL, Green B: The grey scale sonographic appearance of Intra-abdominal mesenchymal sarcomas. Radiology 128:193–197, 1978.
11. Sample WF: A new technique for the evaluation of the adrenal gland with grey scale ultrasonography. Radiology 124:463–469, 1977.
12. Sample WF, Sarti DA: Computed tomography and grey scale ultrasonography of the adrenal gland: A comparative study. Radiology 128:377–383, 1978.
13. Lawson T: Personal Communication.
14. Sample WF, Sarti DA: Diagnostic Ultrasound Text in Cases. Boston, GK Hall and Company, 1980, p 272–274.
15. Bernideno ME, Goldstein HM, Green B: Grey scale ultrasonography of adrenal neoplasms. Am J Roentgenol 130:741–744, 1978.
16. Forsythe JR, Gossink BB, Leopold GR: Ultrasound in the evaluation of adrenal metastases. J Clin Ultrasound 5:31–34, 1977.
17. Lawson AT, Teele R: Diagnosis of adrenal hemorrhage by ultrasound. J Pediatr 92: 423–426, 1978.
18. Yeh HC, Mitty HA, Rose J, et al.: Ultrasonography of adrenal masses: Usual features. Radiology 127:467–474, 1978.

19. Harada K, Igari D, Tanahashi, et al.: Staging of bladder tumors by means of transrectal ultrasonography. J Clin Ultrasound 5:388–392, 1977.

20. Renick MI, Williar JW, Boyce WH: Recent progress in ultrasonography of the bladder and prostate. Trans Am Assoc Genitourin Surg 68:8-10, 1977.

21. Henneberry M, Carter MF, Neiman HL: Estimation of prostatic size by suprapubic ultrasonography. J Urol 121:615–616, 1979.

7 Gynecology

JOHN W. BRECKENRIDGE
ALFRED B. KURTZ

Because of its safety and accuracy, ultrasound is a most important imaging procedure in the evaluation of the pelvis. It avoids the use of intravenous iodinated contrast and, in many cases, makes the use of ionizing radiation unnecessary. This is especially important in adolescent and young adult women, who may be unknowingly pregnant.

Ultrasound has been found to be more accurate than either barium enema or excretory urography in the detection of pelvic masses.[1] It has also been found to provide more important information than computed tomography (CT) primarily because ultrasound can evaluate the pelvis in two planes, demonstrate the ovaries in nearly all cases, and clearly separate the uterus from the adnexae.[2] In addition, the higher cost and the lesser availability of CT are also important reasons for the preferential use of ultrasound.

Recent technologic improvements in gray scale instrumentation have increased diagnostic accuracy. Enhanced soft tissue display and higher frequency transducers have provided more information on each scan. Of the gynecologic masses found at laparatomy, 95 percent can be detected preoperatively by ultrasound.[3] In 91 percent of patients with pelvic masses, important tumor information such as size, location, and echo pattern can be obtained. In addition, in 56 percent of these cases, either a specific histologic diagnosis or correct identification of both a malignant tumor and its organ site could be made.[4] This is especially important when surgery is not immediately contemplated or when the patient is pregnant.

The full-bladder technique is essential in the evaluation of pelvic masses. Bowel has a quite variable ultrasound appearance and can frequently mimic true pathology. While the full urinary bladder displaces most small bowel and omentum away from the reproductive organs, frequently bowel still causes uncertainty. Further workup would then include real-time ultrasound scans to evaluate movement within small bowel loops and the administration of a water enema to provide positive identification of the rectosigmoid colon.

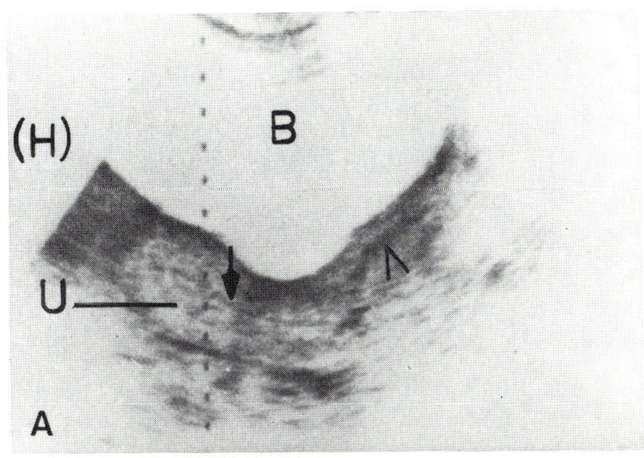

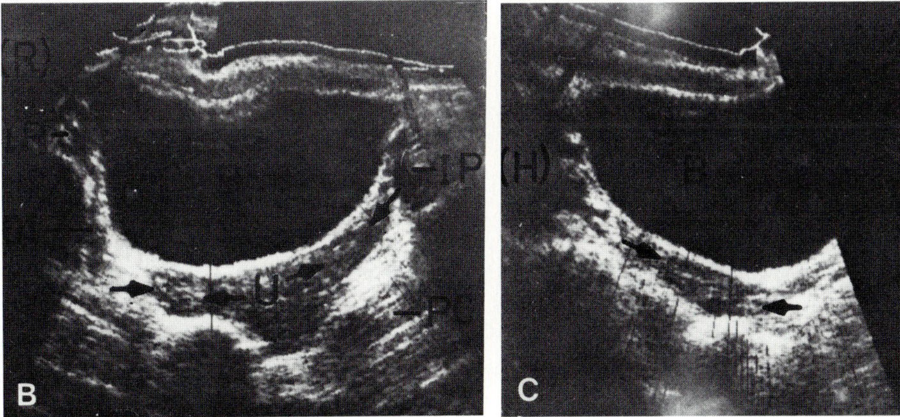

FIGURE 7.1. Normal female anatomy. (a) Midline ultrasound longitudinal scan showing the vagina (open arrowhead), cervix, and uterus. Note the dark horizontal line through the middle of the uterus (arrows) denoting the endometrial lining. (b) Transverse ultrasound scan 2 cm above the pubic symphysis. Note that the ovaries (arrows) are slightly more echogenic than the uterus (U). (c) Longitudinal scan 2 cm to the right of the midline in the same patient as Figure 1(a) showing the ovoid appearance of the normal right ovary (arrows). B = urinary bladder; IP = iliopsoas muscle; OI = obturator internis muscle; PC = pubococcygeal muscle; R = right side of patient; H = head of patient.

NORMAL ANATOMY

Ultrasound scans are usually obtained in both transverse and sagittal planes at 1-cm intervals. Occasionally oblique and decubitus views are also needed. In general the long axis of the uterus is best determined from scans in the sagittal plane (Fig. 7.1a). The vagina, directly posterior to the caudal aspect of the urinary bladder, is recognized as a linear high-amplitude echo. When traced cephalad, another linear structure of moderate to high amplitude will be recognized, corresponding to the central endometrial cavity of the uterus.[5] If searched for, this cavity should be imaged, except when the uterus is retroverted or distorted by tumors, usually submucosal myomas. In addition, bleeding into the endometrial canal causes spreading of the central echo. The normal uterus has an overall homogeneous fine echo pattern and varies in size, depending on age and parity. In the normally menstruating female, the uterus should be 5 to 8 cm in length and 1.6 to 3.0 cm in maximum AP diameter.[6] The uterus becomes small and atrophic after menopause, especially after age 65.[7]

The ovaries are usually situated on either side of the uterus, and in transverse view are frequently imaged at the medial posterior edge of the iliopsoas muscle (Fig. 7.1 b and c). However, since their attachment to the broad ligament is loose, an ovary may, on occasion, be found behind or even above the uterus. The normal ovary measures 1.5 to 3.0 cm in long axis and 3 cm in width.[8] Its echo pattern is uniform and generally coarser than that of the uterus.

The major muscle groups within the pelvis are the iliopsoas, obturator internus, and pubococcygeus (Fig. 7.1b). They are normally imaged in transverse projection, and disruption of the muscles usually implies inflammatory or neoplastic involvement.

TUMORS OF THE UTERINE CORPUS

By far, the most common tumor of the uterus is the myoma.[9] Classically, its ultrasound appearance is often that of an homogeneous solid mass, producing a bulge in the uterine contour. Some fibroids may be quite transonic, particularly if they have undergone estrogenic stimulation.[10] Myomas may undergo hyaline degeneration, usually leading to liquefaction or cystic changes.[9] Rarely, sarcomatous degeneration may occur. Calcification is not infrequently found, especially in older women, producing bright reflectors with distal shadowing. All of these factors make the ultrasound appearance of myomas somewhat variable. In general, they create a fine speckled pattern, disrupting the normal uterine architecture and containing focal areas of increased or decreased echogenicity (Fig. 7.2a).[4] Unfortunately, other solid ultrasound masses including endometrial carcinoma and uterine sarcoma may have similar appearances (Fig. 7.2b).[8, 11] More difficult to interpret are: (1) the pedunculated myomas resembling adnexal masses and (2) the inflammatory or neoplastic extrauterine masses that are inseparable from the uterine contour, resembling myomas.[12]

Occasionally carcinoma of the endometrium or cervix will obstruct the cervical canal. The resulting hematometria or pyometria produces the ultrasound picture of an enlarged uterus with a cystic or complex center[2] (Fig. 7.3). Of course, cervical stenosis may also follow surgery or instrumentation so that the diagnosis of carcinoma causing uterine obstruction must depend on detection of a mass in the cervical region.

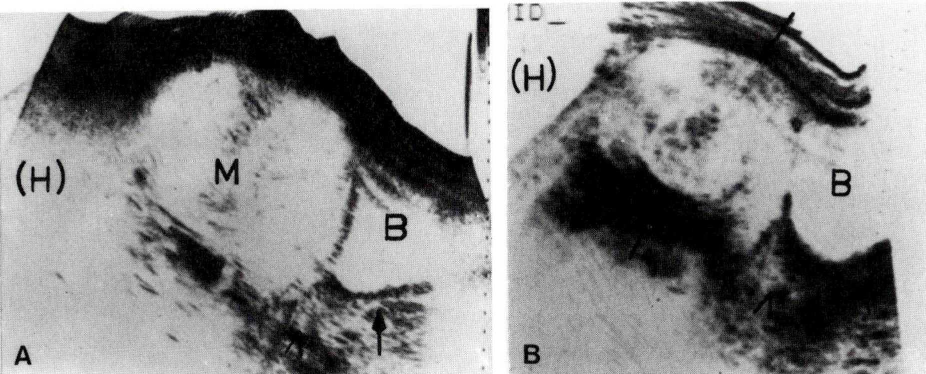

FIGURE 7.2. Uterine abnormalities. (a) Midline ultrasound longitudinal scan showing the normal vagina (arrow) and cervix (open arrowhead). A large solid mass (M) is imaged, contiguous with the cervix. At surgery, this was a leiomyoma (fibroid) of the uterus. (b) Longitudinal midline scan in another patient again showing the normal vagina (small arrows) and cervix (open arrowhead). A large predominantly solid mass with good sound transmission distally is imaged, contiguous with the cervix (large arrows). Note the cavitated portion within. At surgery, a leiomyosarcoma of the uterus was found. B = urinary bladder.

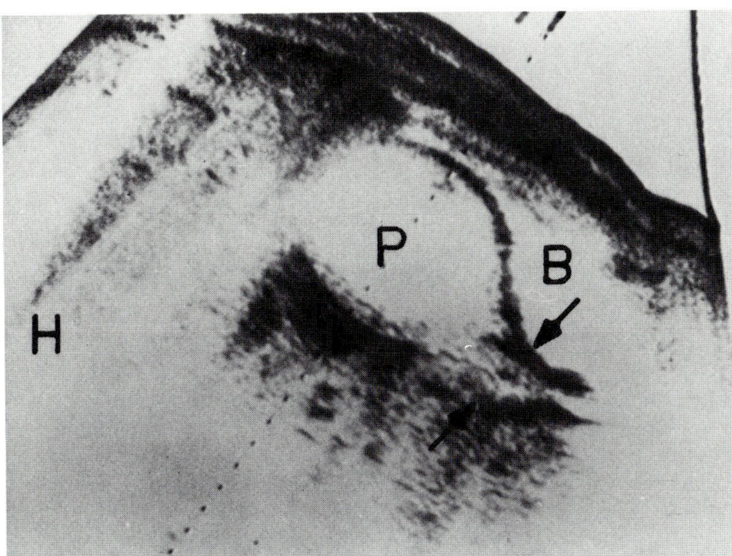

FIGURE 7.3. Cervical cancer. Midline ultrasound longitudinal scan showing a slightly prominent cervix (arrows) without definite mass. Note the large predominantly cystic structure immediately superior and contiguous with the cervix, representing a pyometrium (P) secondary to obstruction by the cervical carcinoma. B = urinary bladder.

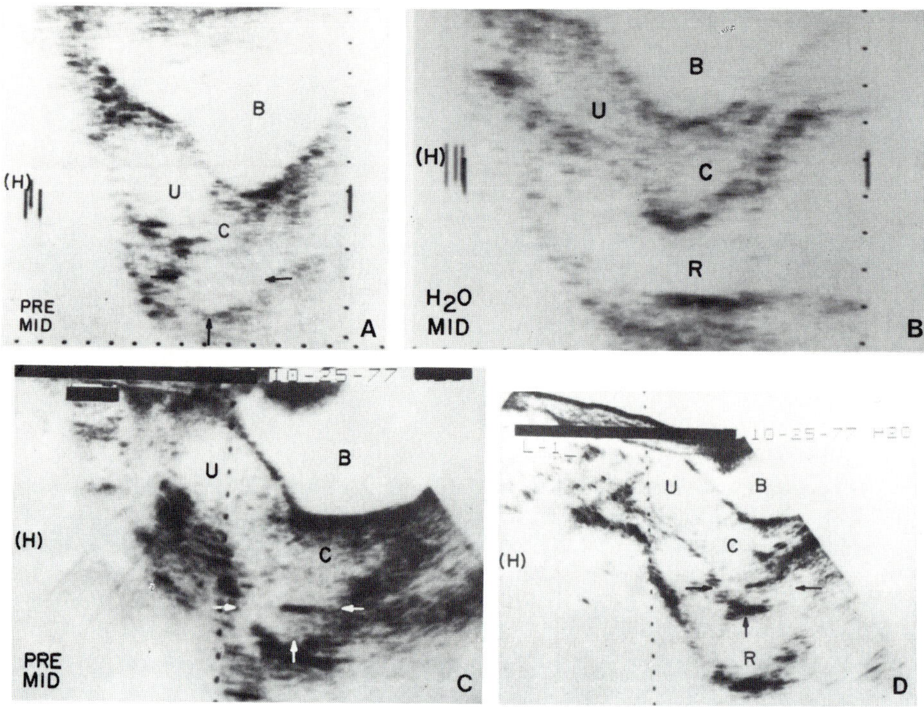

FIGURE 7.4. Pseudotumor of the rectosigmoid colon vs cervical carcinoma. (a) Longitudinal midline ultrasound scan showing a complex mass (arrows) contiguous and extending posteriorly from the cervix (C). Note the similarity between this scan and (c). (b) Same scan as Figure 7.4(a), but with water in the rectosigmoid colon (R). The previously seen mass, a pseudotumor, has disappeared. (c) Longitudinal ultrasound scan 1 cm to the left of the midline, in another patient, showing a solid mass (arrows) contiguous and extending posteriorly from the cervix (C), confirmed by the water-enema image (d). The uterus (U) is otherwise unremarkable. This was a cervical carcinoma. B = urinary bladder; R = rectum.

TUMORS OF THE CUL-DE-SAC

In the female, the area posterior to the uterus and ovaries has been termed the posterior pelvic compartment.[13] Its two major components are the cul-de-sac and rectosigmoid colon. While discussion of specific masses of the rectosigmoid colon is beyond the scope of this chapter, pseudotumors (a variable combination of fluid and feces within the rectosigmoid colon) may mimic true pathology of both the cul-de-sac and colon (Fig. 7.4).

Water distension of the rectosigmoid colon allows definite localization of the colon, with additional evaluation of colon tumors and pseudotumors (Fig. 7.4 a and b). Normally, when both the urinary bladder and rectosigmoid colon are distended, the walls of the interposed cul-de-sac will completely appose. When abnormalities are present within the cul-de-sac, how-

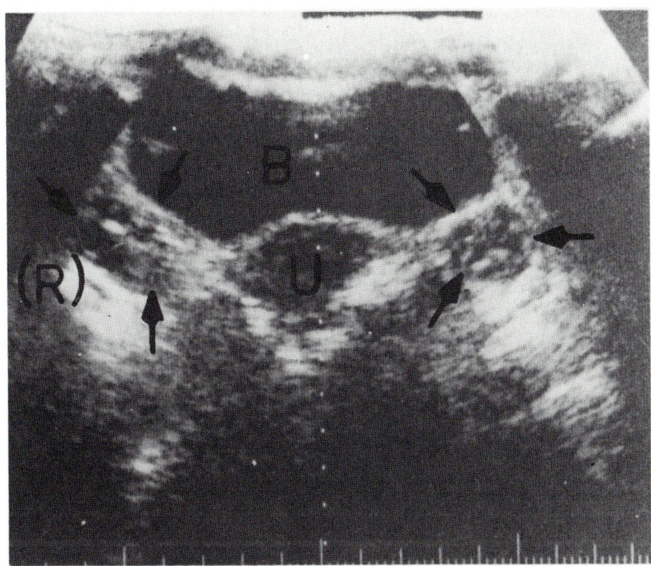

FIGURE 7.5. Cystic ovarian masses. Transverse ultrasound scan 2 cm above the pubic symphysis showing the normal uterus (U) and two enlarged ovaries (arrows) with echo-free areas within. These are multiple follicular cysts. B = urinary bladder.

ever, there will be distortion of the area. The size, shape, and position allows further differentiation of these abnormalities into space-occupying lesions, loculated fluid collections, and free fluid. Space-occupying mass lesions do not change size, shape, or position despite distension of the bladder and rectum. Loculated fluid collections change shape without displacement, while a change in all three implies free intraperitoneal fluid.

Once the space-occupying nature of a cul-de-sac tumor is determined, the differential diagnosis would include either a primary mass of the cul-de-sac or a mass secondarily involving this region. Secondary masses include carcinoma of the cervix (Fig. 7.4c and d), tumors of the uterus, and masses of the ovaries, which may extend posteriorly. Primary lesions, i.e., enlarged lymph nodes, metastatic disease, and benign lesions, such as endometriosis, hematomas, and abscesses, will also distort the cul-de-sac. While the water enema does not allow distinction between these masses, it accurately determines their space-occupying nature, presence within the cul-de-sac, and differentiation from both pseudotumors and fluid collections.

TUMORS OF THE OVARY

With the recent technologic advances in gray scale ultrasound, small nonpalpable physiologic cysts are frequently imaged. One-centimeter follicle cysts have been observed in 75 percent of patients at the time of ovulation, while 2 cm corpus luteum cysts have been imaged in 60 percent of sonograms in the midluteal stage.[14] Since the normal ovaries of young women often con-

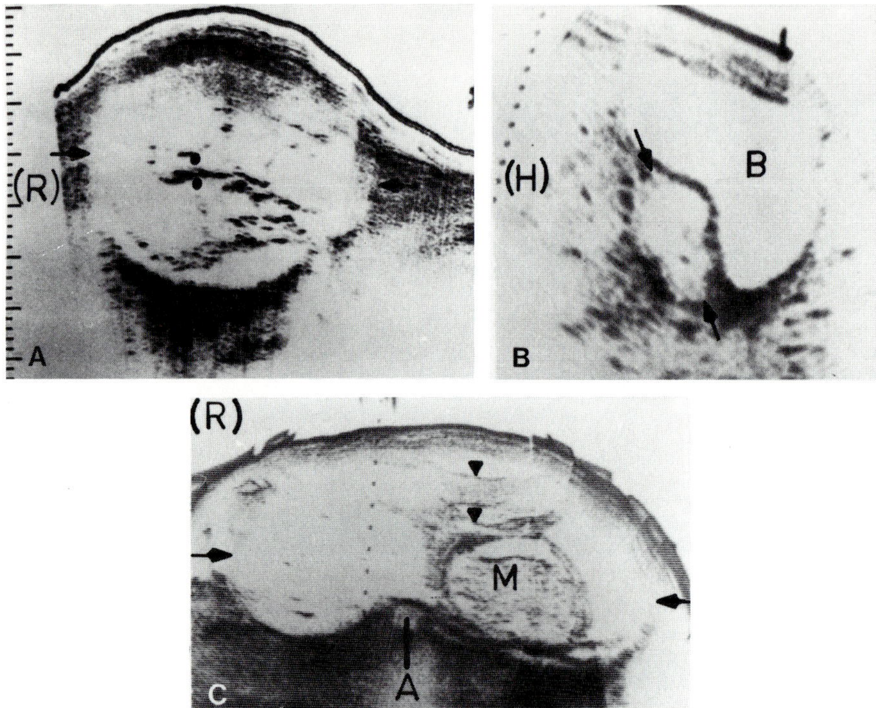

FIGURE 7.6. Cystic ovarian masses. Cystadenoma vs cystadenocarcinoma. (a) Transverse ultrasound scan 6 cm above the pubic symphysis showing a large predominantly cystic mass (arrows) with multiple thin septations (one denoted by dots). This was a cystadenoma. (b) Longitudinal ultrasound scan 3 cm to the right of the midline in another patient showing an enlarged 4 cm ovarian mass (arrows), slightly indenting the urinary bladder (B). Note the mass is predominantly cystic but with some internal echoes. The surrounding echogenic rim is the normal ovarian tissue. This was a serous cystadenocarinoma of the ovary. (c) Transverse ultrasound scan 8 cm above the pubic symphysis in a third patient showing a large ovoid mass (arrows) completely filling the lower abdomen. There are cystic areas, thick septations (arrowheads) and a large solid mass (M). This was a cystadenocarcinoma. A = abdominal aorta.

tain these multiple nonneoplastic follicular retention cysts[15] (Fig. 7.5), the diagnosis of polycystic ovarian disease (Stein-Leventhal Syndrome) should not be made unless uniformly small cysts are imaged at the periphery of the ovaries. Occasionally, a physiologic cyst will become overdistended with fluid, attain palpable size, and usually regress after a few weeks. Hemorrhage into follicular and corpus luteum cysts is not uncommon and may be recognized ultrasonically by internal medium-level echoes. Paraovarian cysts, frequently unilateral, arise from Gartner's duct in the mesosalpinx between the fallopian tube and the ovary and may attain very large dimensions. When they arise near the cervix or vagina, lateral to the uterus, their ultrasound

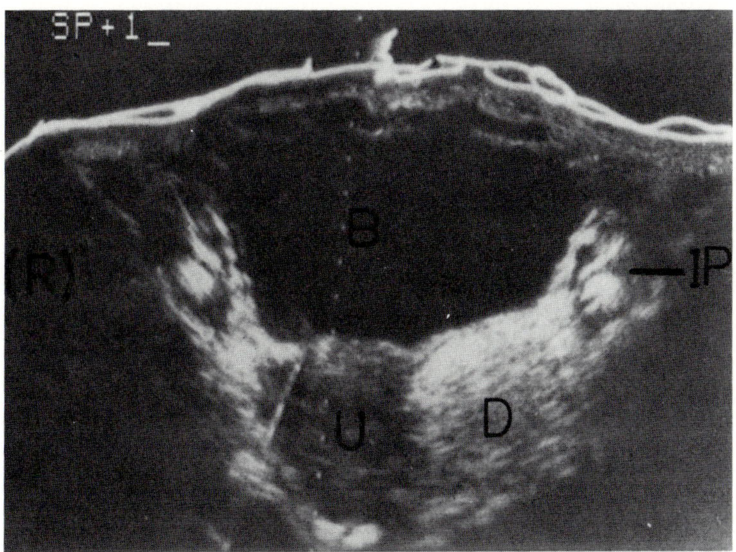

FIGURE 7.7. Dermoid. Transverse ultrasound scan 1 cm above the pubic symphysis showing the uterus (U) to be slightly displaced to the right with a large echo-producing mass (D) to the left, indenting the posterolateral aspect of the urinary bladder (B). Note the normal iliopsoas muscles (IP).

appearance is usually characteristic.[16, 17] Theca lutein cysts, usually complex masses, are seen with trophoblastic tumors[10] or fertility drugs.

Serous and mucinous cystadenomas are true neoplasms and together constitute the most frequent of all ovarian tumors. Serous cystadenomas are usually unilocular and are indistinguishable from other cystic adnexal masses. Larger ones may contain a few septae. Mucinous cystadenomas frequently contain septae and often grow to a very large size (Fig. 7.6a). It is difficult to differentiate cystadenomas from cystadenocarcinomas, since cystadenomas may undergo malignant change and a small focus of malignant cells may be found in the wall (Fig. 7.6b). However, there are certain helpful signs. Cysts under 5 cm and unilocular are almost always benign, particularly if they regress after a few weeks or with estrogen suppression.[18] Of the multiloculated cysts, thick septae, or clumps of solid tissue within the mass, are almost always malignant[4] (Fig. 7.6c). Abdominal metastases, ascites, and hydronephrosis in the presence of a small adnexal mass are highly suggestive of malignancy.[18]

Dermoids (cystic teratomas) are derived from primordial germ cells and may contain a large number of different tissues. Their contents, as well as their ultrasound appearance, are therefore variable.[19] In general, dermoids are uniformly brightly reflective (Fig. 7.7), but may contain cystic or complex areas. Infrequently dermoids may have fluid debris levels. If calcium or bone is present, an ultrasound shadow will be cast.

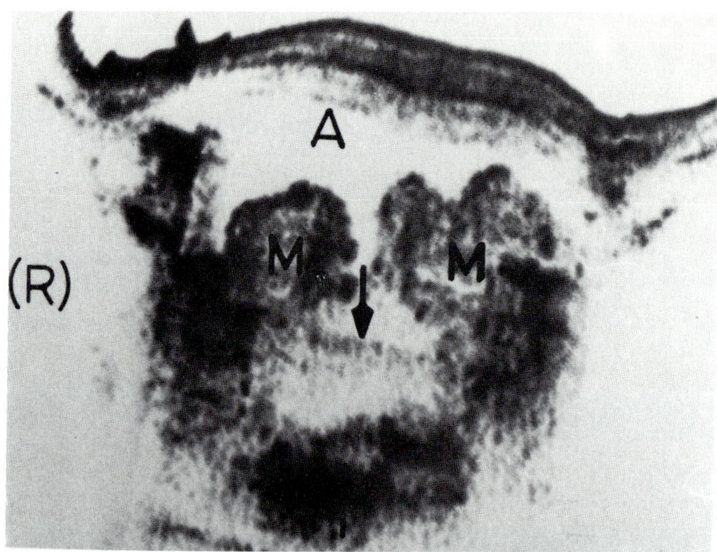

FIGURE 7.8. Bilateral primary ovarian carcinoma. Longitudinal ultrasound scan 5 cm above the pubic symphysis showing two prominent solid masses (M) on both sides of the pelvic walls with a solid mass in the cul-de-sac (arrow). Note the echo-free space representing ascites (A) anteriorly.

In general, solid tumors of the ovary are less frequent than cystic ones[8](Fig. 7.8). A common solid benign tumor of the ovary is the fibroma, which may calcify. Malignant solid tumors, primary ovarian adenocarcinoma and metastases, are sometimes bilateral and often produce ascites. Metastases most commonly arise from the gastrointestinal tract in 50 percent of the cases, the breast in 30 percent, and the genital organs in 20 percent.[20]

DIFFERENTIAL DIAGNOSIS

Diagnostic problems are encountered in mass evaluation in the following situations: (1) when a large cystic mass is centrally located. It may, on occasion, be misinterpreted as the urinary bladder, unless a post-voiding ultrasound scan is obtained. (2) When the uterine borders are ill-defined. This frequently occurs in extrauterine inflammatory lesions adjacent to the uterus, including abscesses and endometriosis, and would be expected in invasive neoplastic masses.[21] In addition, pedunculated uterine fibroids may give a similar ultrasound appearance. (3) When there is more than one mass in the pelvis. While it has been found that 12 percent of patients had two pelvic lesions at surgery, not infrequently one lesion was overlooked on ultrasound evaluation.[4] Presumably this occurred after one mass was imaged, when the observer failed to look carefully for additional abnormalities.

Some palpable pelvic masses are difficult to distinguish by ultrasound. Dermoids, in particular, may cause imaging problems. Not only are their patterns frequently similar to the adjacent bowel and mesentery, but a distended urinary bladder may displace these masses out of the pelvis into the lower abdomen. Two helpful ultrasound hints for defining dermoids are: (1) looking for subtle indentation on the adjacent bladder to confirm that the mass is a true space-occupying lesion and not a fluid-filled bowel (Fig. 7.7), and (2) rescanning after the patient has partially voided to allow the dermoid to redescend into the pelvis. An additional radiograph of the pelvis will frequently demonstrate the fatty or bony components of the dermoid. Similarly, ovarian cysts may be displaced into the lower abdomen by a distended urinary bladder and, on occasion, the patient should be reexamined after partial voiding.

Lastly, suggestive ultrasound shapes and patterns may aid in narrowing some of the more extensive differential diagnoses: (1) if a cystic or complex adnexal mass is of fusiform shape, lateral, and contiguous to the uterus, it is most likely related to sequelae of pelvic inflammatory disease or endometriosis; and (2) if the cystic or complex adnexal mass has thick walls, it is usually an endometrioma, an abscess, a cavitated tumor, tortion of either an ovarian cyst or hydrosalpinx, or, on occasion, a pedunculated fibroid with liquifaction.

References

1. Hogan M, Srichomkuan A: B scan detection of pelvic masses: accuracy compared to the barium enema, intravenous pyelogram. J Clin Ultrasound 6:103–104, 1978.
2. Walsh JW, Rosenfield AT, Jaffe CC, et al: Prospective comparison of ultrasound and computed tomography in the evaluation of gynecologic pelvic masses. Am J Roentgenol 131:955–960, 1978.
3. Cassoff J, Hanna T: Grey scale ultrasonography for assessment of gynecologic pelvic masses. Can Med Assoc J 120:38–46, 1979.
4. Walsh JW, Taylor KJW, Wasson JFM, et al: Gray-scale ultrasound in 204 proved gynecologic masses: Accuracy and specific diagnostic criteria. Radiology 130:391–397, 1979.
5. Callen PW, DeMartini WJ, Filly RA: The central uterine cavity echo: A useful anatomic sign in the ultrasonographic evaluation of the female pelvis. Radiology 131:187–190, 1979.
6. Sample WF, Lippe BM, Gyepes MT: Gray-scale ultrasonography of the normal female pelvis. Radiology 125:477–483, 1977.
7. Miller EI, Thomas RH, Lines, P: The atrophic postmenopausal uterus. J Clin Ultrasound 5:261–263, 1977.
8. Fleischer AC, James AE, Milis JB, Julian C: Differential diagnosis of pelvic masses by gray scale sonography. Am J Roentgenol 131:469–476, 1978.
9. Novak ER, Jones GS, Jones HW: Novak's Textbook of Gynecology. Baltimore, Williams and Wilkins, 1975, p. 246.
10. Hobbins JC, Winsberg F: Ultrasonography in Obstetrics and Gynecology. Baltimore, Williams and Wilkins, 1977, pp 148–150.
11. Lawson TL and Albarelli JN: Diagnosis of gynecologic pelvic masses by gray scale ultrasonography: Analysis of specificity and accuracy. Am J Roentgenol 128:1003–1006, 1977.
12. Bowie JD: Ultrasound of gynecologic pelvic masses: the indefinite uterus and other patterns associated with diagnostic error. J Clin Ultrasound 5:323–328, 1977.

13. Kurtz AB, Rubin CS, Kramer FL, Goldberg BB: Ultrasound evaluation of the posterior pelvic compartment. Radiology 132:677–682, 1979.
14. Hall DA, Hann LE, Ferrucci JT, Black EB, Braitman BS, Crowley WG, Nikrui N, Kelley JA: Sonographic morphology of the normal menstrual cycle. Radiology 133:185–188, 1979.
15. Haller JO, Schneider M, Kassner EG, Staiano SJ, Noyes MB, Campos EM, McPherson H: Ultrasonography in pediatric gynecology and obstetrics. Am J Roentgenol 128:423–429, 1977.
16. Haney AF, Trought W: Parovarian cysts resembling a filled urinary bladder. J Clin Ultrasound 6:53–54, 1978.
17. Scheible FW: Ultrasonic features of Gartner's duct cyst. J Clin Ultrasound 6:438–439, 1978.
18. Meire HB, Farrant P, Guha T: Distinction of benign from malignant ovarian cysts by ultrasound. Br J Obstet Gynecol 85:893–899, 1978.
19. Sandler MA, Silver TM, Karo JJ: Gray-scale ultrasonic features of ovarian teratomas. Radiology 131:705–709, 1979.
20. Rochester D, Levin B, Bowie JD, Kunzmann A: Ultrasonic appearance of the Krukenberg tumor. Am J Roentgenol 129:919–920, 1977.
21. Walsh JW, Taylor KJ, Rosenfield AT: Gray scale ultrasonography in the diagnosis of endometriosis and adenomyosis. Am J Roentgenol 132:87–90, 1979.

8 Pediatrics

MORTON SCHNEIDER

Ultrasound is a very useful technique for examining children.[1, 2] It has the major advantages of being noninvasive and free of ionizing radiation. The use of ultrasound as an initial procedure when an abdominal mass is palpable can help to differentiate cystic from solid masses, as well as determine the organ or site of origin of a mass. Since most cystic masses are benign, examination by ultrasound can eliminate the need for further radiologic procedures. The classical approach of a pediatric mass workup—IVP, UGI, BE—can be altered after an initial sonogram,[2, 3] particularly since not all children need to be subjected to this extensive radiologic workup and radiation.

ABDOMINAL TUMORS

Most pediatric tumors develop in the abdomen.[4] Since most of these tumors are benign, it is important to be able to evaluate these children by a safe, simple method. Ultrasound fulfills this requirement.

Wilms tumor and neuroblastoma, which represents the second most common solid tumor in children, can be easily evaluated by ultrasound.[5, 6] All palpable masses can be sonographically evaluated and categorized as cystic, solid, or mixed tumors. Since most pediatric abdominal masses are renal or retroperitoneal in origin, the use of an excretory urogram as an initial diagnostic examination has been widely accepted. While an excretory urogram can reveal such changes as a mass effect, renal distortion, or displacement, ultrasound can easily supply much more information to these findings.[7, 8] A normal kidney can be easily distinguished from a hydronephrotic or multicystic one. These are the most commonly found benign tumors in children. The finding of a solid intrarenal mass, or a solid mass displacing the kidney, helps to quickly establish the diagnosis of Wilms tumor or neuroblastoma.

A sonogram of Wilms tumor reveals an echogenic mass arising from within the kidney (Fig. 8.1). The mass often distorts the renal outline and internal echo pattern, and, in many cases, secondary hydronephrosis may be present. If the tumor has become necrotic, a complex sonographic pattern

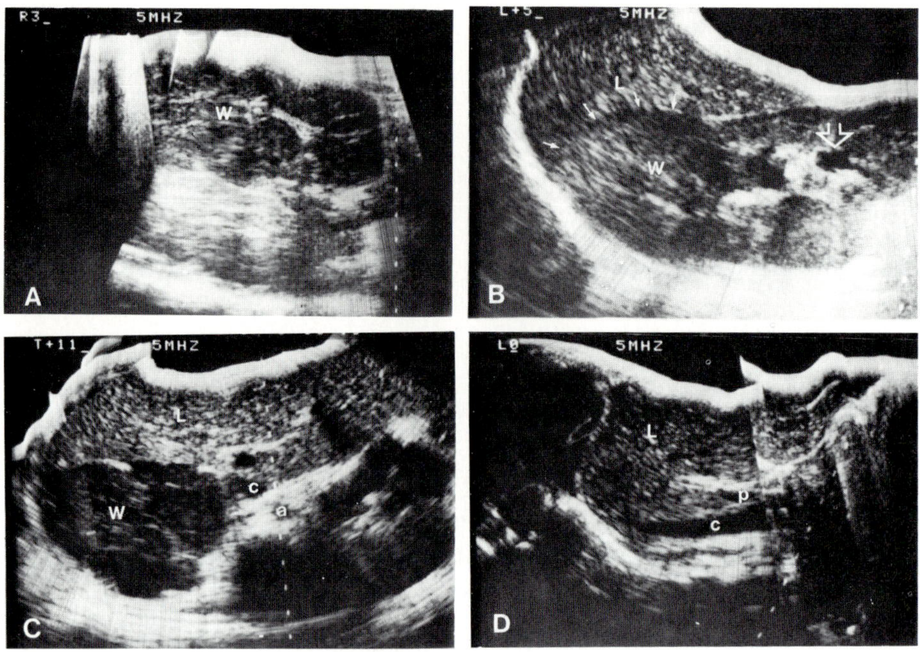

FIGURE 8.1. Wilms tumor. (a) Longitudinal prone sonogram of the right kidney reveals an echogenic mass (W) that distorts the upper half of the kidney. (b) Longitudinal supine sonogram through the liver and right kidney. Note the echogenic mass (W) arising from the superior pole of the right kidney. The open arrowhead shows hydronephrosis of the collecting system. Note the clear cleavage plane (small arrows) between the mass and the liver (L). (c) Transverse supine sonogram through the liver at the level of the tumor. The aorta (a) and the inferior vena cava (c) are identified. (d) Longitudinal supine sonogram through the inferior vena cava (c). No tumor thrombus was identified. The portal vein (p) is seen entering the liver (L).

will be present. Ultrasound should be used to evaluate the inferior vena cava for evidence of tumor thrombus.[9] In addition, a clear cleavage plane should be present between the mass and the liver, which establishes that there is no extension of tumor beyond the retroperitoneum. The opposite kidney can also be evaluated, since bilateral Wilms tumors do occur.

Another important area to evaluate in children is the region of the adrenal gland.[10, 11] It is very difficult to visualize the normal adrenal gland. In neuroblastoma the gland enlarges and usually alters the kidney axis. On the right side, the adrenal gland lies posterior to the inferior vena cava and can occasionally be seen through the liver on a supine scan. Any evidence of elevation of the inferior vena cava and alteration of the right renal axis suggests a neuroblastoma. The tumor itself has a solid pattern with high echo levels often representing microcalcifications (Fig. 8.2). The left adrenal gland, which lies posterior to the splenic vein, is more difficult to visualize since it is often obscured by overlying bowel gas. The left coronal view has been used suc-

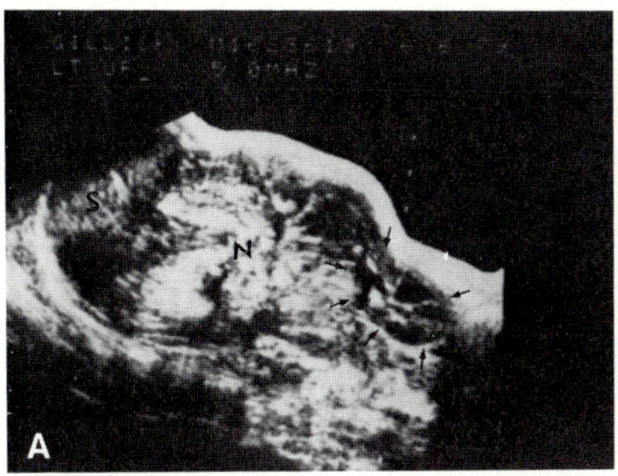

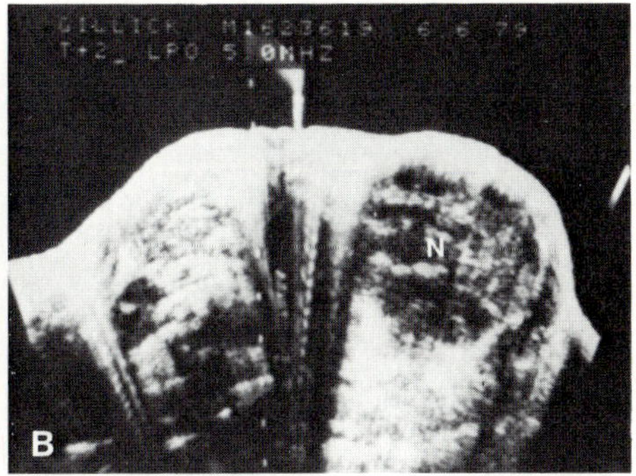

FIGURE 8.2. Neuroblastoma. (a) Sagittal prone scan through the left kidney and mass. The left kidney (indicated by arrows) is clearly separate from the highly echogenic mass (N). The increased echogenicity is presumably produced by the microcalcifications within the mass. It is sonographically important to separate the mass from the kidney and spleen (S). (b) Transverse prone scan through the mass.

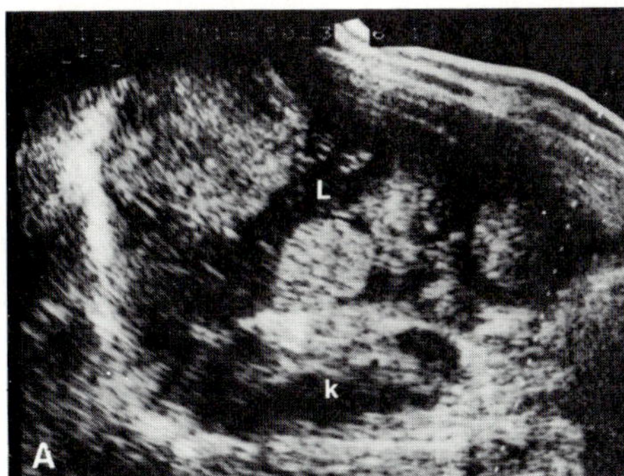

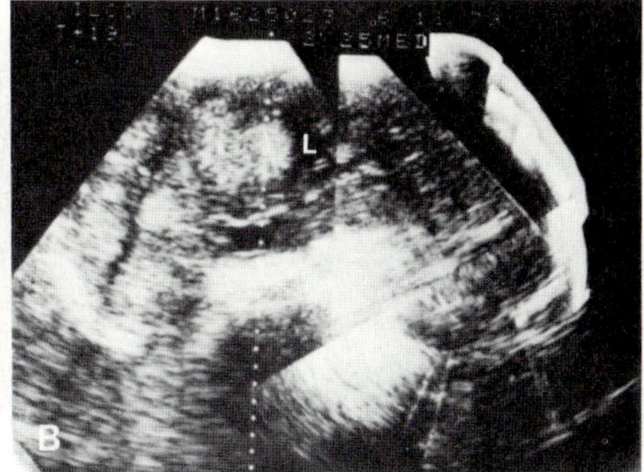

FIGURE 8.3. Liver metastasis—embryonal cell carcinoma. Sagittal (a) and transverse (b) supine scans of a child with an enlarged liver (L). Note the multiple echogenic masses throughout the entire liver. The multiplicity of the masses and the sharp borders suggest metastatic lesions. A primary embryonal cell carcinoma was found.

cessfully for visualization of the left adrenal bed. It is important to completely separate masses in this region from those of the upper pole of the kidney in order to make a correct diagnosis. There is often extension of the tumor into the retroperitoneal nodes and liver.

Primary tumors of the liver are uncommon in children. Hepatoblastoma represents 90 percent of the liver tumors found in children under the age of three. The usual sign of a liver tumor is an enlarging abdominal mass. Ultrasound is very helpful in localizing the abdominal mass to the liver and in differentiating it from neighboring organs.[12] Usually the right kidney is displaced downward by the enlarged liver. This is easily demonstrated by ultrasound. These tumors are sonographically seen as echogenic solid masses within the liver. The presence of multiple masses often suggests metastatic extension of other tumors to the liver (Fig. 8.3). Clinically it is helpful to know alpha-1-fetoglobulin levels to distinguish primary liver cell carcinomas from metastatic tumors. Commonly the liver is involved by Wilms tumor, neuroblastoma, embryonal cell carcinoma, and rhabdomyosarcoma.

LEUKEMIA AND LYMPHOMA

Leukemia and lymphoma occur in children between 2 and 6 years of age. Although the diagnosis can easily be made by blood smears and bone marrow aspirates, ultrasound is helpful in identifying the extent of involvement of the various solid organs of the abdomen (Fig. 8.4). One can easily identify involvement of the liver and spleen by its enlargement and the presence of echo-poor regions within these organs; involvement of the kidneys, testes, and abdominal lymph nodes is also readily observed. In the acute untreated phase, tumor involvement appears as echo-poor areas within the organs. With therapy these echo-poor masses usually decrease in size and/or become more echogenic. In the evaluation of the retroperitoneal para-aortic region, ultrasound is limited by bowel gas and the resolution of the equipment.[13, 14] Use of the coronal view has been helpful in visualizing extensive lymphadenopathy. In addition, distension of the urinary bladder can often help in the evaluation of pelvic lymph nodes by displacing gas-filled bowel (Fig. 8.5). For a more complete evaluation, CT scanning and lymphangiography may be necessary.

PELVIS

Ultrasound can easily evaluate for the presence of a pelvic mass, as well as determine its internal characteristics.[15-17] The only requirement for the examination is a full urinary bladder. It is, of course, necessary to be familiar with the pediatric pelvis and its numerous variations. The uterus varies in size, depending on the age of the patient. In the neonate, the maternal hormones enlarge the uterus for up to 6 weeks. Following this period, the uterus decreases in size and remains small until puberty. Another cause of enlargement of the uterus is rhabdomyosarcoma. This condition represents approximately 10 percent of all solid cancers seen in children.[18] Rhabdomyosarcoma often presents as an echogenic, irregular pelvic mass, distorting or invading the bladder (Fig 8.6). Ultrasound can be used to evaluate for secondary hydronephrosis. In addition, the liver should always be examined for evidence of metastases. While the patient is undergoing therapy, it is easy to follow the effects of treatment on these tumors.

Ovarian enlargement in children is often due to cystic tumors, the most common of these being the cystic teratoma. Frequently these tumors arise from the ovary, but other sites of origin include the testes, retroperitoneum, and sacrococcygeal area. Because of its complex makeup, the sonogram often reveals a mixed pattern with cystic as well as solid components, which are often highly echogenic (Fig. 8.7). This increased echogenicity is due to the

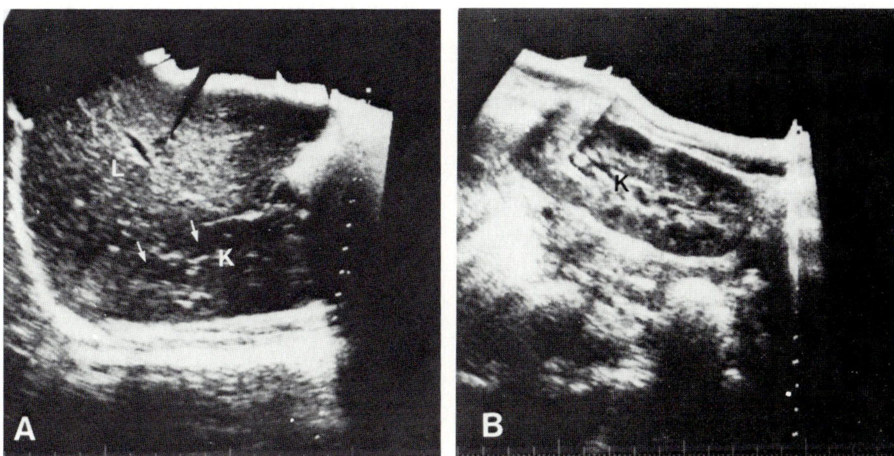

FIGURE 8.4. Leukemia. Longitudinal sonograms (a) through the right kidney (K) supine and left kidney prone (b) in a 28-month-old child. Note the echo-poor areas (arrows) and the enlargement of the kidneys. These findings are typical of leukemic infiltrate (liver = L).

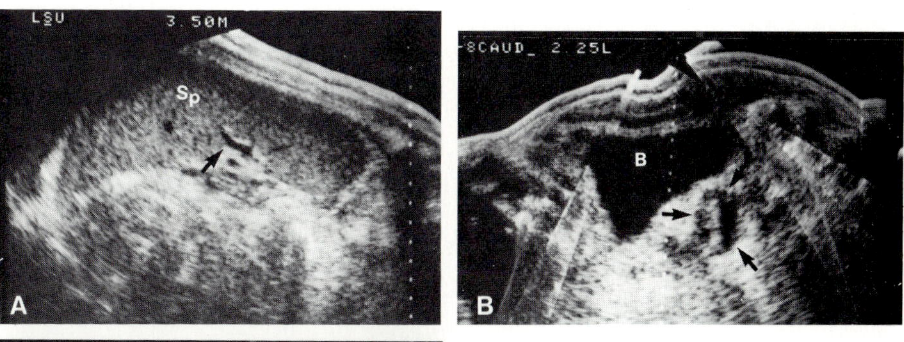

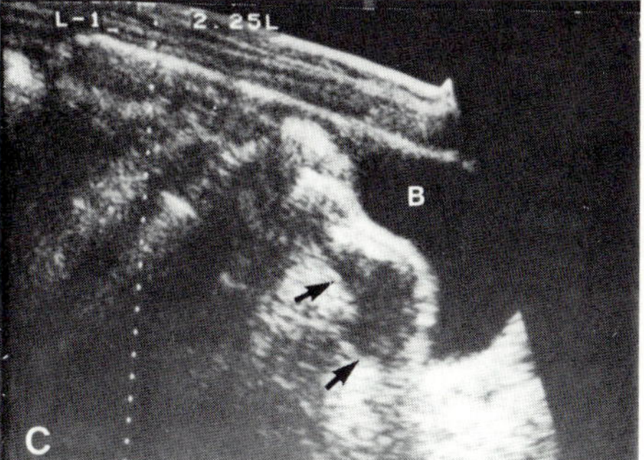

FIGURE 8.5. Lymphoma. (a) Coronal view of the spleen (Sp) revealing enlargement in a 14-year-old boy. The arrow points to the hilum of the spleen with its vessels. No focal defects are seen. Transverse (b) and longitudinal (c) scans through the bladder (B) show enlargement of the left iliac lymph node chain (arrows). This information was helpful in clinically staging this patient with known lymphoma.

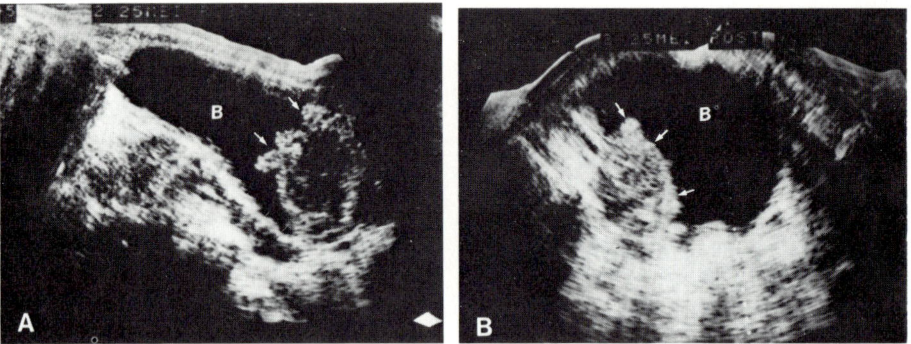

FIGURE 8.6. Pelvic rhabdomyosarcoma. Longitudinal (a) and transverse (b) pelvic sonograms reveal a large irregular echogenic mass (arrows) at the base of a distended bladder (B) in a 4-year-old girl, who presented with symptoms of bladder obstruction. This proved to be rhabdomyosarcoma of the pelvis.

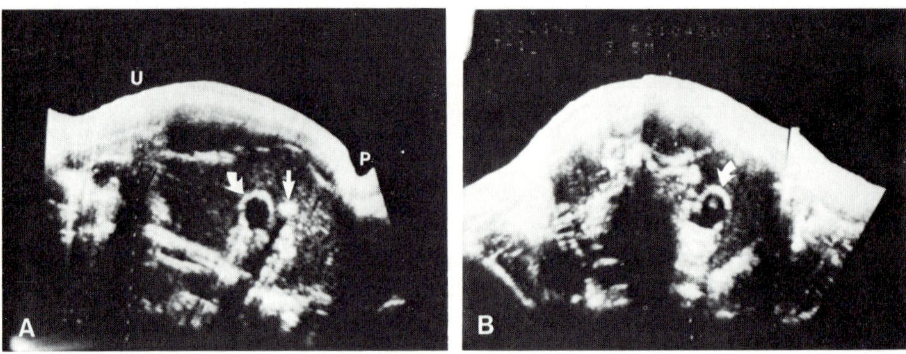

FIGURE 8.7. Cystic teratoma. Longitudinal (a) and transverse (b) pelvic sonograms through a complex-appearing mass. The mass has several different echogenic components, including a cystic area (curved arrow) and an area of acoustic shadowing (straight arrow). The very large mass extends from the pubic symphysis (P) to the umbilicus (U). This 15-year-old girl was thought to be pregnant until the sonogram was performed. The complex mass was a cystic teratoma consisting of fluid, fat, hair, and teeth. The pathology revealed low-grade malignant changes.

high fat content that can sometimes blend with normal pelvic fat, making it more difficult in some cases to detect the mass. The presence of calcification—bone and teeth—results in acoustic shadowing of the ultrasound beam, which can be very helpful in predicting the correct diagnosis.

Solid enlargement of the ovaries may be seen with dysgerminomas. These are rapidly growing tumors that frequently metastasize locally to the pelvic lymph nodes.

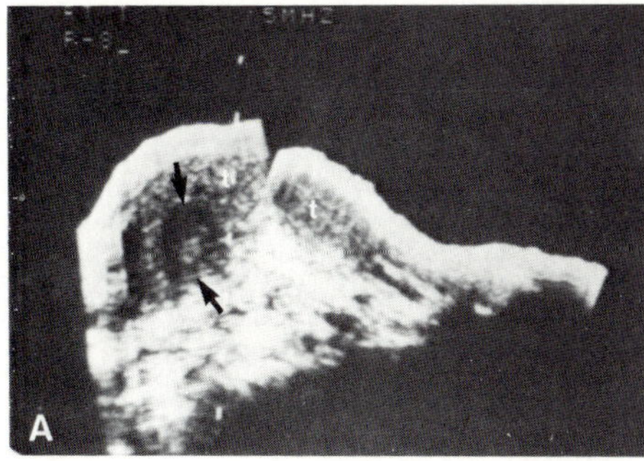

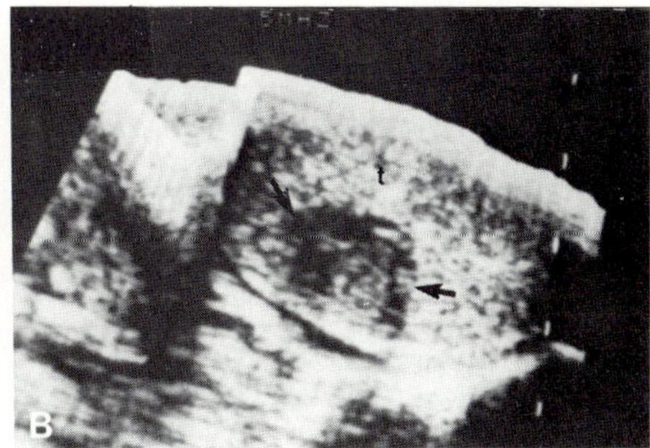

FIGURE 8.8 Scrotal sonogram—Leydig cell tumor. Transverse (a) and longitudinal (b) contact scans of the scrotum demonstrate a discrete echo-poor mass (arrows) in the right testis (t). The mass was suspected in a child with feminizing signs.

TESTICULAR SONOGRAPHY

Ultrasound can be a valuable diagnostic tool in the evaluation of testicular pathology.[19] Alteration of texture has been demonstrated in the presence of neoplasms within the testes (Fig. 8.8). Examinations are easily performed and only require the presence of a high-frequency near-field transducer. Familiarity with the normal testes and its homogenous grandular medium level texture is important. Echo-poor areas are suggestive of leukemic infiltration. Tumors as small as 5 mm have been demonstrated by ultrasound.

CONCLUSION

Ultrasound is used routinely to detect or confirm the presence of masses in children. It has proved to be very helpful in differentiating between the cystic, solid, or complex nature of these masses. Often the only procedure necessary for a child with a mass is a sonogram, thus avoiding unnecessary exposure to radiation. This is especially important if the tumor is thought to be benign.

References

1. Dempsey, PJ, Robinson, AE: Primary abdominal sonography in the neonate. AJR 128: 345, 1977.
2. Haller, JO, Schneider, M: Pediatric Ultrasound, Chicago, Yearbook Medical Publisher, 1980.
3. Gates, GF, Miller, JH: Combined radionuclide and ultrasonic assessment of upper abdominal masses in children. AJR 128:773, 1977.
4. Bloom, HJG, Lamerle, J, et al: Cancer in Children. New York, Springer-Verlag, 1975.
5. McDonald, P: Genitourinary tumors, Prog Pediatr Radiol 3:271, 1970.
6. Proceedings of the National Conference on the Care of the Child with Cancer. New York, American Cancer Society, 1978.

7. Carlson, DH, Carlson, D, Scimin, H: Benign multilocular cystic nephroma. AJR 131:621, 1978.
8. Teele, RL: Ultrasonography of the genitourinary tract in children. Radio Clin North Am 15:109, 1977.
9. Goldstein, HM, Green, B, Weaver, RM: Ultrasonic detection of renal tumor extension into the inferior vena cava. AJR 130:1083, 1978.
10. Beenadino, ME, Goldstein, HM, Green, B: Grayscale ultrasonography of adrenal neoplasm. AJR 130:741, 1978.
11. Yeh, HC, Mitty, HW, et al: Ultrasonography of adrenal masses: Usual features. Radiology 127:467, 1978.
12. Green, B, et al: Gray scale ultrasound evaluation of hepatic neoplasms. Radiology 124: 203, 1977.
13. Brascho, DJ, Durant, JR, Green, LE: The accuracy of retroperitoneal ultrasonography in Hodgkin's disease and non-Hodgkin's lymphoma. Radiology 125:485, 1977.
14. Lee, JKT, Stanley, RJ, et al: Accuracy of computed tomography in detecting intra-abdominal and pelvic adenopathy in lymphoma. AJR 131:311, 1978.
15. Haller, JO, Schneider, M, et al: Ultrasonography in pediatric gynecology and obstetrics. AJR 128:423, 1977.
16. Haller, JO, Schneider, M, et al: Ultrasonic diagnosis of gynecological disorders in children. Pediatrics 62(3):339, 1978.
17. Lawson, TL, Albarelli, JN: Diagnosis of gynecologic pelvic masses by gray scale ultrasonography: Analysis of specifity and accuracy. AJR 128:1003, 1977.
18. Hornback, NB, Shidnia, H: Rhabdomyosarcoma in the pediatric age group. AIR 126: 542, 1976.
19. Sample, WF, Gottesman, JE, Erlich, RM: Gray scale ultrasound of the scrotum. Radiology 127:225, 1978.

9 Superficial Organs

GEORGE R. LEOPOLD

The use of ultrasonography in the diagnosis of deeply situated abdominal and pelvic tumors is well established. More recently, reports have begun to appear touting the value of this technique in the detection of masses involving superficially located organ systems.[1] Since these structures are largely subcutaneous in location, the requirements for penetration by the ultrasound beam are considerably reduced. Consequently, higher frequency beams with much improved lateral resolution may be employed.

While many organ systems are potentially suitable for study by this technique, this chapter will deal with its applicability in studies of the thyroid and testicle. Although these organs have received earlier attention from ultrasonographers, using conventional equipment, the instrumentation described here has produced significant new information of clinical importance.

EQUIPMENT

The equipment used for these studies was developed at the Stanford Research Institute. This device is now being marketed commercially as Picker "Microview", by the Picker Corporation of Northford, Ct. While initially conceived to study the region of the carotid bifurcation,[2, 3] it is apparent that many additional uses exist.

The transducer for this unit is a single 10 MHz element 13 mm in diameter, so that structures approximately 3 cm deep can be studied satisfactorily. The transducer is housed in a small, self-contained water bath that is applied to the skin with suitable contact material. The transducer is mechanically driven back and forth in a linear path within the water bath. This motion permits updating the returning ultrasound information at a frame rate sufficiently rapid to allow display of physiologic motion within the field of view (real time). Since the motion is linear, the eventual display is either square or rectangular—a definite advantage in studying structures just beneath the skin. The operating head of the unit, which contains the water bath-transducer assembly, is mounted on an arm that permits examination in any plane desired.

In the prototype version of the instrument, display was on a conventional cathode ray oscilloscope. A permanent record was obtained by photographing the face of the oscilloscope. In the commercial version, a digital scan converter has been interposed. This feature provides display on a television screen and also allows for some pre and post processing of the ultrasound information. A final record of a digital freeze frame is taken with any convenient multiformat camera. As with conventional contact B-scanners, digital updating has greatly added to the overall stability of this instrument.

While this device provides excellent images, it is highly likely that other "small parts" instruments using other methods will soon be appearing, and that the present device will also continue to improve technologically.

THYROID

To examine this structure, the patient is placed supine, with a pillow behind the neck to produce extension. Careful palpation and correlation with other studies (plain films, nuclear medicine studies) will often help to direct the examination. Although examination in almost any plane is possible, it is best to begin with sagittal or transverse sections to obtain orientation. Since the study is in real time, the area in question can be surveyed quickly. Because of the small field of view, the two halves of the neck are done separately. Areas of interest are recorded in at least two planes to allow spatial orientation. Each recorded frame should be immediately identified by the examiner since the image frequently will not contain recognizable anatomic landmarks.

In the normal individual, the initial transverse scans show the thyroid gland as a medium gray-level echogenic structure that is quite homogeneous (Figs. 9.1 and 9.2). On occasion, small echo-free structures are noted within the gland, which appear to continue into other transverse planes and almost certainly represent vessels. Considerable variation in size and shape of the individual lobes is common. The parathyroid glands to date have not been identified in the normal state—probably because their texture is similar to that of normal thyroid and the glands are in close apposition to the posterior aspect of the thyroid. Lateral to the thyroid, the circular lumen of the common carotid artery is clearly visible. The artery is easily recognized by its highly echogenic elastic lamina and characteristic pulsations. The internal jugular vein is situated just lateral and slightly anterior to the carotid. It is easily distinguished by its respiratory variation, triplicate pulsation, and marked enlargement following Valsalva maneuver. Just anterior to the gland, the sternothyroid, sternohyoid, and sternocleidomastoid muscles are noted. In longitudinal orientation, the same structures are demonstrable, and the course of vessels may be more readily appreciated.

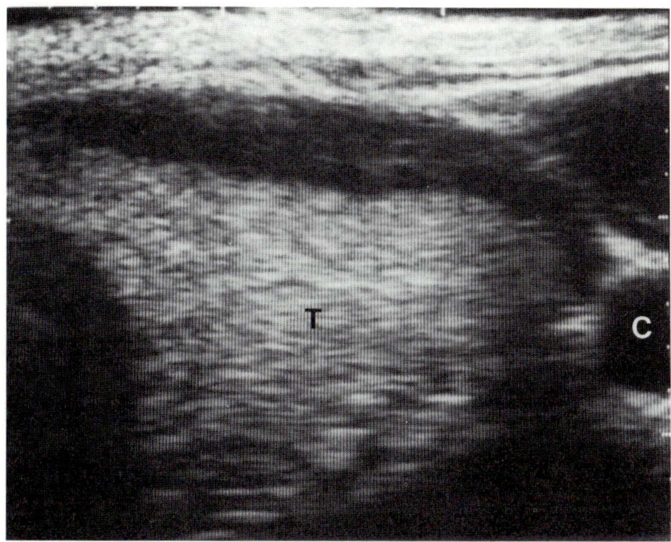

FIGURE 9.1. Transverse scan, left lobe of thyroid (smallest scale division = 2 mm). The shape and consistency of the normal thyroid (T) are well demonstrated. A portion of the common carotid artery (C) is seen lateral to the thyroid.

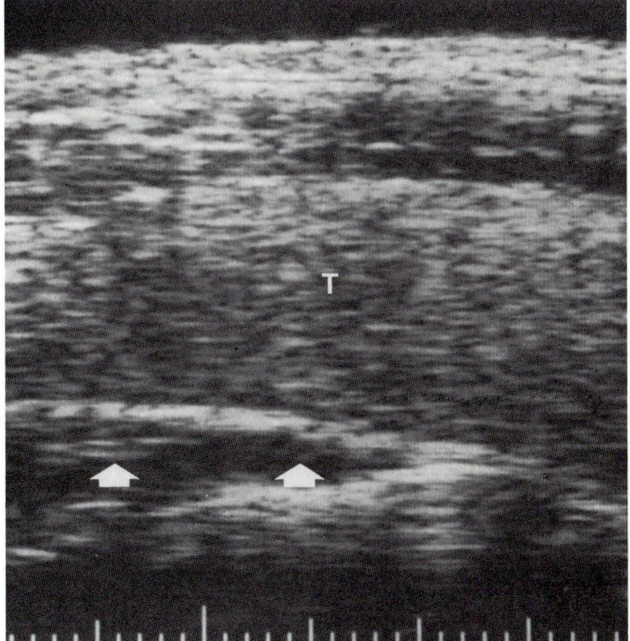

FIGURE 9.2. Sagittal scan, left lobe. The thyroid is again well seen. The sonolucent band posterior to it (arrows) is the longus colli muscle.

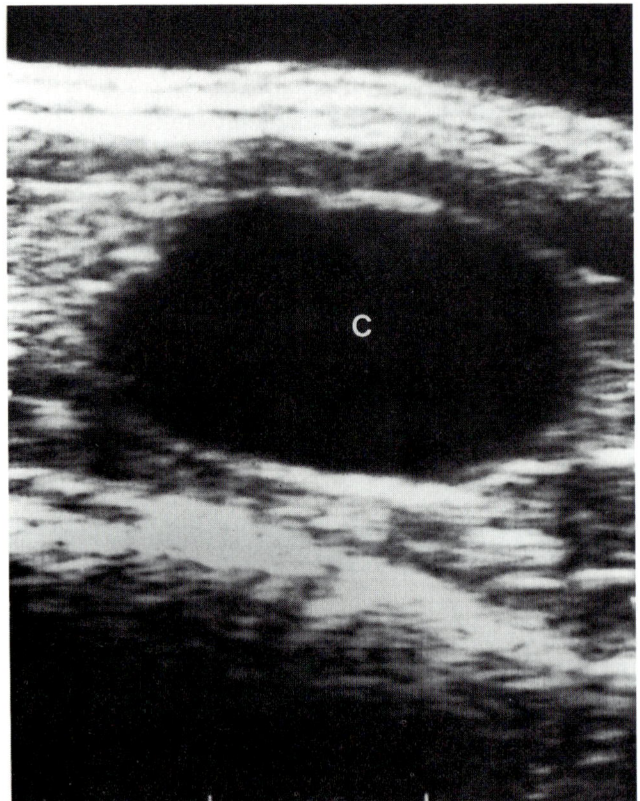

FIGURE 9.3. Sagittal scan, right lobe. This 2-cm nodule has the typical ultrasonic characteristics of cysts elsewhere in the body.

Thyroid Masses

Recent studies point to the effectiveness of this technique in assessing thyroid nodules.[4] Masses as small as 3 mm are easily visualized. Since this far exceeds the resolving capability of clinical nuclear medicine studies, it is not surprising to find multiple nodules—even though other studies suggested the patient had a single lesion.

Cysts

Of all lesions presenting as "cold" on radionuclide examination, only 20 percent will ultimately prove to be cysts. While congenital cysts of the thyroid do occur, most of these lesions probably represent adenomas that have undergone extensive cystic degeneration. It is not surprising then that their sonographic appearance exhibits considerable variability. While some have characteristics of cysts elsewhere in the body (Fig. 9.3)—absence of internal echoes, exquisitely sharp margins—many do show internal structure at 10 MHz examination. This can be the result of hemorrhage or liquefaction necrosis of a preexisting adenoma, or from hemorrhage into a congenital cyst. Recent hemorrhage appears as diffuse, very low-level echogenicity, while a more chronic hemorrhage usually progresses to septation or synechial formation within the lesion. Small cystic areas are sometimes noted within carcinomas of the thyroid, but major cystic degeneration is very rare. Thus, the presence of large amounts of fluid within a thyroid nodule suggests it is benign. When thyroid cancer metastasizes to adjacent lymph nodes however, extensive cystic change in those nodes is common.

Many endocrinologists and surgeons elect to treat suspected cysts by percutaneous aspiration. As indicated above, bloody aspirate will be obtained from many of these lesions and obviously does not have the same ominous significance as it does with renal cyst puncture. Careful cytologic analysis of the fluid is crucial in ruling out malignancy. This may be greatly facilitated by discussing the situation in advance with the laboratory in order to ensure correct handling and preparation of the specimen.

Cysts treated in this fashion may or may not recur, and the course of events is easily documented by serial ultrasound studies.

Adenomas

This is by far the commonest thyroid nodule. Most authors report that 60 percent of nodules that show no radioiodine uptake are adenomas. As mentioned previously, marked cystic degeneration renders the lesion indistinguishable from a complicated cyst. The majority of these lesions, however, are chiefly solid and possess echogenicity very similar to that of normal thyroid parenchyma. They may be recognized by the lucent "halo" found at the periphery of the lesion (Figs. 9.4 and 9.5). The thinness of this halo suggests that the capsule is the most likely source of this finding. However, other factors, such as hemorrhage around the lesion, may undoubtedly contribute to this appearance. Considerable interest has arisen in the specificity of this finding, as to its reliability in differentiating benign from malignant nodules of the thyroid.

Our early clinical experience indicates that a thin halo completely surrounding a lesion is a highly reliable indicator of benignancy. We have, however, encountered such a finding in a single patient with pure follicular carcinoma. This lesion is characteristically encapsulated and grossly resembles a follicular adenoma (Fig. 9.6). Differentiation depends on demonstrating capsular penetration or vascular invasion microscopically. It is, therefore, to be expected that this relatively infrequent tumor will continue to be difficult or impossible for ultrasonographers to recognize.

Peripheral rim-like calcification of a nodule (producing uniform shadowing) is also characteristic of adenoma, just as it is in plain radiography (Fig. 9.7). Internal calcification is of no diagnostic significance, since it may be seen in carcinomas, adenomas, and post inflammatory states.

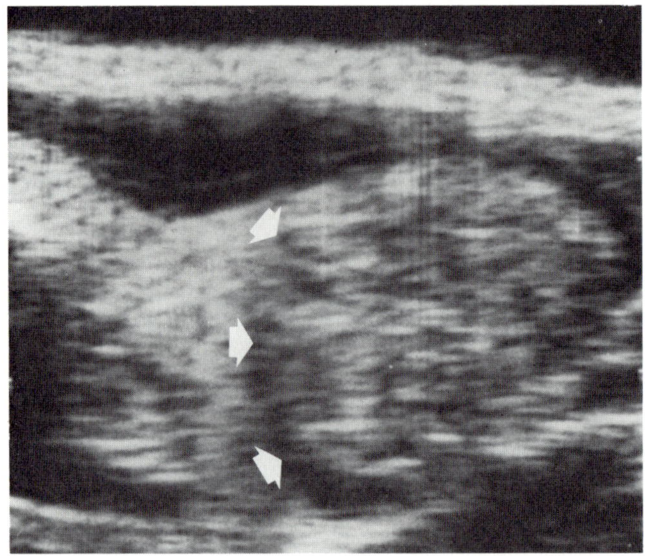

FIGURE 9.4. Transverse scan, left lobe. This echogenic nodule is surrounded by a thin sonolucent halo (arrows), a common finding in benign adenomas.

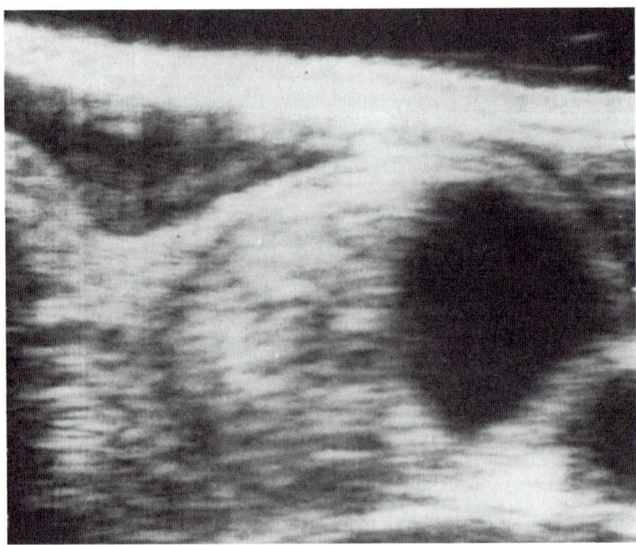

FIGURE 9.5. Transverse scan, left lobe. Another section taken of the nodule shown in Figure 9.4 reveals a sizeable cystic component. This is also a common finding in benign nodules.

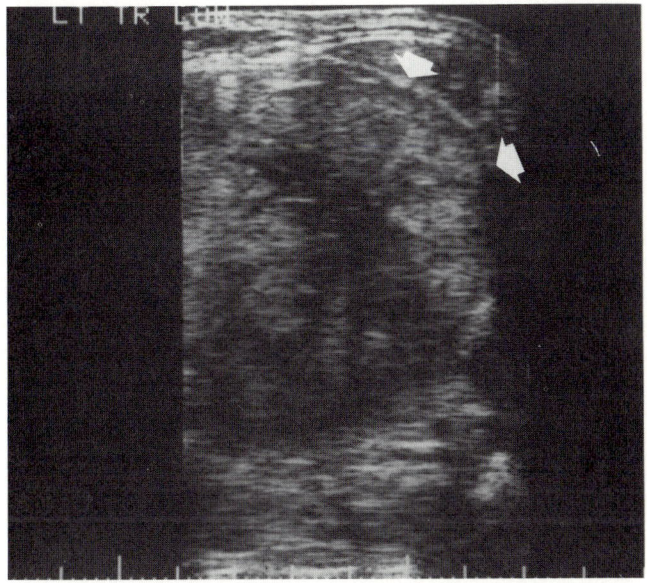

FIGURE 9.6. Transverse scan, left lobe. A large weakly echogenic lesion is seen. Although there is a thin halo (arrows), this nodule proved to be a pure follicular carcinoma.

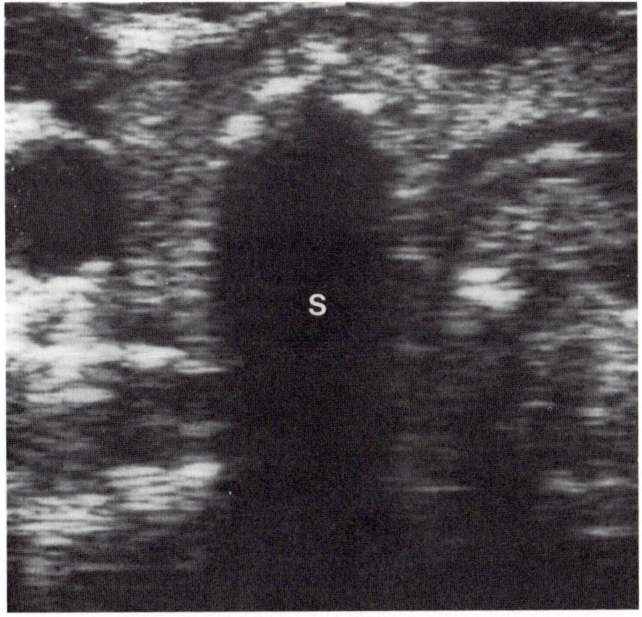

FIGURE 9.7. Transverse scan, right lobe. This nodule has peripheral calcification which produces acoustic shadowing (S), an indicator of benign adenoma.

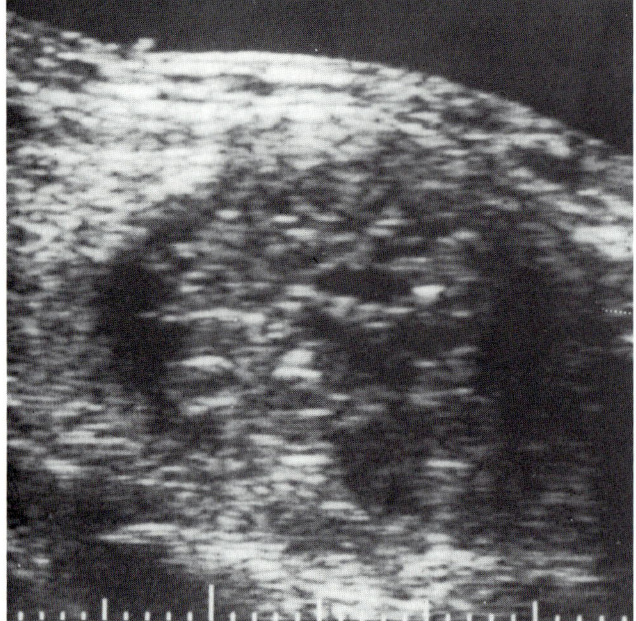

FIGURE 9.8. Longitudinal scan, left lobe. Large echo-poor lesion with no surrounding halo. At surgery, a mixed papillary-follicular carcinoma was discovered.

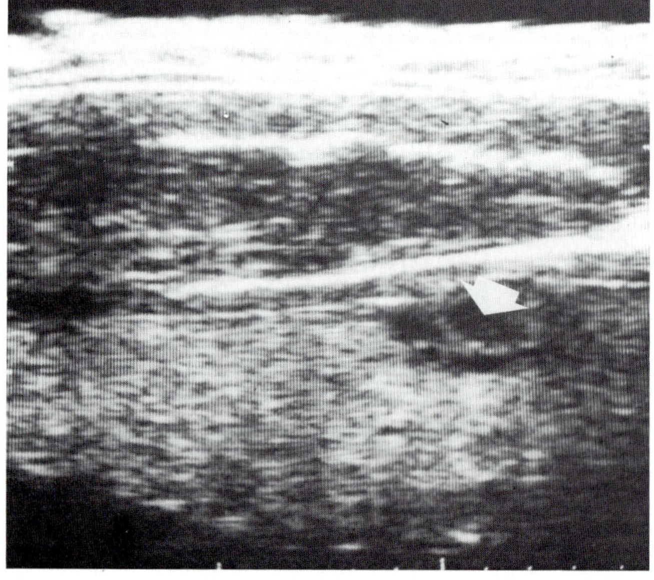

FIGURE 9.9. Longitudinal scan, left lobe. This 4-mm nodule (arrow) proved to be a papillary carcinoma. Physical examination and radionuclide examination were normal.

Carcinoma

Carcinoma accounts for 20 percent of cold nodules in the nonirradiated population. Our experience to date, with the exception of the follicular carcinoma mentioned previously, has been with papillary and mixed papillary-follicular lesions. Medullary and undifferentiated carcinomas also exist and may have a totally different appearance. With the former, there may be other associated endocrine adenomata, while in the latter case, the tumor is so rapidly progressive that diagnostic studies are of limited use.

Our series of carcinomas have manifested low-level echogenicity and the absence of a surrounding halo (Fig. 9.8). The smallest lesion detected and proved to be a carcinoma measured 4 mm in diameter (Fig. 9.9). As previously noted, small areas of degeneration may be seen, but marked cystic changes are unusual.

While it is clear that these devices afford a new dimension to studies of the morphology of thyroid nodules, they also are disclosing new areas of controversy. Pathologists frequently note the presence of small foci of carcinoma within the thyroid gland at autopsy. It seems reasonable to wonder whether these lesions would ever have become clinically significant. By identifying such masses with high resolution ultrasonography, we may, in fact, be subjecting the patient to other unnecessary diagnostic and therapeutic procedures. Nevertheless, we believe that instruments such as this are necessary to establish the relationship of these "mini-cancers" to clinical thyroid carcinoma.

One must also consider the fact that in patients with a previous history of head and neck irradiation, a much higher percentage of cold nodules (perhaps 50 percent) will be carcinomas. Under these circumstances, many advocate surgical excision regardless of the ultrasound or nuclear medicine findings. We have, however, altered our diagnostic approach to such patients. If the ultrasound study, which is performed first, fails to demonstrate a focal thyroid mass, no nuclear medicine study is performed. The patient is simply requested to return at approximately 3-year intervals for further study. If a mass is identified, a radionuclide study is requested to assess its functional status. The decision for or against surgery is then based on the combined results of all tests, as well as on the history and physical examination.

TESTICLE

Small parts scanning of the contents of the scrotal sac can frequently be helpful in the diagnosis of both inflammatory and neoplastic disease.[5] The examination is usually conducted with the patient in the supine position. Each half of the scrotal sac is examined separately because of the limited field of view. The examiner gently supports the side being studied against the membrane of the scanning head. By manipulating the testicle in mediolateral direction, the real-time nature of the study allows a quick survey assessment of anatomy. Views in both the transverse and sagittal planes are usually photo-

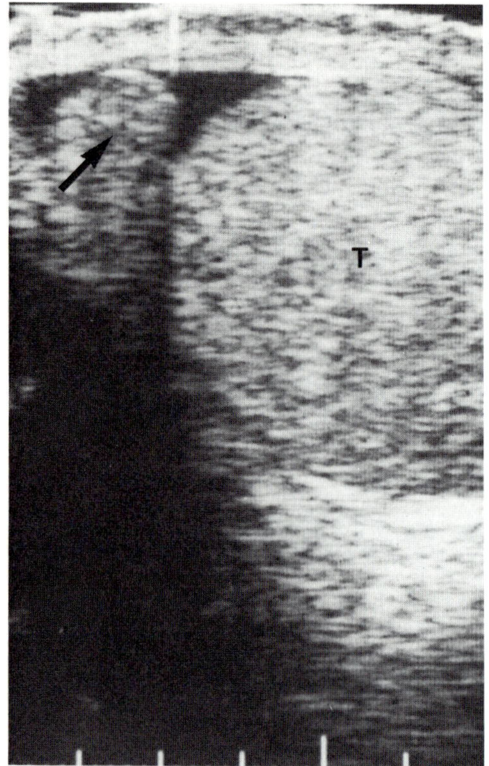

FIGURE 9.10. Longitudinal scan, left testicle. The even internal texture of the testicle (T) is seen. The somewhat coarser epididymis (arrow) and a small amount of fluid (normal) are also noted.

graphed for permanent record. The entire study takes about 5 minutes to perform and is usually not attended by any discomfort to the patient.

In the normal testicle, the parenchyma appears as a uniform midlevel gray echogenicity—similar to that of normal thyroid. The epididymis may be seen as a vertical band of tissue of marked echogenicity on the posterior aspect of the testicle, but is easier to recognize at the cephalad pole where its enlargement (head) caps the gland (Fig. 9.10). In many normal individuals, a small amount of fluid is seen surrounding the testicle. This should not be mistaken for the reactive hydrocele that frequently accompanies both inflammatory and tumorous conditions of the testicle.

Scrotal Masses

One of the major benefits of this technique is the ability to sort out the anatomy in a patient presenting with scrotal swelling. In many cases it is difficult,

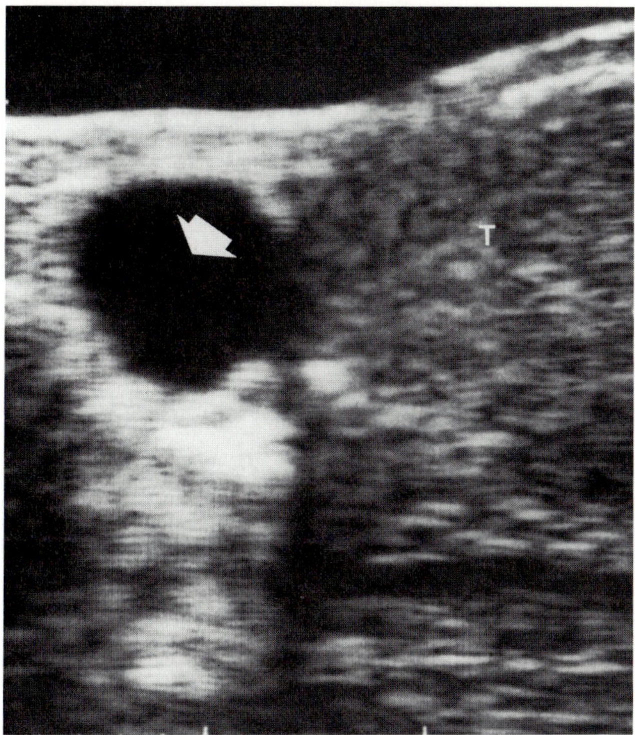

FIGURE 9.11. Longitudinal scan, right testicle. A small cystic mass (arrow) is seen within the epididymis, clearly separate from the testicle. This proved to be a spermatocele on aspiration.

even for an experienced examiner, to determine the origin of such masses. Ultrasonography is nearly always capable of localizing the lesion to epididymis, testicle, or a combination of the two.

Epididymis

Most masses that involve the epididymis are inflammatory in nature (Fig. 9.11). The epididymis enlarges and takes on a more lucent character. Focal abscesses present as sonolucent areas within the epididymis. On occasion, tumors of the testicle secondarily involve the epididymis, but it is usually possible to determine the site of origin by the relative involvement of both structures.

Testicle

Most testicular tumors present as areas of decreased echogenicity, compared with normal parenchyma (Fig. 9.12). Some authors report that teratocarcinomas commonly exhibit areas of cystic degeneration and septation, al-

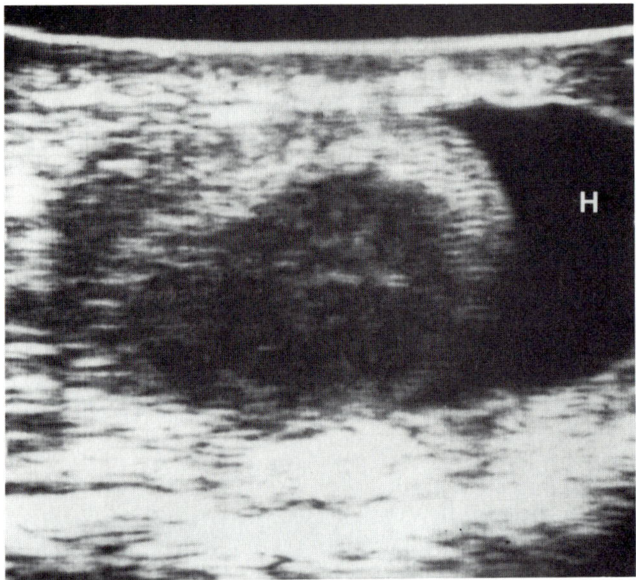

FIGURE 9.12. Sagittal scan, right testicle. The echo-poor mass within the testicle is an embryonal carcinoma. A reactive hydrocele is also present (H).

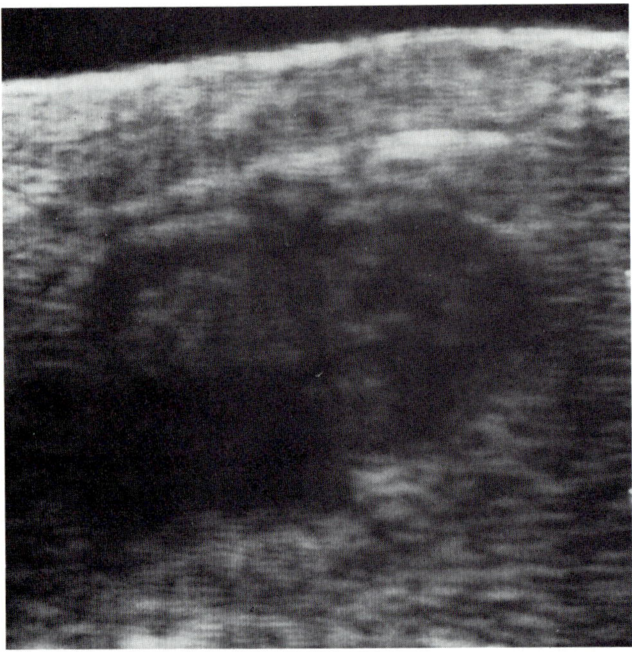

FIGURE 9.13. Transverse scan, right testicle. Although very similar in appearance to the mass in Figure 9.12, this lesion turned out to be a chronic testicular abscess.

though we personally have not had the opportunity to study such a case. The smallest tumor diagnosed thus far has been a 6-mm seminoma. This lesion was not palpable and was discovered on survey scanning in a young patient who presented with unexplained retroperitoneal adenopathy.

While inflammatory masses of the testicle are usually easy to differentiate from tumor on a clinical basis, we have encountered at least one case in which a chronic abscess was found in an older patient, was totally nontender, and was mistakenly diagnosed as a tumor (Fig. 9.13). This case demonstrates that while instrumentation of this sort is an excellent tool for studying the gross morphology of a lesion, it is not a substitute for the microscope.

CONCLUSIONS

High resolution ultrasonography has significant potential for the study of superficial organ system pathology. In addition to the two systems discussed here, it is possible to study tumors of other organs, such as the eye, breast, parotid, and parathyroid. Further refinements in equipment and increasing clinical experience will undoubtedly result in expansion of this technique into additional areas.

References

1. Leopold G: Ultrasonography of superficially located structures. Radiol Clin N Am 18:161–173, 1980.
2. Green P, Taenzer J, Ramsay S, et al: A real-time ultrasonic imaging system for carotid arteriography. Ultrasound Med Biol 3:129, 1979.
3. Leopold G, Humber P, Wickbom I, et al: Ultrasonic imaging for carotid occlusive disease. In Noninvasive Diagnostic Techniques in Vascular Disease, 2nd Edition, ed. Bernstein EF. St. Louis, CV Mosby Co, 1980.
4. Scheible W, Leopold G, Woo V: High resolution real-time ultrasonography of thyroid nodules. Radiology 133:413–417, 1979.
5. Leopold G, Woo V, Scheible W: High resolution ultrasonography of scrotal pathology. Radiology 131:719–722, 1979.

10 Eye and Orbit

RICHARD L. DALLOW

The eye and its surrounding adnexal tissues have the potential for development of a large variety of tumors. The globe itself contains epithelial, neural, and vascular elements, each of which can produce neoplasia. Additionally, metastases occur commonly to the choroid layer of the eye. Fibroproliferative disease in the eye can produce mass lesions that may also simulate true tumors.

The globe, however, represents only one component of the tissues encompassed by the bony orbit. It is surrounded anteriorly by the eyelids, with epithelial and glandular tissues, and more posteriorly by the lacrimal gland, extraocular muscles, fat, optic nerve, and other major vascular and neural components. Tumor potential of these surrounding tissues is greater and more varied than within the eye and affects visual functioning indirectly. The orbit may be invaded by tumors from the sinuses, which line three of its four walls, and from the adjacent intracranial spaces.

TECHNICAL REQUIREMENTS

For the eye, as in other medical diagnostic ultrasound applications, a pulse-echo technique is used with A-mode, B-scan, and M-mode display systems.[1,2] Echoes relate closely to anatomic boundaries of the eye and orbital structures. B-scan images serve as two-dimensional sections through the eye and orbit for topographic analysis of the location, size, and shape of lesions.[3,4] A-mode is used to characterize tissue types more fully by depicting the entire range of echo amplitudes. M-mode is used for physiologic studies of lens changes and choroidal pulsations and, occasionally, for magnet tests on foreign bodies.[5]

Unique features of the eye are its small size (24 mm diameter), cystic composition, and fine anatomic details, often measuring less than 0.1 mm. The orbit is about 40 mm deep and filled primarily with heterogeneous fat. Because of the requirement for high resolution of 0.1 mm of tissue differentiation and the relatively shallow penetration needed, as well as the cystic character of an exposed organ, making penetration easier, high frequency ultrasound transducers are used. The commonly used frequencies for eye ultrasound are 8 to 10 MHz, although 15 or 20 MHz is common for high resolution and biometry. A 5 MHz transducer may be used occasionally for deeper penetration to the orbital apex or for higher sensitivity to weaker echoes. The transducers generally are weakly focused with a 1.0 mm beam width between 10 and 30 mm from its surface.

B-scan images may be produced in several different manners, which influence results considerably. Gray scale images are produced with an automated real-time sector scanner with the transducer encased in a small fluid-filled compartment.[6] The smooth anterior surface of this compartment is placed directly on the eyelids or the topically anesthetized eyeball. Most such sector scanners have sweep rates of 10 to 30 frames per second. Gray scale is of only minimal value in eye diagnosis. The A-scan is utilized primarily for tissue characterization instead of relying on B-scan gray scale information.[7,8] B-scan eye images can be enhanced by complete outlining, with high contrast imaging and compound scanning patterns. This requires a different scanning system—a water immersion system.[9] This is achieved by using a bistable ultrasound unit with a hand-operated transducer that is moved across the eye in a combined linear and sector pattern, thus producing echoes from all aspects and contours of the eye. The image is compounded from many beam directions on a storage oscilloscope. The eye is surrounded by a saline-filled plastic bag with a large aperture over the eye. The transducer is submerged in the saline about 1 cm above the eye and manipulated on a cantilevered carriage. Thus, there are two methods of B-scan ultrasound examination of the eye and two corresponding equivalent assemblies: (1) the *contact method* with an automated, real-time, sector scanner, and (2) the *immersion method* with a hand-operated transducer and selective scanning patterns, transducer frequencies, and signal processing. The immersion system is more flexible and more sophisticated and produces the best results in B-scan imaging.

A-scan for application to the eye has the same unique features described for B-scan.[10] A-scan can be performed with a separate direct contact method or in combination with B-scan either by contact or immersion techniques. Receiver sensitivity is reduced to characterize echo intensities on a relative scale, usually using the highly reflectile scleral coat of the eye as a reference echo. Some controversy exists over the type of amplifier system best suited for A-scan machinery. Linear, logarithmic, and S-shaped amplifiers are available, each tending to emphasize a different part of the echo intensity spectrum.

Commercially available ultrasound units with combinations of these features are marketed by several different manufacturers specifically for eye applications. In general, ultrasound units used for abdominal and other body areas have not been adaptable to eye studies, as they lack high resolution, compound scanning, etc.

Other techniques have been devised to accentuate features of B-scan images, notably the color-coded scans[11] and the isometric scans.[12] The latter permits one to tilt the image on edge and view A-scans superimposed on the B-scan image. The most promising development in ophthalmic ultrasound appears to be computer signal analysis of spectral components of the returned echoes. It is hoped that this technique will lead to more precise tissue differentiation in the future.

OCULAR TUMORS

The most common intraocular tumors in adults are malignant melanoma, metastatic tumors to the uveal tract, and choroidal hemangioma.[13] In children, retinoblastomas and gliomas are more likely. Some cysts and other abnormalities may simulate the appearance of tumors clinically. Ultrasound is extremely useful in detecting and differentiating such lesions and has become one of the most useful tests in evaluating eyes with suspected tumors.[14-19] Ultrasound assumes a crucial role when opacities of the lens or vitreous obscure the view for clinical examination of the posterior portions of the eye. Ultrasound findings in these conditions will be described separately for each tumor type.

Malignant melanoma, a potentially fatal tumor, is the most frequent tumor of the eye in adults. Melanomas arise in the uveal tract (choroid, ciliary body, and iris), are usually located along the inner globe surface, and protrude into the acoustically clear vitreous cavity. They vary in size from a barely detectable 0.1 mm mass to a tumor that fills the entire eye and even erodes outside it into adjacent tissues. The tumor contour is usually smoothly convex on B-scan, with a high-density lead echo seen on A-scan (Fig. 10.1). The internal echo pattern of melanomas is characteristically one of a gradual decay slope of closely spaced spikes down to the baseline. Echoes come from the cellular aggregates, fibrous septa, and vessels within the mass. This can vary, of course. Most melanomas are seen as compact masses of similar cells, but occasionally a necrotic center or a fungating growth pattern will alter the ultrasound findings.

Certain topographic pattern variations are associated with melanomas. The smooth convex contour pattern is distorted once the tumor breaks through Bruch's membrane and the retina and begins a less contained growth within the vitreous cavity. A polypoid or "collar-button" appearance is produced. Other tumors do not generally show this pattern. While melanomas expand primarily inward within the eye, they also frequently produce an apparent shallow "excavation" of the surrounding coats of the eye. This appears as a concave indentation of the normal globe contour posterior to the tumor. It does not imply extension through the eye, however. This excavation is seen in approximately 40 percent of smaller melanomas, and it is virtually pathognomonic of melanoma. Sound attenuation through large compact melanomas produces a relative shadowing artifact in the fat pad posterior to the lesion (Fig. 10.3). This appears as an artifactually blank area in the fat, which is usually completely filled in with echoes in the normal unaltered state. Some melanomas are so cellularly compact and homogeneous that they appear echo-free internally, similar to some lymphomas.

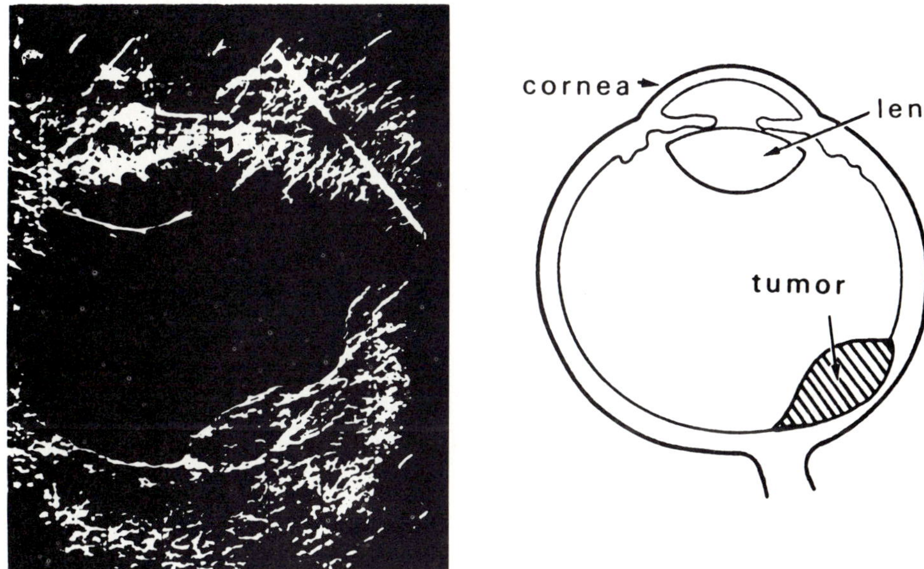

FIGURE 10.1. Choroidal melanoma located in the posterior pole with a smooth, convex contour, internal tissue echoes, and choroidal excavation sign present.

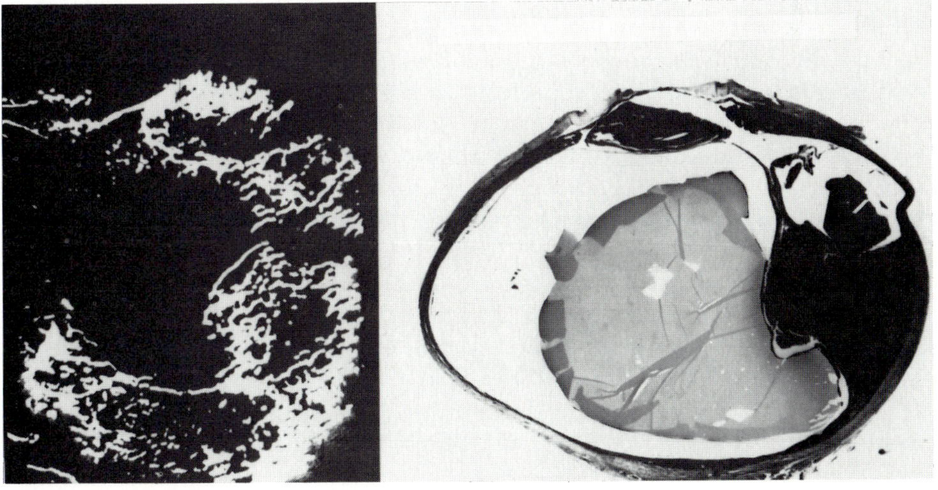

FIGURE 10.2. Large choroidal melanoma associated with total retinal detachment forcing anterior displacement of the lens and iris (left). Histopathology section of same eye (right).

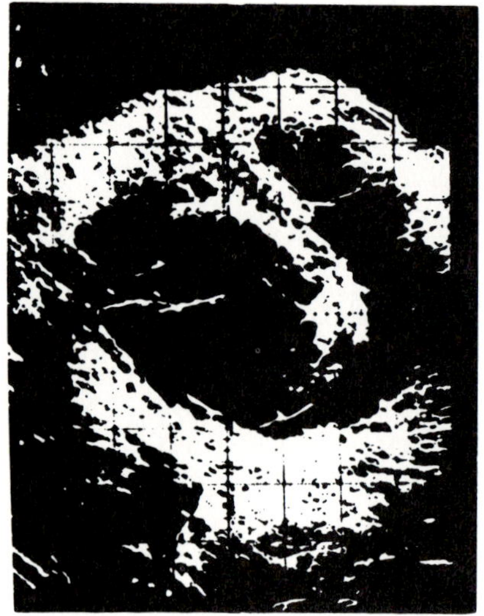

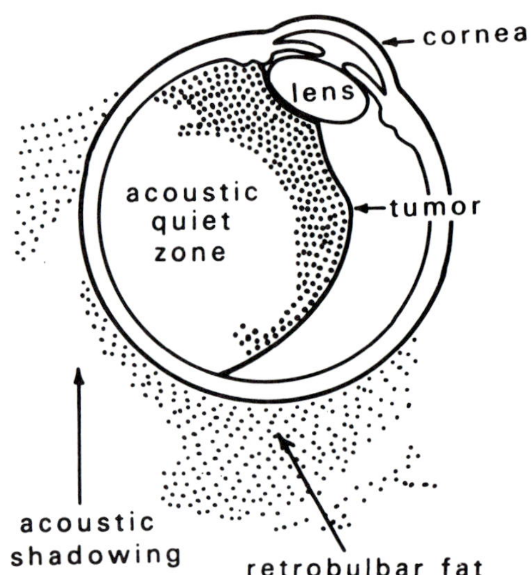

FIGURE 10.3. Internal tumor quiet zone and acoustical shadowing result from greater sound energy absorption within the choroidal melanoma with less penetration of orbital tissues behind the mass.

A-scan can be critical in differentiating lesions, especially when the B-scan image is equivocal.[20] A localized vitreous hemorrhage can appear compact enough on B-scan to resemble a tumor mass. A-scan amplitudes show a high lead echo for a tumor with a gradual decay of amplitudes (Fig. 10.4), whereas amplitudes from a hemorrhage are much lower, more closely arranged, and scintillating, because of slight motion of the red cell aggregates producing the echoes (Fig. 10.5). A retinal detachment may at times resemble a melanoma with the anechoic pattern, especially if the retina is elevated only in one quadrant. A-scan of retinal detachment shows only a solitary high spike with no underlying tissue echoes (Fig. 10.6). B-scan images of hemorrhage or retinal detachment show no posterior excavation and no shadowing. Ultrasonic features of melanomas are summarized in Table 10.1.

Tumors may be measured by ultrasound to document size and growth. Many of the melanomas of the eye are observed for years before they show sufficient growth to warrant enucleation of the eye. Biometry is best performed with high-resolution transducers (15 or 20 MHz). Resolution and accuracy of 0.1 mm is necessary in this application, since many of the tumors are less than 1 mm high. Maximal tumor height is measured by arranging the A-scan for highest lead in terminal echoes, or by coordinating it with a simultaneous B-scan image. Base diameter of tumors cannot be accurately measured because of the ultrasound beam width. Measurements also serve the purpose of following tumor regression after proton beam or cobalt plaque therapy.

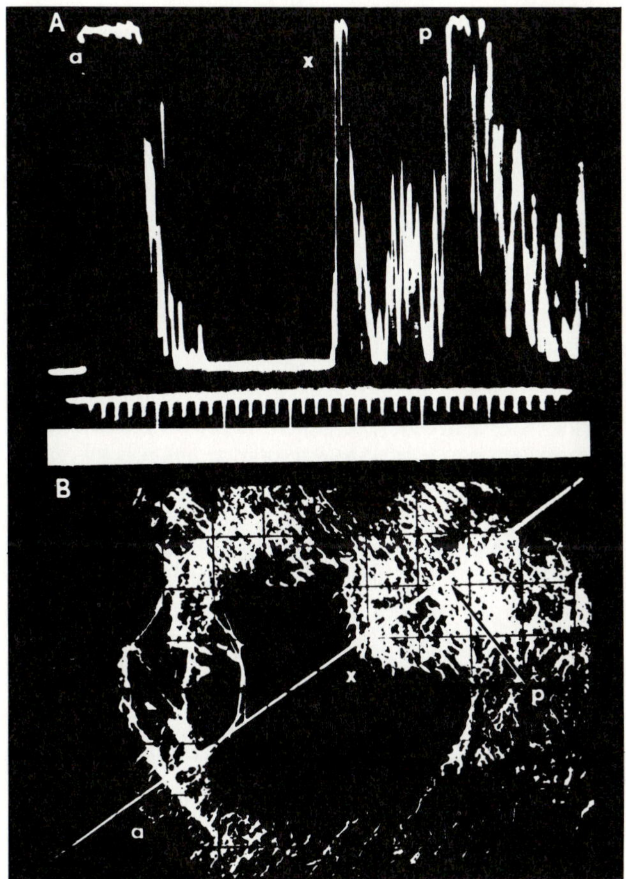

FIGURE 10.4 Metastatic uveal tumor exhibiting a high leading echo on A-scan (arrow).

Metastatic tumors in the eye have the same characteristic locations as do melanomas, i.e., within the uveal tract, most frequently the posterior pole. They may come from any source, including tumors of the breast, gastrointestinal system, lung, or prostate. In contrast to melanomas, metastatic tumors tend to have a flatter configuration on B-scan, appearing as a low, undulating mass elevated only 1.0 mm, but having a broad-based diameter (Fig. 10.7). Metastatic tumors may be multiple, whereas melanoma is almost always a solitary lesion. Metastases lack the excavation sign, quiet internal echo pattern, and the attenuation sign sometimes seen with melanomas. In many cases, their A-scan patterns do not differ significantly from the melanoma pattern. However, since metastatic tumors are usually heterogenous and vascularized, they are filled with midamplitude echoes and show less decay pattern than do melanomas.

Hemangiomas also arise within the choroid component of the uveal tract.

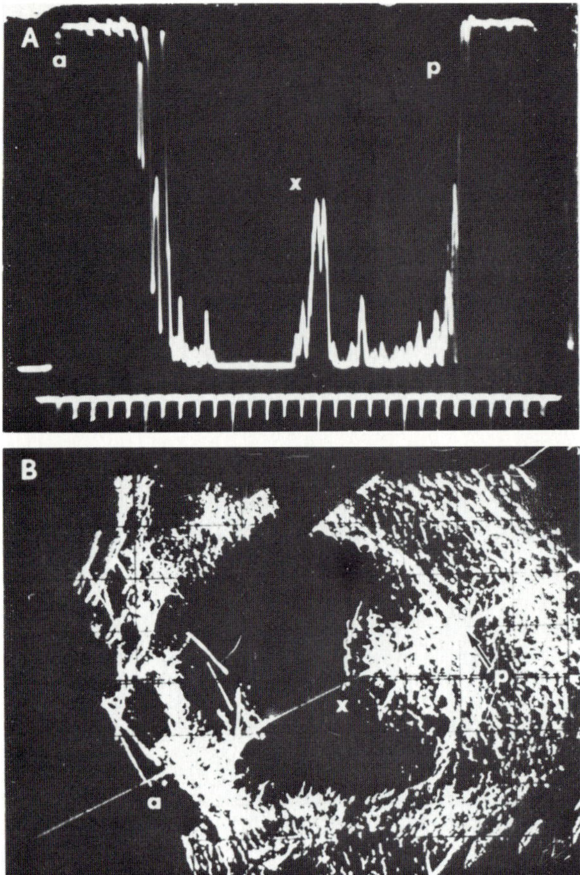

FIGURE 10.5. Vitreous hemorrhage does not appear as high amplitude lead echo (arrow) on A-scan.

This benign and generally nonprogressive tumor has a very low elevation and a broad base dimension. The tumor composition of multiple small vascular channels and blood-filled spaces produces a characteristic A-scan appearance of sustained high amplitude echoes throughout the lesion. There is no decay pattern, no excavation, no shadowing, and no quiet zone. If the lesion is large enough, it can usually be differentiated from solid tumors.

Retinoblastoma is the most common intraocular malignancy in children, but it is often masked by opacities, such as cataract, hemorrhage, or vitreous membranes. Retinoblastoma is seldom seen when it appears initially as a small lesion along the inner globe surface, except in hereditary cases when routine examinations are done for it. More often it appears as a fairly large fungating lesion, often with necrotic foci, calcium deposits, and associated vitreous debris and retinal detachment. The ultrasound pattern is thus quite

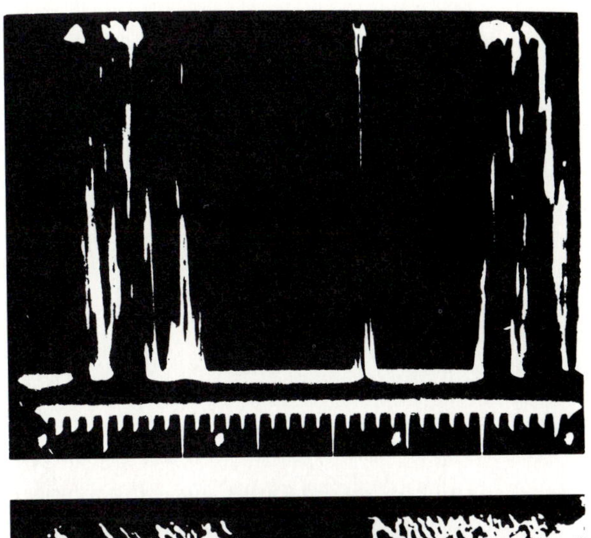

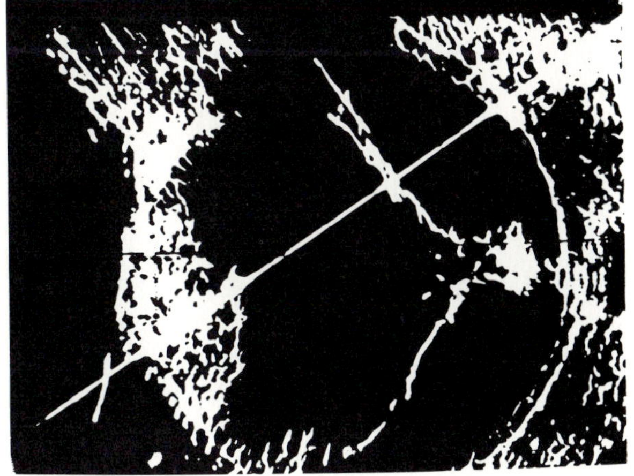

FIGURE 10.6. Retinal detachment appears on A-scan as a high amplitude echo with an echo free subretinal space.

variable.[21] It always shows an irregular pattern of high amplitude echoes and membranes. The detection of multiple, "foreign body" type, very high echoes, reflected from the calcium within the tumor, is virtually pathognomonic for retinoblastoma. However, this sign is not always present.

Other conditions may simulate the appearance of intraocular tumors, both clinically and ultrasonically. Vitreous hemorrhages and retinal detachments have been mentioned previously and their differentiation by ultrasound described. One particularly difficult lesion to differentiate is an organized subretinal hemorrhage, or disciform maculopathy, which is a common finding in elderly patients. It appears on B-scan as an elevated mass in the posterior pole and has a size, shape, and configuration resembling a small melanoma. The A-scan pattern may also be indistinguishable from melanoma. Subreti-

TABLE 10.1 Ultrasonographic features of choroidal melanoma.

Contour	B-scan
Tissue characteristics	A-scan
Choroidal excavation	B-scan
Acoustic quiet zone	B-scan
Acoustic shadowing	B-scan

nal hemorrhage does lack the signs of excavation, quiet zone, and attenuation, and it does not show growth on serial examinations over time, whereas a melanoma is likely to increase in size.

Cystic lesions can also simulate tumors. Cysts are common in the ciliary body region, which is a locus for melanoma as well. Both appear clinically as dark masses because of the heavy pigmentation of the uvea in this region. B-scan outline of the two lesions is similar, with a rounded mass appearance (Fig. 10.8). Because of the anterior location, the other B-scan signs are not applicable.[22] A-scan demonstrates no internal echoes for a cyst, but at least some internal tissue echoes are evident in all melanomas located this anteriorly, no matter how homogeneous they are.

Many other lesions can resemble tumors on ultrasound examination of the eyes.[13] A partial list includes: vitreous hemorrhage, subretinal hemorrhage, retinal detachment, choroidal detachment, ciliary body cysts, brawny scleritis, lymphoid hyperplaisa, melanocytoma, dislocated cataract, scleral buckling implant, other foreign bodies, phthisis bulbi, and optic nerve head elevation from papilledema or tumor.

The reliability of ultrasonic diagnosis and tumor differentiation has been documented by several investigators, with a general consensus of better than 90 percent accuracy regardless of the specific technique employed.[17, 19] Occasionally, it may be difficult to identify an ocular tumor on the basis of a single examination alone. In an eye with complex findings or equivocal results, the importance of serial examinations over time cannot be stressed enough. Most tumors will show a progressive increase in size, while others may resolve, or at least remain static. The major limitations of ultrasound diagnosis in this area are related to the size and location of lesions. Lesions under 0.5 mm in elevation may be missed entirely, and difficulty in acoustic tissue differentiation may occur with tumors less than 2 mm in elevation. Very large tumors filling the vitreous may also be difficult to evaluate because of tumor breakdown from necrosis.

ORBITAL TUMORS

The orbit can harbor virtually any type of tumor, and all may have similar clinical presentations of a proptotic eye with no direct evidence of the responsible process. The most common causes of exophthalmos are, in fact, inflammatory diseases (Graves' disease, pseudotumor, cellulitis) rather than

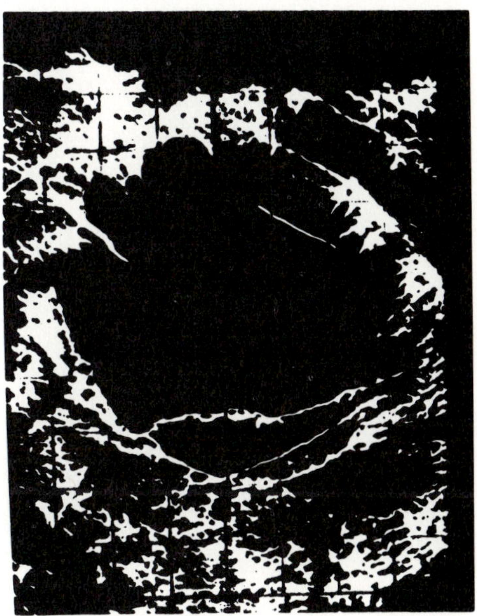

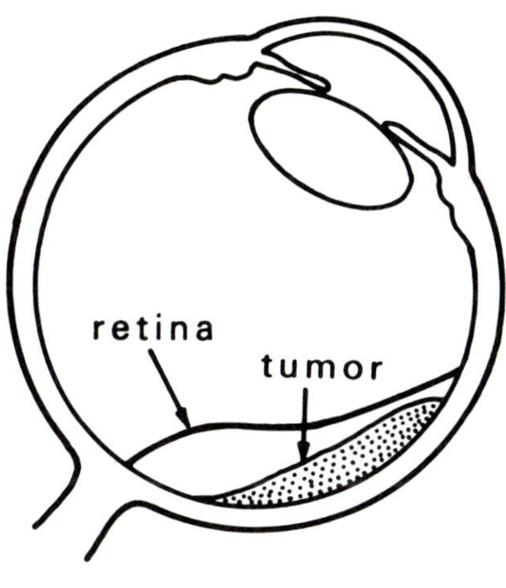

FIGURE 10.7. A metastatic uveal tumor often appears as a flattened choroidal tumor with overlying retinal detachment.

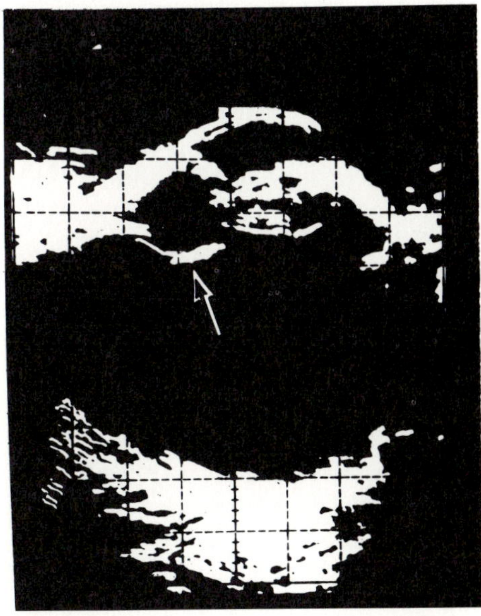

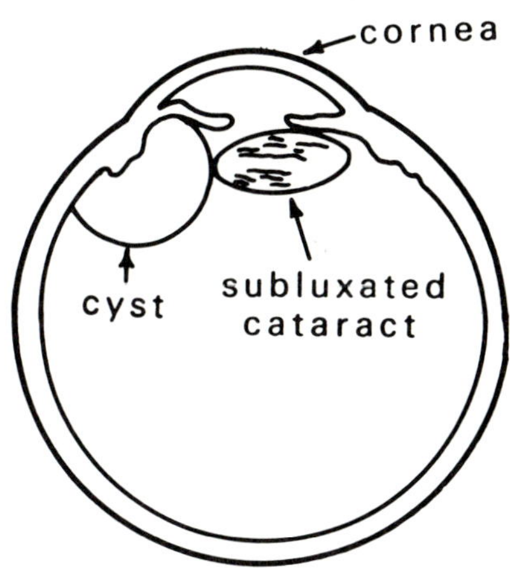

FIGURE 10.8. Ciliary body cyst (arrow) with a smooth, rounded contour and acoustically clear internal space.

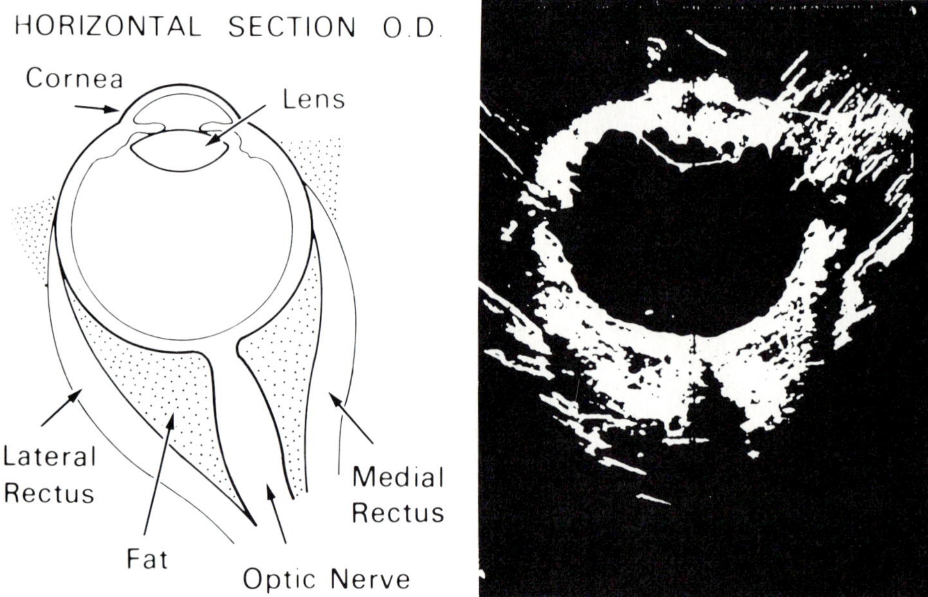

FIGURE 10.9. B-scan ultrasonic representation of normal orbit (right) with diagram of major components (left).

true neoplasms. The incidence of specific tumors varies in different series and for different age groups. A rough descending order of frequency is as follows: metastatic neoplasms, secondary neoplasm (from adjacent sinuses, lids, or intracranial space) hemangioma, lacrimal gland tumors (benign or malignant), lymphoma, glioma, meningioma, dermoid cysts, mucocele, rhabdomyosarcoma, leukemia, etc. Some arteriovenous anomalies can simulate orbital tumors, including varices and shunts. Radiography, computerized tomography, and ultrasound are essential tests for defining orbital abnormalities and for guiding surgical approaches.[23-25]

Normal orbits produce a consistent picture on B-scan ultrasonography.[26-28] The scan produces a thin section through the entire orbit about 1 mm thick and with 0.3 mm anteroposterior resolution in the deeper aspects of the orbit (Fig. 10.9). The eye portion of the scan shows clear delineation of the cornea, lens, and globe contour. The retrobulbar pattern is derived primarily from the large fat pad, which has a triangular shape and is bounded anteriorly by the globe and on the sides by the extraocular muscles. The fat is quite heterogeneous, being composed of fat globules, fibrous septa, vessels, and nerves. High amplitude echoes are produced throughout the fatty tissue complex, giving it a "filled-in" appearance on the B-scan image and a decaying high amplitude pattern on A-scan (Fig. 10.10).

The extraocular muscles and optic nerve are more compact, well-organized, and homogeneous tissues compared to the fat pad. These structures appear

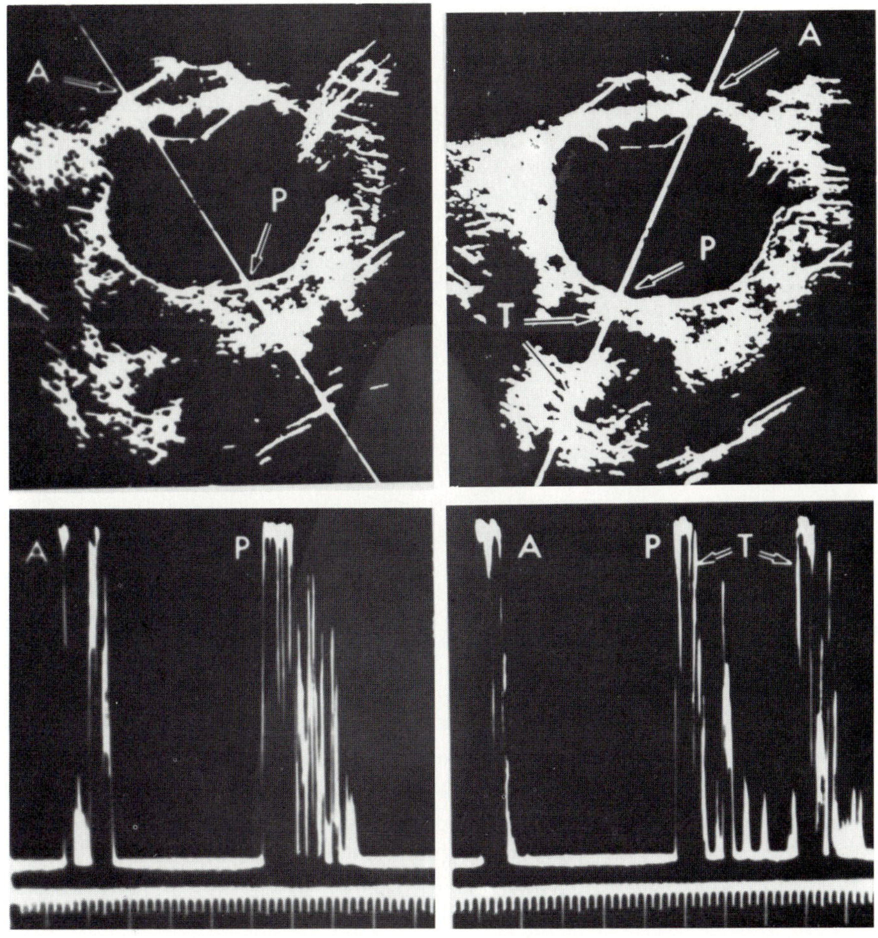

FIGURE 10.10. Combined A-mode and B-scan ultrasound display of orbit containing lymphangioma tumor. B-scan image (top) illustrates morphology of eye (A to P) and irregular tumor mass (T) within muscle cone. A-mode analysis (bottom) corresponds to bright lighted axis on B-scan image above. Anteroposterior direction runs from left to right on A-mode images. Lower left image represents normal A-mode pattern of eye (A to P) and retrobulbar fat (following P). Lower right image depicts A-mode pattern with axis shifted through abnormal portion of orbit. Typical A-mode tumor pattern (T) replaces retrobulbar fat. (Dallow RL: Ultrasonography in the diagnosis of orbital diseases. In Controversy in Ophthalmology, eds. Brockhurst RJ, Boruchoff SA, Hutchinson BT, Lessell S. Philadelphia, WB Saunders, 1977.)

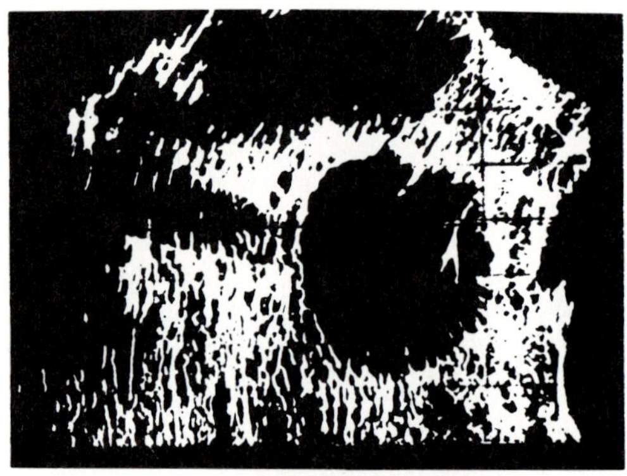

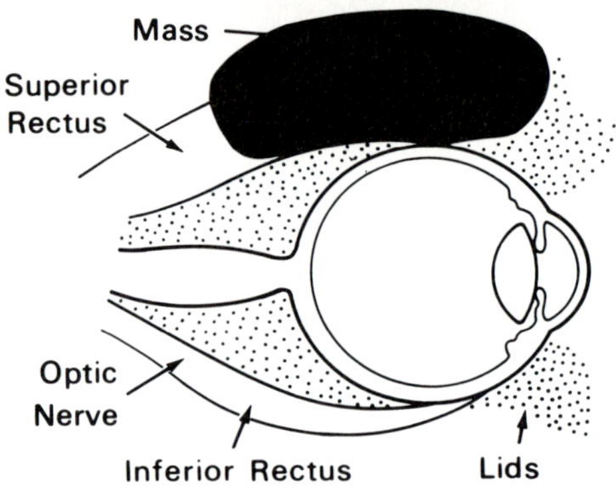

FIGURE 10.11. Mucocele adjacent to globe equator and indenting it slightly. Lesion has smooth, circumscribed contour, good sound transmission, and no internal echoes.

as relatively echo-free areas in contrast to adjacent fat. Hence a B-scan section at the level of the optic nerve produces a W-shaped area of echoes posterior to the globe, with muscles and optic nerve seen in negative contrast. The bony orbital wall is represented by only a few low-amplitude echoes, partly because the beam is not perpendicular to its surface and does not receive a maximum echo from the wall, and partly because the sound undergoes a shearing effect when it strikes bone.

Orbital abnormalities may be classified by ultrasonic criteria into four major categories: pseudoproptosis, mass lesions, inflammatory disorders, and traumatic changes.[29, 30] Each of these categories is further subdivided into several specific types of lesions. Each category will be described separately with examples.

Mass lesions are evidenced on B-scan images as a distinct distortion of the normal retrobulbar pattern of fat, optic nerve, and rectus muscles.[27] Any abnormal contour intruding into this pattern must be suspected as representing a tumor. Four general tumor types are easily identifiable: cystic, solid, angiomatous, and infiltrative. These patterns are defined by ultrasonic evidence of contours, sound transmission, internal tissue echoes, and location of the lesions.

Cystic tumors seen on B-scan have a smoothly rounded contour that is sharply defined from adjacent structures and often causes some distortion of normal tissues by compression (Fig. 10.11) Cystic masses demonstrate good sound transmission, so that the posterior wall of these lesions is clearly defined. Internally, cysts are generally devoid of echoes because there are no significant tissue interfaces within the lesion. These findings are characteristic of a fluid-filled cystic lesion, such as mucocele or a retention cyst. Dermoid tumors produce similar ultrasound findings but usually have low amplitude echoes derived from the internal structures and debris within the mass.

Solid tumors also demonstrate well-defined contours ultrasonically that contrast with adjacent tissues (Fig. 10.12). The tumor contour may be smoothly rounded or somewhat irregular. In contrast to cystic lesions, solid tumors produce significant sound attenuation, so that penetration is poor and the posterior margin of the tumor may not be well defined. Tissue interfaces within the tumor produce multiple low amplitude to midamplitude echoes within its substance, indicating a moderately heterogeneous tissue. These ultrasound findings indicate circumscribed, solid tumors, such as neurogenic tumors, lacrimal gland tumors, and some metastatic tumors.

Location of the lesion within the orbit on ultrasonic scanning gives further clues about its probable tissue type. A lesion of this kind, within the muscle cone and involving the optic nerve, is most likely to be one of the neurogenic tumors (glioma, meningioma, or neurofibroma). A similar lesion located in the upper temporal aspect of the orbit is most likely a lacrimal gland tumor. Ultrasonography defines the amount of posterior extension of such tumors, thereby helping the surgeon to choose his best approach for excision of the lesion.

Angiomatous tumors studied by ultrasonography may demonstrate an irregular contour with fingerlike protrusions extending into the orbital fat pad, usually with a larger mass more posteriorly. The tumor contour may or may not be well defined from adjacent tissues. The internal structure of angiomatous tumors presents many dense acoustic interfaces, from the vessel walls and blood-filled spaces comprising the tumor. Ultrasonically, this highly heterogeneous tissue appears as multiple, irregular, high-amplitude echoes throughout the mass (Fig. 10.13). Because it is largely fluid, the mass transmits sound very well so that the entire mass is seen. The irregular contour and heterogeneous structure are a marked contrast to the cystic and solid tumors described previously.

Infiltrative tumors share ultrasonic characteristics with both solid and angiomatous tumors. They usually have an irregular contour that may be located anywhere in the orbit, but often appear along the bony orbital walls (Fig. 10.14). The mass may appear to invade adjacent fat. As with other solid tumors, low-amplitude internal echoes are present within the lesion, and sound attenuation is high, often making the posterior tumor margins indistinct. The size of infiltrative tumors is quite variable, but they are frequently

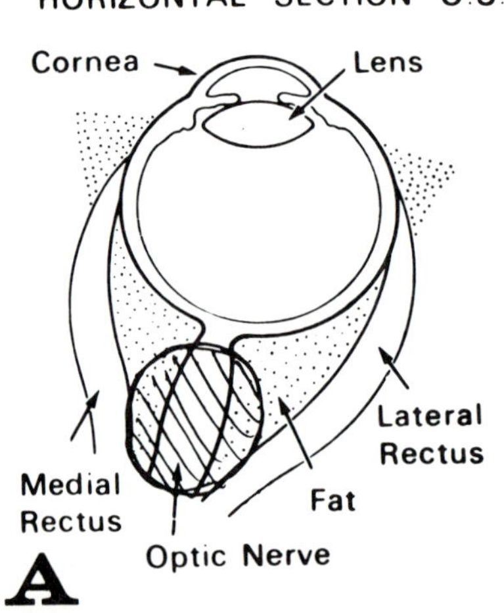

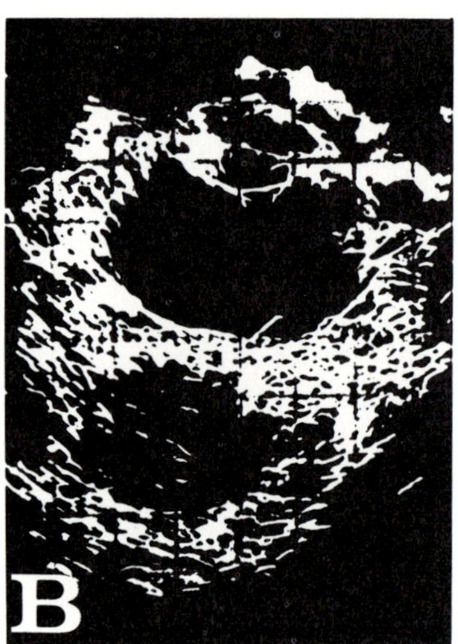

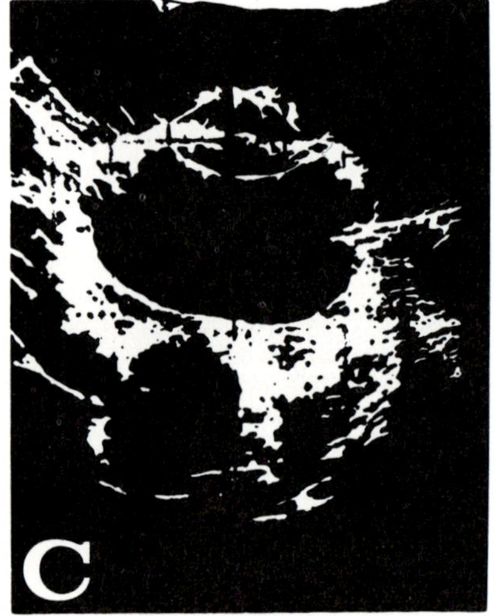

FIGURE 10.12. Solid tumor within muscle cone having circumscribed appearance, low irregular internal echoes (seen at 5 mHz in B), and poor sound transmission (seen at 10 mHz in C). Optic nerve glioma was found surgically. (Dallow RL, Coleman DJ: Ultrasonic evaluation of orbital disorders. In Ocular and Adnexal tumors, ed. Jakobiec FA. Birmingham, Aesculapius, 1978.)

large when first examined. This ultrasonic pattern is associated with lymphomas, sarcomas, and metastatic tumors.

Tumors extending into the orbit from the intracranial space or from adjacent sinuses may have a very flat configuration that follows the contour of the orbital walls. Such en plaque tumors are difficult to demonstrate by ultrasonography; they constitute one category of orbital disease in which this test produces false negative reports. Once the tumor enlarges sufficiently to appear as a 3 mm, circumscribed mass within the orbit, it becomes detectable by ultrasonography. A sphenoid wing meningioma is one tumor that characteristically progresses in this fashion.

It is not always possible to classify orbital tumors ultrasonically into the four categories noted before, since tumors that are similar pathologically do

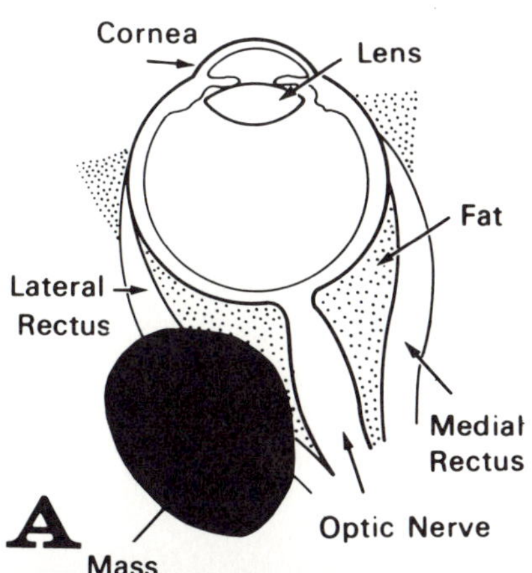

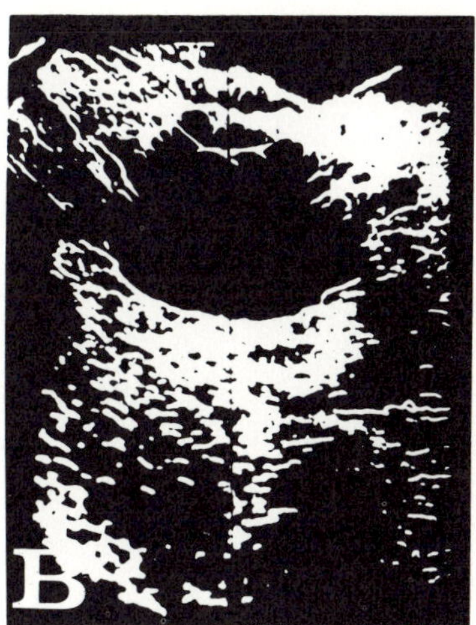

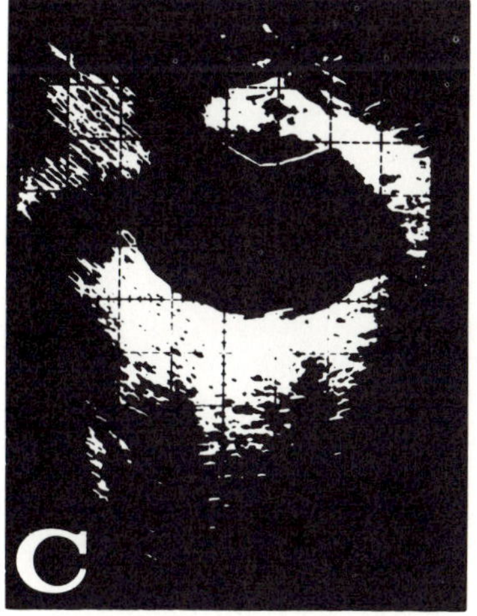

FIGURE 10.13. Hemangioma in orbital apex appears poorly circumscribed (b) with relatively frequent midamplitude internal echoes, considering its posterior location (C). (Dallow RL: Ultrasonography in the diagnosis of orbital diseases. In Controversy in Ophthalmology, eds. Brockhurst RJ, Boruchoff SA, Hutchinson BT, Lessell S. Philadelphia, WB Saunders, 1977.)

not always appear similar anatomically, and vice versa. In general, however, the ultrasonic patterns and absorption characteristics described have been highly consistent for the types of tumors noted.

Tumors cause distortion of the normal orbital ultrasound patterns by intruding as new structures. Tumors also have ultrasonic characteristics derived from their own tissues. Inflammatory and congestive processes of the orbit, by contrast, tend to involve structures normally present in the orbit, sometimes causing only subtle changes of the normal ultrasonic patterns. Inflammatory ultrasound findings may be diffuse or localized to a particular area or tissue in the orbit, depending on the specific inflammatory process involved. A wide range of diseases produces orbital inflammation, including infections, lymphoid or granulomatous processes, or secondary passive congestion of tissue. The etiologic history of inflammatory changes can only be inferred from ultrasonography, since the same findings may be present in

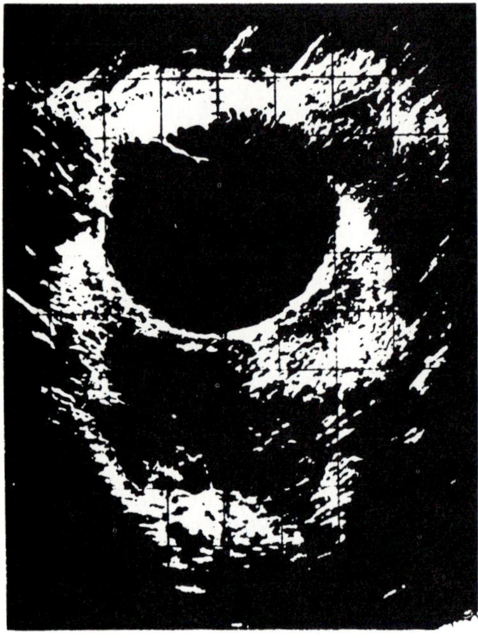

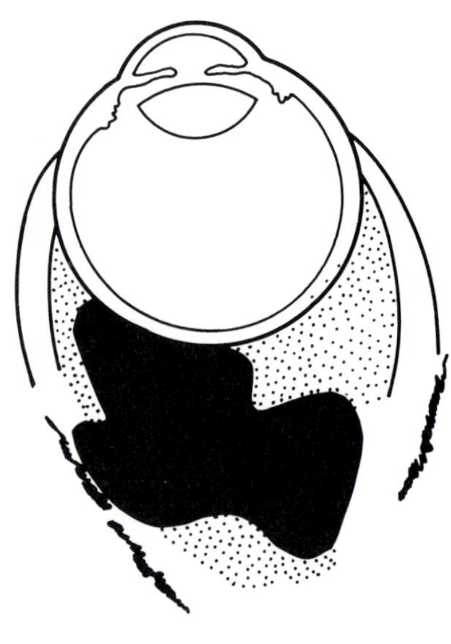

FIGURE 10.14. Infiltrative orbital neoplasm (lymphoma) exhibits irregular contour invading several tissue planes and moderately good sound transmission, but very low internal echoes. (Dallow RL, Coleman DJ: Ultrasonic evaluation of orbital disorders. In Ocular and Ednexal Tumors, ed. Jakobiec FA. Birmingham, Aesculapius, 1978.)

several different pathologic disorders. Of major importance is the fact that inflammatory changes are clearly distinguished from the findings associated with tumors.[31, 32]

Cellulitis, or *idiopathic orbital inflammation*, produces diffuse orbital ultrasound findings. The fat pad is generally the most involved tissue, with a diffuse, mottled texture identified ultrasonically by widening of spaces between echoes. These changes probably result primarily from interstitial edema separating fat globules and connective tissue abnormally. A granuloma or abscess area may be identifiable ultrasonically as a focal mottled area, which is usually more evident after the area has become partially walled off from adjacent tissues. Edema in the posterior sub-Tenon's space encircling the globe and around the optic nerve sheath is particularly characteristic of pseudotumor.

Dysthyroid exophthalmos (orbitopathy of Graves' disease) causes diffuse orbital edema and inflammation with particular involvement of the extraocular muscles. Accentuation and enlargement of the extraocular muscles is seen ultrasonically in nearly all patients with this disorder. On B-scan images, dysthyroid exophthalmos appears as a generalized widening of the echo-free area between the retrobulbar fat pad and the bony orbital wall (Fig. 10.15).

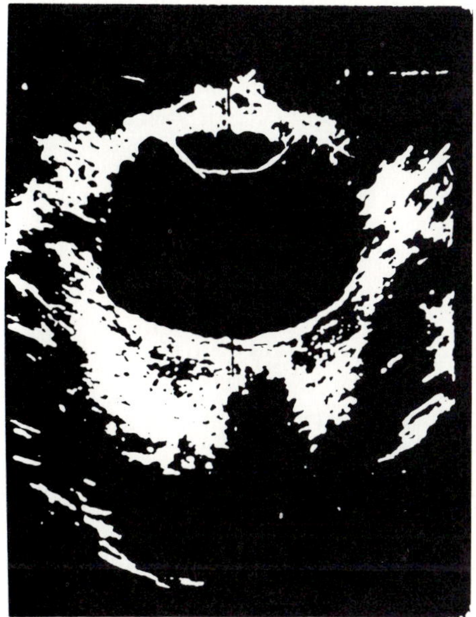

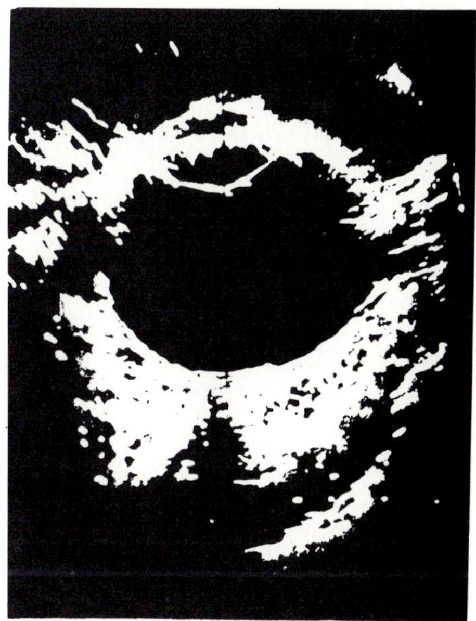

FIGURE 10.15. Dysthyroid exophthalmos. Marked enlargement of extraocular muscles is highly suggestive of thyroid orbital disease, even though it may be quite asymmetrical. (Dallow RL: Ultrasonography in the diagnosis of orbital diseases. In Controversy in Ophthalmology, eds. Brockhurst RJ, Boruchoff SA, Hutchinson BT, Lessell S. Philadelphia, WB Saunders, 1977.)

The muscle contours are much better defined than normally, and abnormal echoes may be seen within the disorganized muscle tissue. The four rectus muscles may be visualized ultrasonically by scanning in both the horizontal and vertical meridians. The degree of muscle enlargement varies considerably from subtle to marked, depending on the amount of soft tissue edema from the disease process. Bilateral changes are often evident, even when exophthalmos appears unilateral clinically.

Although these ultrasound signs are highly suggestive of dysthyroid exophthalmos, they are not pathognomonic for it. Passive congestion of the orbit secondary to arteriovenous anomalies may produce similar ultrasound findings. Other inflammatory processes may produce edematous muscles, fat, and perineural sheaths, including myositis and pseudotumors. Pseudotumors of the orbit often present a clinical and pathologic enigma. The term pseudotumor is used commonly to include such diverse processes as idiopathic inflammation, chronic granuloma, lymphoid infiltration, and myositis, as well as many other more specific disease entities. Ultrasonic signs of pseudotumor are likewise diverse but are often helpful in identifying the process as inflammatory rather than tumorous.

Acute proptosis of an eye after blunt *trauma* is usually attributable to orbital hemorrhage, which resolves during a period of 1 to 2 weeks. When the

TABLE 10.2. Ultrasonic orbital diagnosis.

Pseudoproptosis	Mass lesion	Inflammatory change	Traumatic effect
Large globe	Cystic	Enlarged muscles	Foreign body
Shallow orbit	Solid	Focal granuloma	Hemorrhage
	Angiomatous	Edema/inflammation	
	Infiltrative	Optic neuritis	

trauma is minimal, or when the proptosis does not resolve rapidly, a hemorrhaging tumor must be suspect. Ultrasonography provides a means of distinguishing hemorrhage from neoplasm. A diffuse orbital hemorrhage produces only a vague mottling of the orbital fat where blood has extravasated. A compact hematoma, however, may resemble a neoplasm in many respects, appearing as a circumscribed solid mass. Repeat ultrasonography at appropriate intervals will establish a gradual diminution in the size of the lesion if it is, indeed, a resolving hematoma. An increase in the size of the lesion, demonstrated by ultrasonography, implies a true neoplasm and justifies surgical exploration.

Foreign bodies of all types, including metal, glass, plastic, and even biologic matter, are detectable with ultrasonography. The object can be localized precisely with reference to adjacent anatomic structures. It can be determined definitively whether the foreign body lies in the eye; a determination that cannot always be made by radiographic analysis. Foreign bodies may be missed by ultrasonography if they are not oriented in such a way that they reflect echoes along the beam pathway so that it may be detected by the transducer. Objects as small as 1 mm are detectable with optimal orientation of the examining ultrasonic beam. However, orbital foreign body echoes are often lost in the highly reflective retrobulbar fat pad.

Vascular intercommunications, intracranially or intraorbitally, can cause exophthalmos. These disorders produce no specific signs on ultrasonography but often demonstrate the congestive changes described previously. With careful study, a dilated superior ophthalmic vein can be detected in many orbits so affected. Vascular contrast studies are necessary to document the abnormal vascular channels. The role of ultrasonography in these situations is to narrow the possibilities by failing to show gross tumor or specific inflammatory changes. Ultrasonic orbital diagnosis is summarized in Table 10.2.

The *diagnostic accuracy* of ultrasound for orbital diseases, as demonstrated in different series, lies between 80 and 90 percent. This approximates the accuracy of computerized tomography, and both tests far exceed the correct positive yield of other radiographic studies. Ultrasound is actually the most versatile of all of the tests, because it not only detects tumors, but also characterizes them in terms of general tissue type with high reliability. Ultrasound also is the most effective test for defining inflammatory changes in the orbit.

Computerized tomography is less effective in both respects, but it has the distinct advantage of showing the periorbital and intracranial tumors that ultrasound cannot, because they lie beyond the bony walls of the orbit. Computerized tomography has problems in distinguishing inflammatory masses from tumors, with a resulting significant false positive tumor diagnostic rate of about 10 percent. Ultrasound generally identifies these inflammatory problems properly. Ultrasound resolution exceeds that of computerized tomography for smaller lesions in the orbit. Thus, the two tests are actually quite complimentary, and both are essential to a full, careful orbital evaluation.

References

1. Coleman DJ, Lizzi FL, Jack RL,: Ultrasonography of the Eye and Orbit. Philadelphia, Lea and Febiger, 1977.
2. Dallow, R.L. (ed.): Ophthalmic ultrasonography: comparative techniques. Int Ophthalmol Clin 19(4):1–310, 1979.
3. Baum G, Greenwood I: The application of ultrasonic locating techniques to ophthalmology. Part 1. Reflective properties. Am J Ophthalmol 46:319, 1958.
4. Purnell EW: Ultrasound in ophthalmological diagnosis. In Diagnostic Ultrasound, eds. Grossman C, et al. New York, Plenum Press, 1966, pp 95–109.
5. Coleman DJ, Weininger R: Ultrasonic M-mode technique in opthalmology. Arch Ophthal 83:475, 1969.
6. Bronson NR, Fisher YL, Pickering NC, Trayner EM: Ophthalmic Contact B-scan Ultrasonography for the Clinician. Westport, Virginia, Intercontinental Publications, 1976.
7. Oksala A, Lehtinen A: Diagnostic value of ultrasonics in ophthalmology. Ophthalmologica 134:387, 1957.
8. Ossoinig KC: Quantitative echography—the bases of tissue differentiation. J Clin Ultrasound 2:33, 1974.
9. Coleman DJ, Konig WF, Katz L: A hand operated ultrasound scan system for ophthalmic evaluation. Am J Ophthalmol 68:256, 1969.
10. Ossoinig KC: Preoperative differential diagnosis of tumors with echography. Part II. Instrumentation and examination techniques. In Current Concepts in Ophthalmology, vol 4, ed. Blodi FC. St Louis, CV Mosby, 1974, pp 280–296.
11. Coleman DJ, Katz L: Color-coding of B-scan ultrasonograms. Arch Ophthalmol 91: 429, 1974.
12. Coleman DJ, Katz L, Lizzi FL: Isometric, three dimensional viewing of ultrasonograms. Arch Ophthalmol 93:1362, 1976.
13. Chang S, Dallow RL, Coleman DJ: Ultrasonic evaluation of intraocular tumors. In Ocular and Adnexal Tumors, (ed.) Jakobiec FA. Birmingham, Aesculapius, 1978, pp 281–310.
14. Baum G: Use of ultrasonography in the differential diagnosis of ocular tumors. In Ocular and Adnexal Tumors, ed. Boniuk M. St Louis, CV Mosby, 1964, pp 308–321.
15. Buschmann W: Ultrasonic diagnosis of intraocular tumors. Wiss. Z. Humboldt University, Berlin (Math. Naturwis), 14:163–1965.
16. Coleman DJ: Reliability of ocular and orbital diagnosis with B-scan ultrasound. Part I: Ocular diagnosis. Am J Ophthalmol 73:501, 1972.
17. Coleman DJ: Reliability of ocular tumor diagnosis with ultrasound. Trans Am Acad Ophthalmol Otolaryngol 77:677, 1973.

18. Coleman DJ, Abramson DH, Jack RL, Franzen LA: Ultrasonic diagnosis of tumors of the choroid. Arch Ophthalmol 91:344, 1974.
19. Ossoinig KC, Bigar F, Kaefring SL: Malignant melanoma of the choroid and ciliary body. A differential diagnosis in clinical echography. In Ultrasonography in Ophthalmology, eds. Francois J, Goes F. Basel, S Karger AG, 1975, pp 141–154.
20. Hodes BL, Choromokos E: Standardized A-scan echographic diagnosis of choroidal malignant melanomas. Arch Ophthalmol 95:593, 1977.
21. Sterns GK, Coleman DJ, Ellsworth RM: The ultrasonographic characteristics of retinoblastoma. Am J Ophthalmol 78:606, 1974.
22. Sullivan SF, Dallow RL: Intraocular reticulum cell sarcoma: its dramatic response to systemic chemotherapy and its angiogenic potential. Ann Ophthalmol 9:401, 1977.
23. Bilaniuk LT, Dallow RL: Diagnostic techniques in orbital surgery. In Complications of Ophthalmic Plastic Surgery, ed. Soll B. Aesculapius Publishing Co, Birmingham, 1976.
24. Dallow RL, Momose KJ, Weber AL, et al: Comparison of ultrasonography, computerized tomography (EMI scan), and radiographic techniques in evaluation of exophthalmos, Trans Am Acad Ophthalmol Otolaryngol 81:305–322, 1976.
25. Dallow RL: Reliability of orbital diagnostic tests: Ultrasonography, computerized tomography, and radiography. Ophthalmology 85:1218, 1978.
26. Coleman DJ: Reliability of ocular and orbital diagnosis with B-scan ultrasound. II. Orbital diagnosis. Am J Ophthalmol 74:704–718, 1972.
27. Coleman DJ, Jack RL, Franzen LA: High resolution B-scan ultrasonography of the orbit. I. The normal orbit. II. Hemangiomas. III. Lymphomas. IV. Neurogenic tumors. Arch Ophthalmol 88:358–384, 1972.
28. Dallow, RL, Coleman DJ: Ultrasonic evaluation of orbital diseases. In Ocular and Adnexal Tumors, ed. Jakobiec FA. Birmingham, Aesculapius, 1978, pp 311–340.
29. Dallow RL: Evaluation of unilateral exophthalmos with ultrasonography: analysis of 258 consecutive cases. Laryngoscope 85:1905–1919, 1975.
30. Purnell EW: Ultrasonic interpretation of orbital disease. In Ophthalmic Ultrasound, eds. KA, Keeney AH, Sarin LK. St Louis, CV Mosby, 1969.
31. Coleman DJ, Jack RL, Franzen LA, et al.: High resolution B-scan ultrasonography of the orbit. V. Eye changes of Graves' disease. Arch Ophthalmol 88:465–471, 1972.
32. Coleman DJ, Jack RL, Jones IS, et al: High resolution B-scan ultrasonography of the orbit. VI, pseudotumors of the orbit. Arch Ophthalmol 88:472–480, 1972.

11 Breast

CATHERINE COLE-BEUGLET
BARRY B. GOLDBERG

When a lump is detected in the breast, either by the patient or by a clinician during physical examination, various imaging modalities have been employed to further evaluate the mass. At present, x-ray mammography is the imaging modality of choice, with established diagnostic criteria for carcinoma of the breast.[1, 2] However, a significant percentage of palpable lesions, when imaged by x-ray mammography do not demonstrate the classic diagnostic features that allow one to differentiate between a benign or malignant lesion. Usually, biopsy is then recommended for a specific diagnosis. In a small percentage of cases, the masses are not imaged on the x-ray mammogram because they are located in dense breast parenchyma.

Ultrasound two-dimensional imaging of palpable breast masses has been used as an adjunct to the diagnosis of breast lesions. Water path techniques, developed by Kossoff and Jellins in Australia, have proved successful for the sonic imaging of breast masses.[3, 4] A 98 percent accuracy for the detection of fluid-filled cysts has been reported by Jellins and Kossoff.[5] An automated multitransducer water bath system in which the patient's breast is immersed in water heated to body temperature detects fluid-filled masses as small as a few millimeters in diameter. An enclosed water path system developed by Kobayashi in Japan is positioned over the breast as the patient lies supine.[6] This technique is reported to have an 85 percent diagnostic accuracy for breast carcinoma.[7] The smallest nonpalpable carcinoma detected by Kobayashi was 5 mm in diameter.[8] Teixidor and associates in the United States, used contact B-scanning for palpable masses, and found that its diagnostic accuracy for breast mass differentiation improved when ultrasound B-scan imaging was used in conjunction with x-ray mammography.[9]

The value of contact B-scanning in the supine patient is limited because transducer-skin contact is difficult to maintain and because of mobility. Real-time techniques, using contact methods in the supine patient, with or without an intervening water bath, have also been used to examine the breast. Linear array or sector transducers are moved across the breast, and the im-

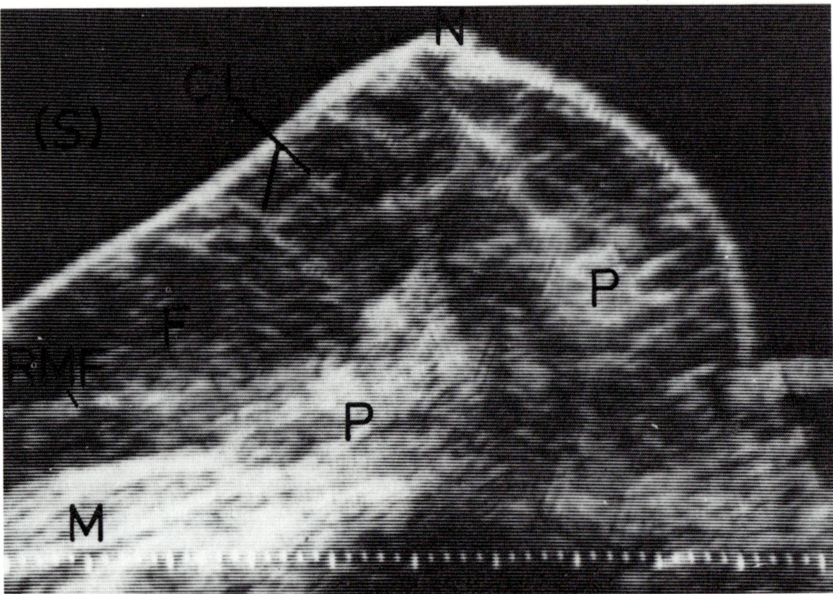

FIGURE 11.1. Normal breast of a postmenopausal 56-year-old asymptomatic patient with no palpable breast masses. Sagittal B-scan at the level of the nipple; superior (S) to the left. (N=nipple; CL=Cooper's ligaments; F=fat lobules; P=breast parenchyma; RMF=retromammary fascia; M=muscle) Graticule 1 to 1.5 cm (same scale on all prints).

ages obtained are recorded on videotape, movie, or disc format. With the real-time automated water path directed breast scanning equipment that recently became available, the patient is examined in the prone position. Real-time imaging allows rapid viewing and the video images can be replayed to evaluate suspicious areas further. The reported diagnostic accuracy of real-time B-scan imaging of palpable masses compared favorably with x-ray mammography.[10] Automated water path static and real-time scanners image the total breast parenchyma ultrasonically, not just areas of palpable mass lesions.

To interpret multiple two-dimensional B-scan images or to review real-time examinations, knowledge of the normal architecture of the breast is essential. It is composed of variable amounts of glandular parenchyma, stroma, and adipose tissue. The amount of fat present is related to a variety of factors, including age, obesity, and hormonal status, and is maximal in older postmenopausal women (Fig. 11.1). The premenopausal breast contains mainly glandular elements and only a small amount of fat, often confined to a thin layer of subcutaneous fat (Fig 11.2). Any alteration in the expected normal ultrasound pattern of glandular tissue must be viewed as suspect. When a mass is imaged, its marginal and internal echo characteristics, as well as its

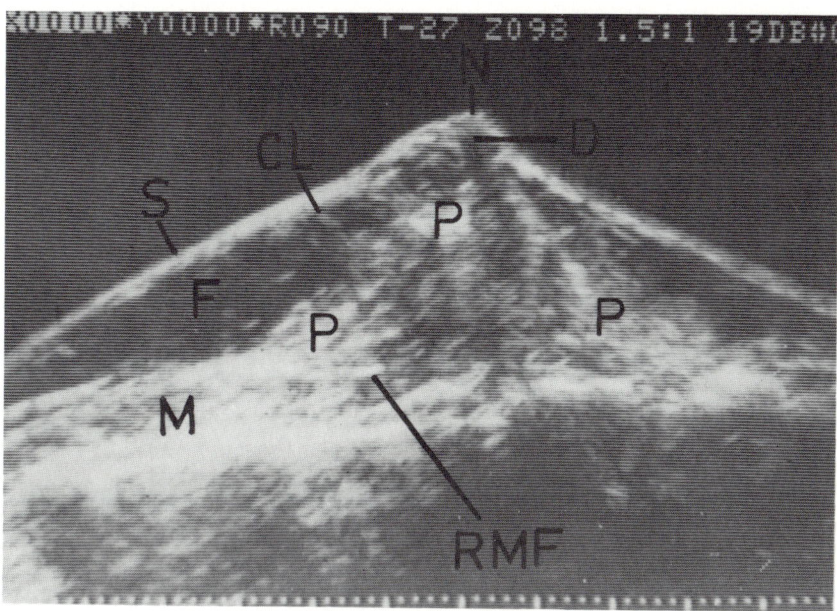

FIGURE 11.2. Normal breast of a premenopausal 32-year-old asymptomatic woman with no palpable breast masses. Sagittal B-scan at the level of the nipple; superior to the left. (S=skin; N=nipple; D=subareolar duct confluence; CL=Cooper's ligaments; F=fat, P=parenchyma; RMF=retromammary fascia; M=muscle.)

TABLE 11.1. Typical breast mass ultrasound criteria.

Criterion	Fluid Filled	Solid	
		Benign	Malignant
Contour	Smooth	Smooth	Irregular
Shape	Round or oval	Round or oval	Round lobulated, tubular
Internal echoes	None	Weak, uniform	Weak, non-uniform
Boundary			
Anterior	Strong	Strong to intermediate	Intermediate
Posterior	Strong	Strong to intermediate	Weak to absent
Distal echoes	Enhanced, lateral wall shadows	Intermediate	Shadowing (either central or partial)
Attenuation effect	Minimal	Minimal to intermediate	Intermediate to great

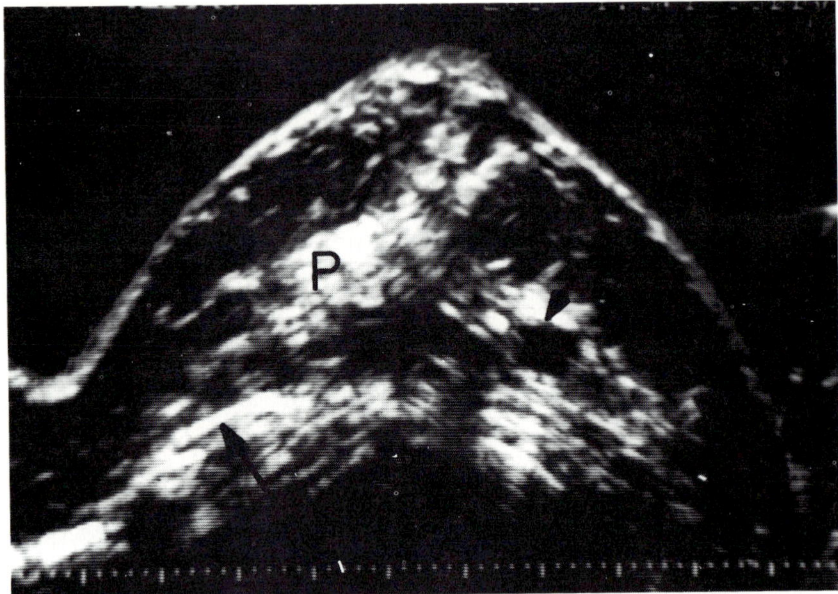

FIGURE 11.3. Fluid-filled cyst, confirmed at aspiration, in 41-year-old woman with a small palpable nodule in the left upper outer quadrant of the breast. Transverse B-scan, 10 mm superior to the nipple (N). Lateral to the right is a 12 mm, echo-free area (arrow) within the breast parenchyma (P) , with well-defined margins and enhanced sound transmission through the retromammary fascia (RMF) and muscle layer. (F=subcutaneous fat.) Diagnosis: Fluid-filled cyst.

echo-attenuating properties, are analyzed to determine whether it is benign or malignant (Table 11.1). Fluid-filled areas are diagnosed according to standard ultrasound criteria: smooth, strongly echogenic margins, echo-free centers, and enhanced echogenicity distal to the fluid-filled areas (Fig. 11.3). Solid mass lesions are analyzed for irregular or smooth margins, nonuniform or uniform internal echo distribution, and echo attenuation properties in an attempt to distinguish malignant from benign appearing masses (Figs. 11.6 and 11.7).

If a mass lesion is not present but there is an alteration in the expected normal architecture of the breast, this area is correlated with the patient's past history of breast disease, present symptoms, and physical examination. As sites of previous biopsies can cause scarring with resulting fibrosis and retraction, the exact location of the scars must be correlated with sites of ultrasonic architectural disruption. Abnormal ultrasound patterns may also be caused by infection, hematoma, or fat necrosis, and must be distinguished from malignant lesions. Clinical information is often needed to make such a distinction.

A tumor may produce an area of strong echo attenuation (shadowing).

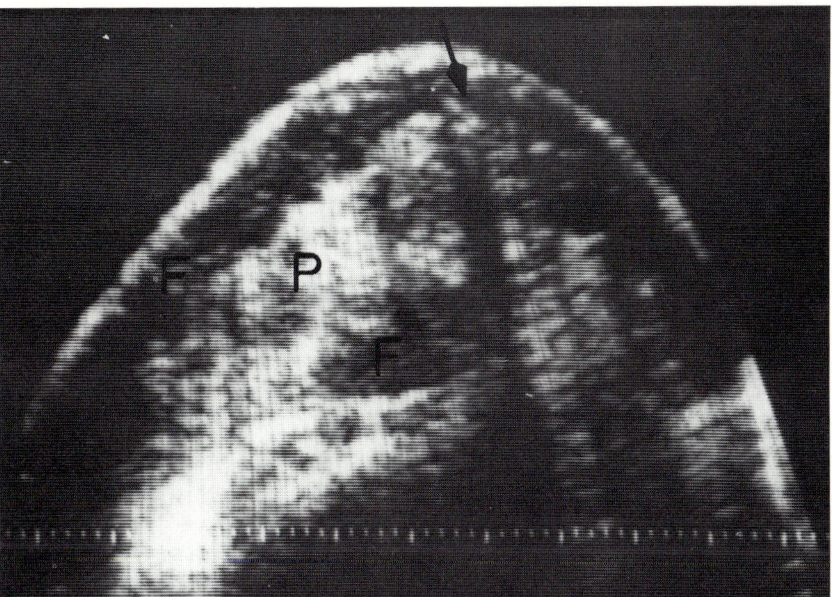

FIGURE 11.4. Clinically occult infiltrating duct carcinoma in a 44-year-old patient with a family history of breast carcinoma who was sent for mammography for a breast checkup. No palpable masses. Ultrasound: right breast transverse B-scan 24 mm above the nipple. Lateral to the left. Area of echo attenuation images as a 1 cm wide shadow in the central breast, which begins distal to several small bright echoes just below the subcutaneous fat and extends through the chest wall (arrow). This disrupted architecture proved to be caused by an infiltrating duct carcinoma. (P = Parenchyma; F = Fat.)

However, care must be taken in differentiating this pattern from similar patterns arising from scars or fibrous tissue. Tumor shadowing is usually more localized. For example: a 44-year-old patient presented for a breast examination. She had a family history of breast carcinoma, but no symptoms and no evidence of palpable abnormalities. An ultrasound examination demonstrated an area of architectural disruption, with a prominent acoustic shadow emanating from the subcutaneous area. (Fig. 11.4). The scan was reported as suspicious of malignancy. X-ray mammography showed a small area of clustered microcalcifications in the lateral aspect of the left breast, for which biopsy was recommended to rule out carcinoma. The specimen, taken after needle localization, demonstrated an infiltrating duct carcinoma measuring less than 2 cm in diameter in the area designated by ultrasound and x-ray. A subsequent modified radical mastectomy showed no residual tumor and no evidence of metastasis in the axillary lymph nodes.

The investigation of women suspected of being at high risk has posed some problems with the recent controversy concerning screening for breast cancer using x-ray mammography.[11, 12] A family history of breast cancer may

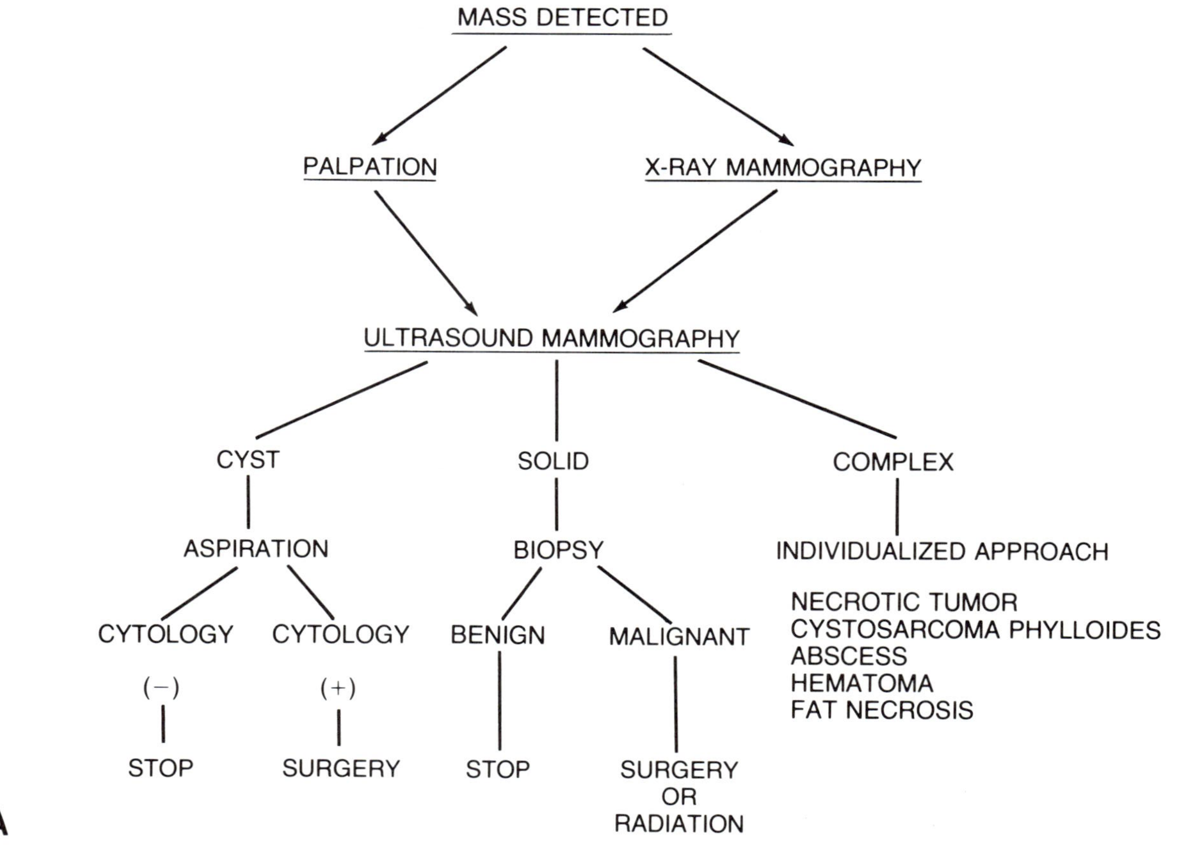

FIGURE 11.5 (a) Flow chart outlining steps in the diagnosis and treatment of breast disease in symptomatic patients.

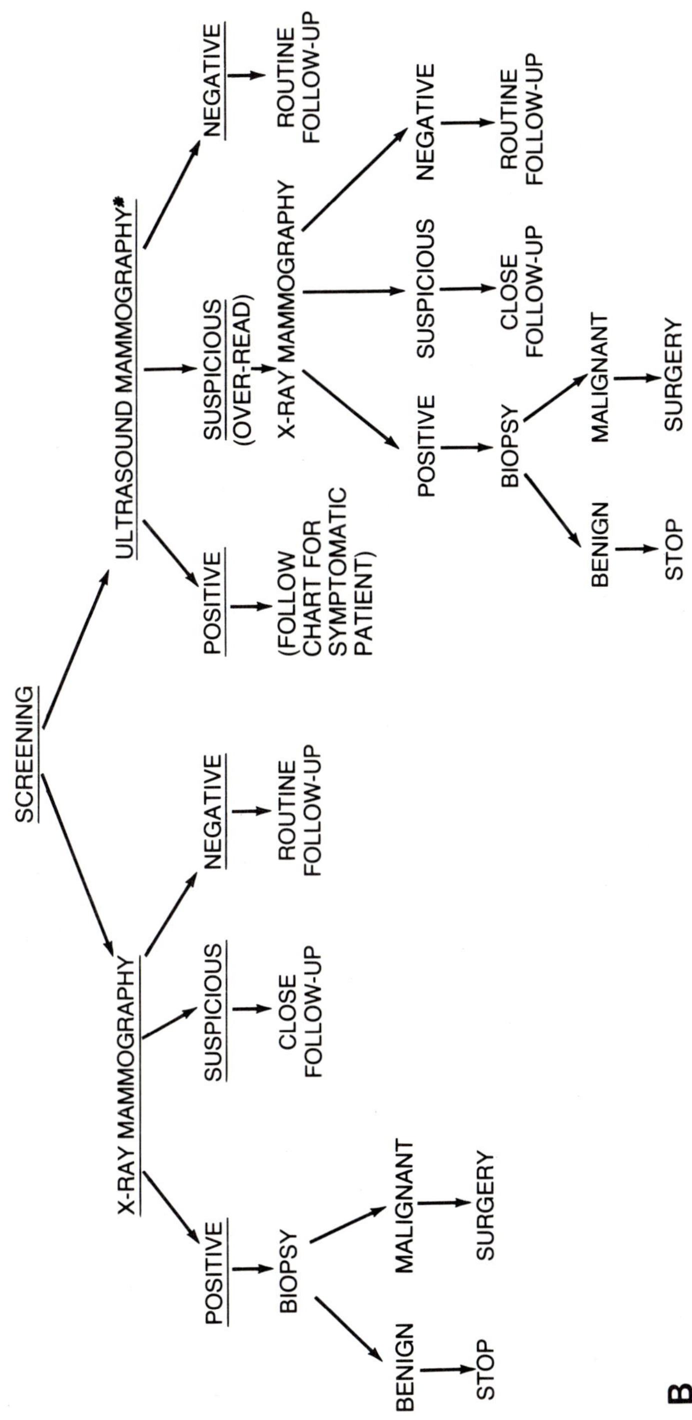

FIGURE 11.5. (b) Flow chart outlining steps in the diagnosis and treatment of breast disease in asymptomatic patients.* Efficacy not established; research in progress.

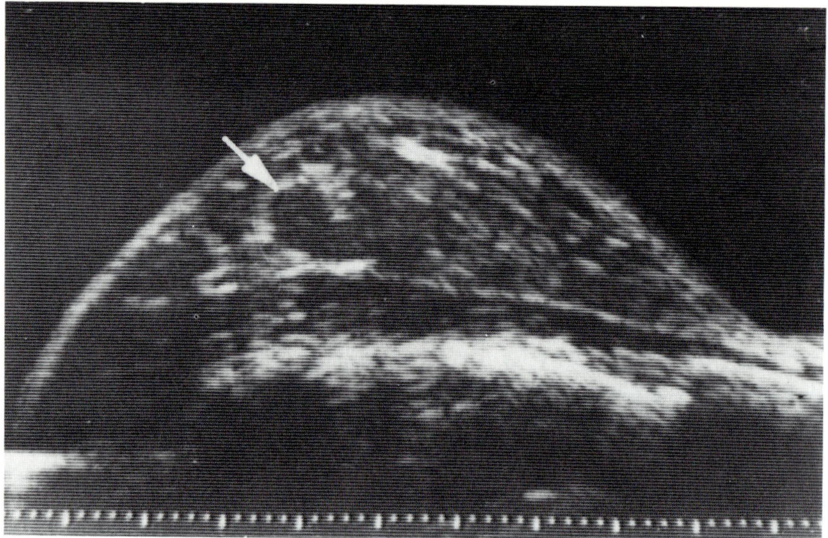

FIGURE 11.6. Benign, solid fibroadenoma in a 20-year-old woman with a mobile 2 cm mass in the upper inner quadrant of the left breast. No x-ray mammogram was obtained. Ultrasound of the left breast, transverse B-scan, 12 mm above the nipple; medial to the left. A 1.8 cm lobulated, smooth-walled solid mass (arrow) with strongly echogenic margins and weak uniform internal echoes represents a benign solid mass that proved to be a fibroadenoma.

place a woman at an increased risk for the development of breast carcinoma.[13, 14] Currently, routine x-ray mammography for the detection of breast carcinoma in asymptomatic women has been advised only for patients over the age of 50. Therefore, asymptomatic women at high risk, who are below this age, must rely on physical examination. Automated ultrasound mammography may offer an alternative method for investigating these asymptomatic women.

Figures 11.5(a) and (b) are flow charts outlining the present use of ultrasound mammography in the diagnosis of breast disease. The symptomatic patient with a palpable mass, detected on physical examination or x-ray mammography, may benefit from an ultrasound mammogram. The mammogram will show whether the mass is fluid-filled, solid, or complex. Fluid-filled structures can be aspirated and if cytologic examination of the fluid is negative for atypical cells, the patient can be followed clinically. If blood or atypical or cancer cells are present in the fluid, surgery is then recommended to rule out the rare disease, intracystic carcinoma.

Solid mass lesions on ultrasound mammography are analyzed according to the criteria in Table 11.1 in an attempt to differentiate benign from malignant appearing solids. Fibroadenomas comprise the majority of benign solid masses (Fig. 11.6), while infiltrating duct carcinoma comprise most malignant masses (Fig. 11.7). Ultrasound can also image complex areas; that is, mixed

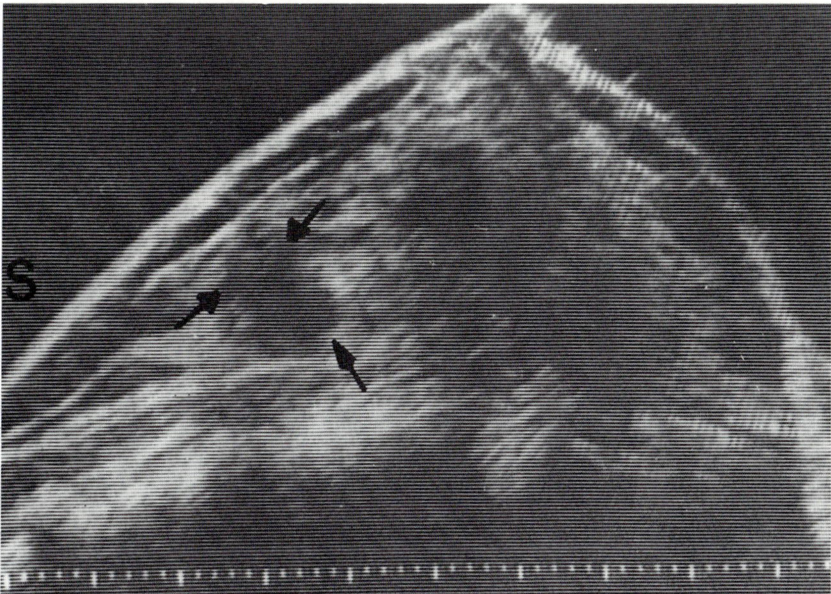

FIGURE 11.7. Malignant, solid, infiltrating duct carcinoma. A 2-cm palpable mass at the 12 o'clock position in the left breast of a 42-year-old woman. Sagittal B-scan 5 mm lateral to the nipple shows a 2 cm, irregular marginated solid mass with weak internal echoes (arrows). Diagnosis, malignant mass. S = Superior.

solid and fluid-containing abnormalities. Abscess formation in cases of mastitis, hematoma formation, or fat necrosis can present as a complex ultrasound pattern. Necrotic tumors or cystosarcoma phylloides may have a similar pattern. Thus, complex structures often require an individualized approach for specific diagnoses.

For the asymptomatic patient with no breast complaints or palpable masses, x-ray mammography is still the established diagnostic imaging modality for the detection of occult carcinoma. Although ultrasound mammography is presently being evaluated for this purpose, a large number of patients must be examined to established the efficacy of this imaging modality for the detection of occult breast carcinoma. Research into the potential usefulness of ultrasound for breast screening is in progress at many medical centers in this country and throughout the world.

References

1. Witten DM: The Breast. An Atlas of Tumor Radiology. Chicago, Year Book Medical Publishers, 1969, p 330.
2. Wolfe JN: Xeromammography. Springfield, Charles C Thomas, 1975, pp 111–128.
3. Kossoff G, Carpenter DA, Robinson DE, et al: Octoson—a new rapid general purpose

echoscope. In Ultrasound In Medicine, eds D. White, R. Barnes, New York, Plenum Press, 1976, Vol. 2, p 333.

4. Jellins J, Kossoff G, Reeve TS, et al: Ultrasonic Gray Scale Visualization of Breast Disease. Ultrasound Med Biol 1:393–404, 1975.
5. Jellins J, Kossoff G, Reeve TS, et al: Detection and classification of liquid filled masses in the breast by gray scale echography. Radiology 125:205–212, 1977.
6. Kobayashi T: Gray-scale echography for breast cancer. Radiology 122:207–214, 1977.
7. Kobayashi T: Clinical Ultrasound of the Breast. New York, New York Plenum Press, 1978.
8. Kobayashi T: Clinical ultrasound in neoplastic diseases: echography for tumor diagnosis. J UOEH 1:167, 1979.
9. Teixidor HS, Kazam E: Combined mammographic-sonographic evaluation of breast masses. Am J Roentgenol 128:409–417, 1977.
10. Cole-Beuglet C, Beique RA: Continuous ultrasound B-scanning of palpable breast masses. Radiology 117:123–128, 1975.
11. The Effects on Populations of Exposure in Low Levels of Ionizing Radiation (BEIR Report). Advisory Committee on the Biological Effects of Ionizing Radiation, National Academy of Sciences, National Research Council, 1972.
12. Simon N: Cancer of the breast induced by radiation. JAMA 237:789–790, 1977.
13. Knudson, AG: Genetic susceptibility to cancer. In Proceedings of the Eleventh Canadian Cancer Research Conference, National Cancer Institute of Canada, Toronto, Canada, 1976, p 93.
14. Petrakis NL: Genetic factors in etiology of breast cancer. Cancer 39:2709, 1977.

12 Treatment Planning

ALFRED KRATOCHWIL

A high radiation dose can be delivered to any anatomic structure of the body by means of high-voltage therapy. Because of the problems with dose distribution in the radiation field, radiation therapy cannot be standardized and must be planned individually for each patient.[1] The aim of radiation therapy planning is to attain an even dosage within the target volume, sparing the surrounding healthy tissue as much as possible.[2-4] For individual treatment planning, one has to consider not only individual variation but also differences in the radiation sources.[2] It is now generally agreed that the radiation field is best described by graphic isodose distribution.[5]

A major advance toward individual treatment planning accompanied the introduction of automatic isodose plotters and computers which complete treatment planning in a fraction of the time that was once necessary.[5-9]

Until recently, however, a big gap existed between these sophisticated methods of calculating dosage and the relatively poor knowledge of the location of individual tumors and their extent in anatomic terms. Tumor location, based simply on clinical findings and direct or indirect radiologic signs, cannot be regarded either as individual or exact. The same statement applies as well to the use of simulators fed with standardized anatomic scans. Between these projected scans and the individual patient's anatomy, large discrepancies could be noticed, comparing these results with ultrasonic scans.[4, 10, 11]

The use of transverse X-ray tomographs to obtain individual treatment planning has to be regarded as inconvenient, as the differentiation of soft tissues in these scans is sometimes impossible. There is often distortion and magnification of the portrayed area.[12, 13] Exact topographic orientation of the tumor target in its relation to the surrounding tissue and towards the body surface can be obtained with a high degree of accuracy either by computerized or ultrasonic tomography.[14] Because ultrasonic waves are almost totally reflected from gaseous interfaces, such as the lungs and intestine, such organs are inaccessible to ultrasonic examination. Another limiting factor is the high absorption of ultrasonic energy by bone, so that the skeleton also cannot be examined by ultrasound. For ultrasonic examination, two different methods are used today. An image in real-time can be produced either by multiarray systems or by mechanical or rotating probes. These scanners produce linear or sector scans of the region of interest. The advantage of these systems is their easy handling and the possible observation of physiologic organ movements caused by respiration, pulsation or peristalsis. The disadvantage of this system is that it cannot produce a picture of the entire region of interest, as is necessary for treatment planning. This is due to the size of the probes used.

Ideal transverse scans of the entire area can be produced, however, by compound scanners. The produced image is static and does not allow one to observe physiologic movements. The image needs some seconds to be produced. For this overlap of application, a combined examination with both systems is in common use today. For quick orientation and tumor localization, the examination is started with a real-time scanner. In the tumor region, compound scans are performed for treatment planning.[15] Using a series of transverse and longitudinal scans, a three-dimensional image can be formed in one's mind.

Of primary interest is the location of the primary tumor and the extension of the mass.[4, 15, 16] By means of ultrasonic tomography, tumors of the following organs, measuring at least 2 cm in diameter, can be outlined: liver, gallbladder, pancreas, kidney, spleen, adrenals, paraaortic lymph nodes, uterus, ovaries, breast, prostate, thyroid, and limbs.[17, 18]

Tumor extension can be assessed by ultrasound. Penetration of the organ's border can be seen in pancreatic and kidney tumors as can infiltration of the vena cava. In genital tumors, especially prostatic cancers,[18, 19] the tumor-extension towards the bladder and rectum can be observed.

In the evaluation of tumor extension to the lymphatic system, ultrasonic examination is of special value.[20] A systematic search for involved lymph glands should be performed in all cases suffering from Hodgkin disease, testicular tumors, tumors of the uterine neck, bladder, kidney, pancreas, and colon.[21-25] Although lymphoangiographic methods give excellent results in the diagnosis of sacral and ileolumbar lymph node involvement, its diagnostic value is limited in the paraaortic and subdiaphragmatic regions. This limitation occurs because the lymphatic duct may branch off below the third lumbar segment, thus avoiding the paraaortic and subdiaphragmatic region.[26] Another limiting factor is the angiographic demonstration of lymph nodes, which depends on the undisturbed function of the system. This function can, however, be damaged severely or interrupted by radical therapy, such as irradiation or surgery.[18, 23] Although X-ray films can demonstrate the point at which lymphatic flow ceases, it cannot evaluate the region beyond this area. As sonography is independent of function, involved lymph nodes can be detected if they are larger than 2 cm in diameter. Sonography therefore is an excellent additional method for the diagnosis of lymphatic lesions.

The accuracy of ultrasound in localizing involved lymph nodes, compared with angiography and the findings during surgery, is as high as 90 to 98 percent. In every second case, the ultrasonic examination demonstrated that the extension of the mass was larger than assumed by lymphography. This compares favorably with the results obtained by a comparison between cavo- and lymphangiography.[4, 23, 26, 27]

Blood bone tumor dissemination to the brain, lungs, and liver is important in the management of tumor patients. Structural changes of the liver can be detected by ultrasound if the lesion is larger than 1 cm in diameter. Metastatic lesions are irregular in outline and vary in their echogenicity.

Tumor extension to the pleural or peritoneal cavity can be diagnosed by demonstrating pleural effusion or ascites.[17, 18, 21] Ascites has the same ultrasonic characteristics as pleural effusion. In peritoneal carcinosis, the intestinal loops adhere to each other and are fixed at the mesenteric root. They are not able to float on the surface of the fluid, as in benign ascites.[28]

TREATMENT PLANNING

For treatment planning, the patient is examined in therapy position. Initially, the region of interest is located by real-time scanner. Once the tumor is localized, a static scanner is used. At least three different scans should be performed.[8] These scans should be located at the center of the tumor and at its upper and lower margins. The images obtained may be supplemented by longitudinal scans (Fig. 12.1).

Ideally, a full 360° scan of the region of interest should be achieved.[29] As this is not possible in every case, for many reasons it was agreed that scans of 180° to 270° for each port of treatment would be sufficient.[5, 29] Each of these scans should be related to a fixed reference point, such as the symphysis, femoral heads, iliac crest, spine, etc.[8]

Each of these ultrasonic scans should contain the following essential information for treatment planning:[30] (1) body circumference and contour, (2) distance of the tumor from the surface, (3) tumor volume, (4) tumor relationship to radiosensitive organs, (5) position of radiation ports relative to the tumor, and (6) possibilities to check the therapeutic response and to rearrange the treatment plan as indicated.

Body Contour and Circumference

Using an ultrasonic static scanner, the patient contour can be accurately outlined at any level and at any plane. If only surface contour information is needed, the gain is reduced. By moving the transducer gently, without pressure, across the body, a contour is built-up on the video screen.[10, 31-35] To obtain surface images from more complicated anatomic structures, such as the face and neck, special probes of small diameter are used.[3, 5]

Previously, the body contours for treatment planning were recorded using shaping solder wire, plaster, or thin plastic sheets formed to the body surface.[5, 12, 36] These techniques are not only cumbersome but they are often inaccurate due to significant distorsion of the outline. By comparing conventional and ultrasonic imaging of body contours in a series of patients, differ-

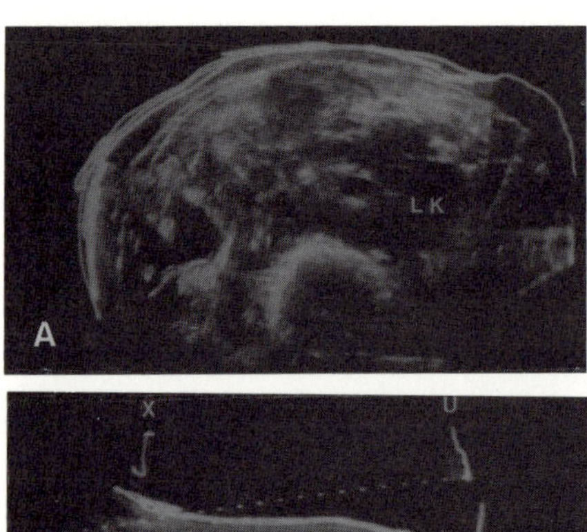

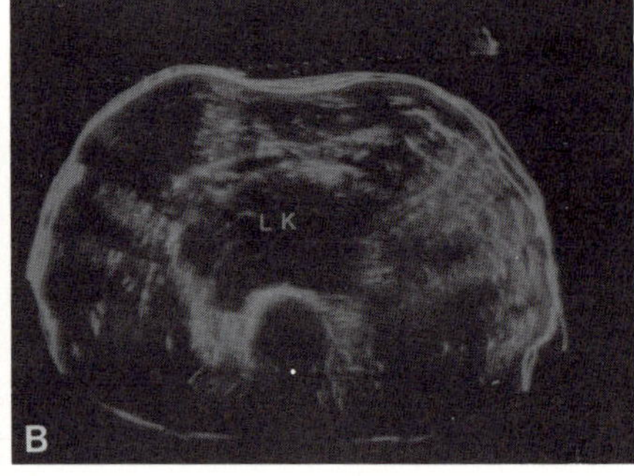

FIGURE 12.1. Enlarged lymph nodes in a case of seminoma. (a) transverse scan; (b) transverse scan; (c) longitudinal scan. LK = lymph node; X = xyphisternum; U = umbilicus.

ences of up to 3 cm in favor of the ultrasonic method could be observed. For these reasons, mechanical methods for obtaining body contours should be abandoned.[8]

Depth of the Radiation Target

Since the amount of ionizing radiation that reaches a deep tumor is decreased by absorption by overlying tissue, it is extremely important to determine the depth of the tumor.[5] This information is contained in every ultrasonic tomogram that displays the entire body circumference in the plane of scanning. The distance from the surface can be measured with electronic calipers, calibrated to the specific propagation velocity of the ultrasonic beam. As the beam transverses tissues of different propagation velocities, an average tissue velocity is assumed for calibration.

Tumor Volume

By performing scans at standardized intervals, the tumor area in each image can be calculated by planimetry.[27, 37] Employing microprocessors, the volume of even very irregular masses can be obtained. In a test using models of known volume, the difference, by ultrasound, was less than 5 percent.[9]

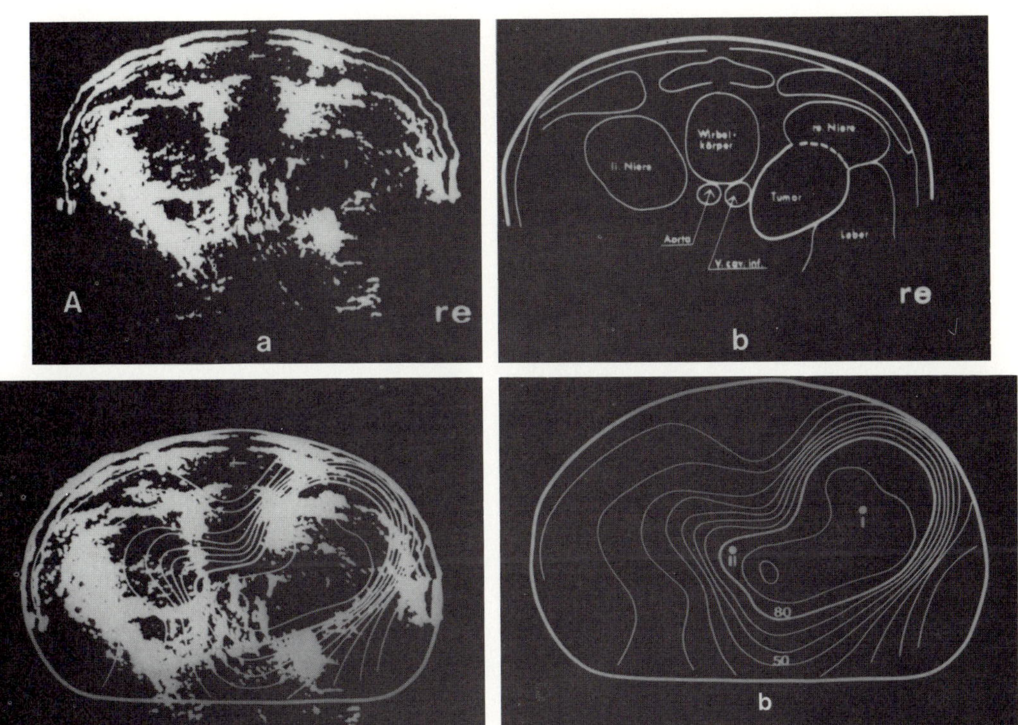

FIGURE 12.2. (a) Treatment planning in a case of hypernephroma of the right kidney. a = ultrasonic bistable scan in prone position; b = schematic drawing. (b) Same case as (a). The isodose curves are superimposed on the ultrasonic scan. (Friedrick M, Fiegler W, Scheffler A, Ernst A: Die ultraschalltomographie und strahlentherapie. Strahlentherapie 146:298, 1973.)

Location of Radiosensitive Organs

Complications caused by radiotherapy are dose-dependent. Therefore, radiotherapists are very interested in the location of radiosensitive organs in the radiation field. One of the limiting factors in abdominal radiotherapy is caused by renal sensitivity.[38] An exact location of the kidney is therefore important since intravenous urography and scintography are too inaccurate in this respect, and they have now been replaced by ultrasonic tomography. The kidneys can be located either in the supine or prone position (Fig. 12.2 a and b). The depth of the organ can be simply determined. The outline of the kidneys, in both inspiration and expiration, can be traced on the skin. This information is used to calculate and locate lead blocks helping to reduce damage to the kidneys.[21] Similar information is used to localize the liver.

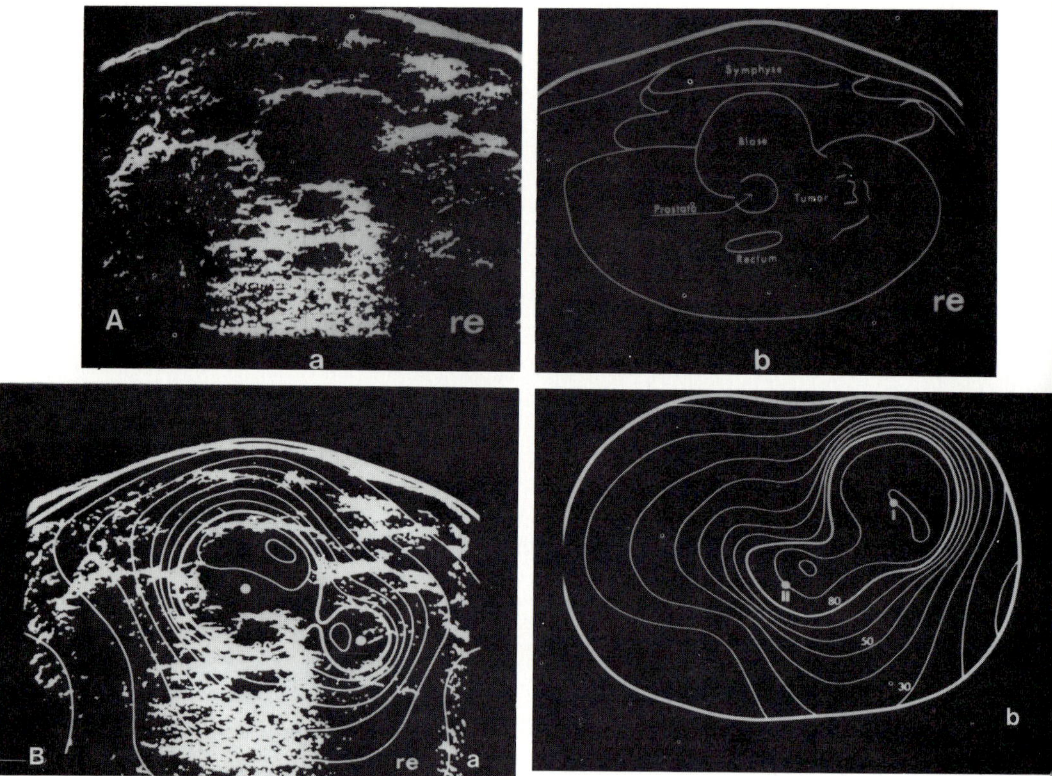

FIGURE 12.3. (a) Treatment planning in prostatic cancer. a = ultrasonic scan; b = schematic drawing. (b) Same case as (a). The isodose curves are superimposed on the ultrasonic pictures. (Friedrick M, Fiegler W, Scheffler A, Ernst H: Die Ultraschalltomographie und Strahlentherapie. Strahlentherapie 146:298, 1973.)

Longitudinal scans allow for easy demarcation of the diaphragm.[21] In thin patients and young children even the spinal canal can be localized.

Dosimetry

Individual treatment plans can be established from the information contained in the ultrasonotomograms (Figs. 12.2, 12.3, 12.4, and 12.5). Polaroid photographs provide the matrix for dosage calculation and distribution. To fulfill requirements for treatment planning, this information must be magnified to life size. Keep in mind that the 1-cm grid on the oscilloscope is reduced in the Polaroid to 0.68 cm. Working with a scale factor of 1:3, the magnification factor has to be 1:4.4.[36, 39] Life-size magnification can be obtained more simply by using opaque projectors.[13, 29, 40] The goal of life-size magnification can be achieved just as well by using hard copy units.

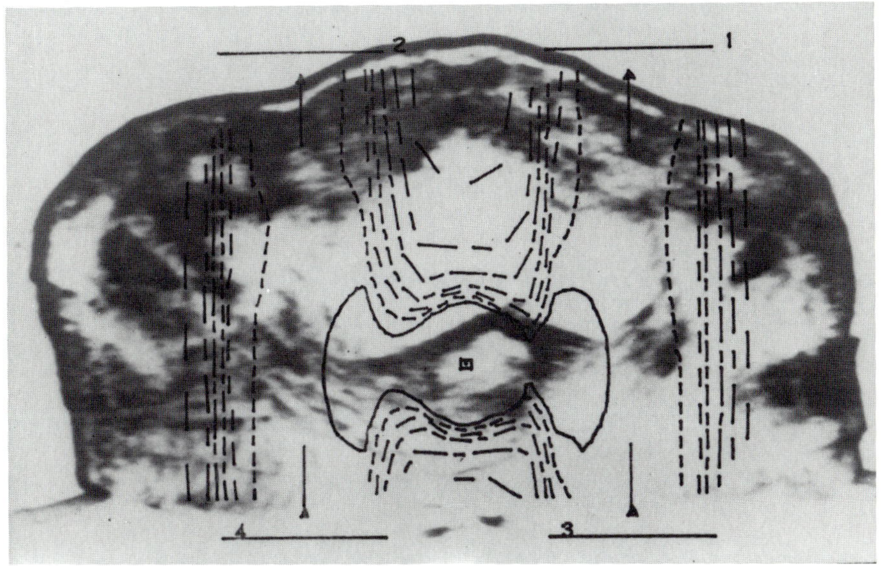

FIGURE 12.4. Carcinoma of the cervix stage III; combined brachytherapy.

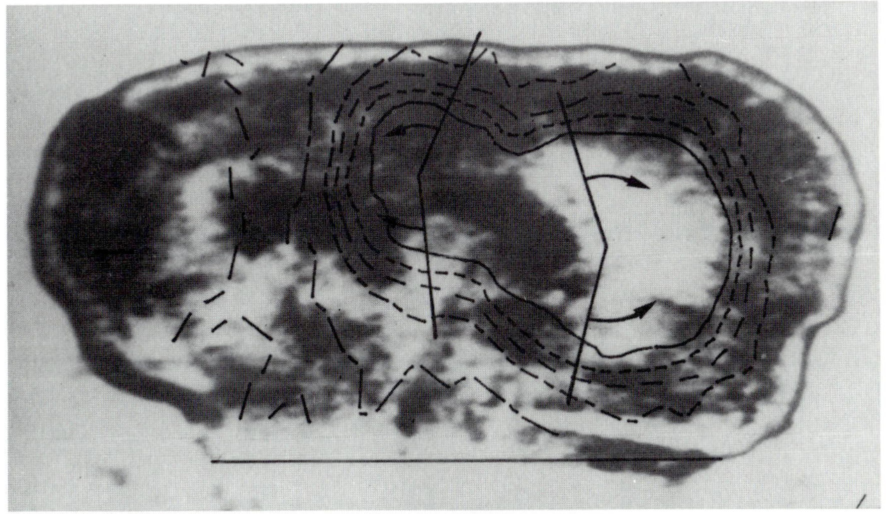

FIGURE 12.5. Tumor of the left kidney, patient in prone position. Bi-axial pendulum treatment.

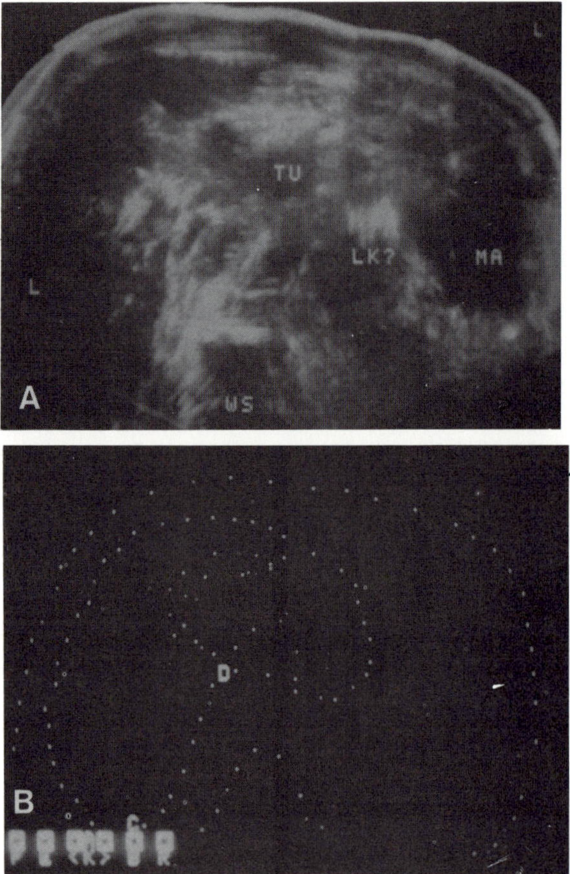

FIGURE 12.6. Pancreatic carcinoma with enlarged paraaortic lymph node (TU). a = ultrasonic scan; b = marcation of the body surface, liver, and tumor extension with the lightpen.

The most reliable way to calculate dose distribution is to interface the sonograph directly to a computer that contains all relevant data for treatment planning[6, 40] (Fig. 12.6). Using a digitized lightpen, the necessary information for body contour, location of the tumor, and its relationship to radiosensitive organs can be fed directly into the computer.[7] Data acquisition can be performed as well with two lightpens and a color videomonitor. Anatomic information is extracted from the ultrasonic image and displayed in one color. The computer isodose curves are displayed in a second color and superimposed on the image of the anatomic structure. With the patient in treatment position, the plan can be modified until it fits individual demands (Figs. 12.7 and 12.8). The final plan is recorded on paper or color film.[41] In combination with a plotter, the plan may be printed or stored on a videotape.

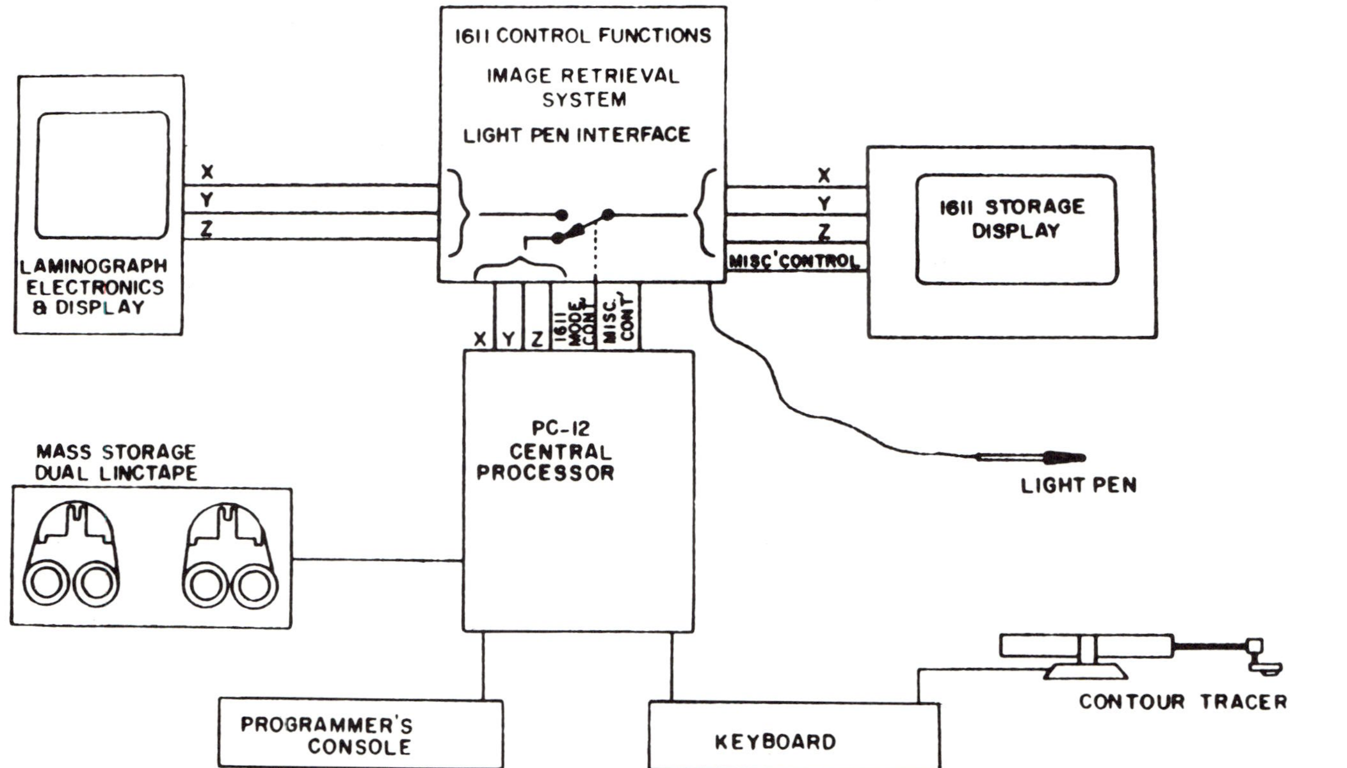

FIGURE 12.7. Using the ultrasound machine interfaced with the computer for treatment planning according to Braschо.[7] (Brascho DJ: Computerized radiation treatment planning with ultrasound. Am J Roentgenol 120:213–223, 1974. © American Roentgen Ray Society, Williams & Wilkins.)

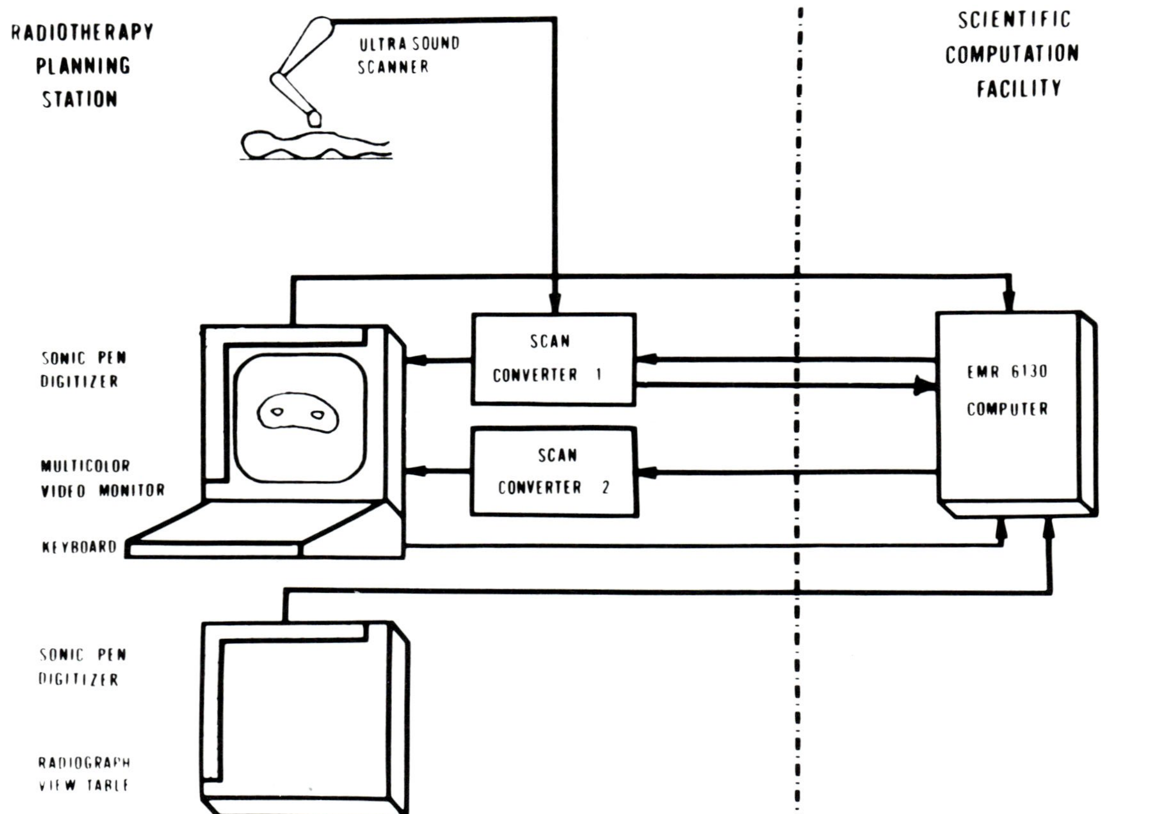

FIGURE 12.8. Radiotherapy treatment planning according to Slater.[41] (Slater JM, et al: Radiotherapy treatment planning using ultrasound graph pen computer system. Cancer 34:96–99, 1974.)

Location of Radiation Ports and Pendulum Axis

As the examination is performed with the patient in therapy position, the ports of the radiation fields and the position and length of the pendulum axis[5] can be transferred immediately to the patient's skin.[12, 16, 29, 42] If less-sophisticated instrumentation is available, the position of these ports in relation to the tumor may need to be checked.[10, 43] After the radiation ports are marked on the skin, the patient is reexamined, and the transducer lifted at the skin marks. Should the examination show that the entire tumor is not encompassed by the radiation field, the margins may have to be reestablished based on the ultrasonic findings.[10, 42, 43]

Determination of Chest Wall Thickness

Due to the high risk of pulmonary complications from irradiation in patients with known breast tumors, the chest wall thickness must be known to avoid complications.[5, 12, 44, 45] For this situation, special treatments such as tangential fields, high energy electrons, and control of the depth of beam penetration have been developed. The application of these fields is facilitated by ultrasonic examination. Echoes are produced at the skin, the pleural surface, and the sternum.[44] The ultrasonic record is incorporated in the usual way into the treatment plan (Fig. 12.9).

INTRACAVITARY TREATMENT PLANNING

Since radiation damage to the bladder and rectum can be caused by intracavitary treatment depending on the distance of the radiation source, this information is important,[46] and can be obtained by ultrasound. The bladder wall and its relationship to either the uterus or prostate[18, 19] can be outlined by allowing the bladder to fill with urine. The position of the rectum can be determined by inserting a rectal catheter or by filling the rectum with barium.[46, 47] This information is particularly important for the treatment of cervical cancer. The position of the uterine body will vary with varying degrees of filling of the bladder or rectum. Since intracavitary irradiation is performed when the bladder is drained by a catheter, ultrasonic examination of the pelvic organs is performed under the same conditions, even if the results are not as clear as normally achieved with a full urinary bladder technique.[12]

For better evaluation of dose distribution, unloaded applicators can be inserted into the uterus under local anesthesia, the bladder filled with 200 ml, and the position of the tandem localized by ultrasonic examination.

Diagnostic ultrasound can also assist in the management of patients with bladder malignancies. The exophytic tumor can easily be demonstrated and infiltration of the bladder wall determined.[48] Using a full-bladder technique, the prostate gland can be outlined in both transverse and longitudinal scans, facilitating treatment planning.

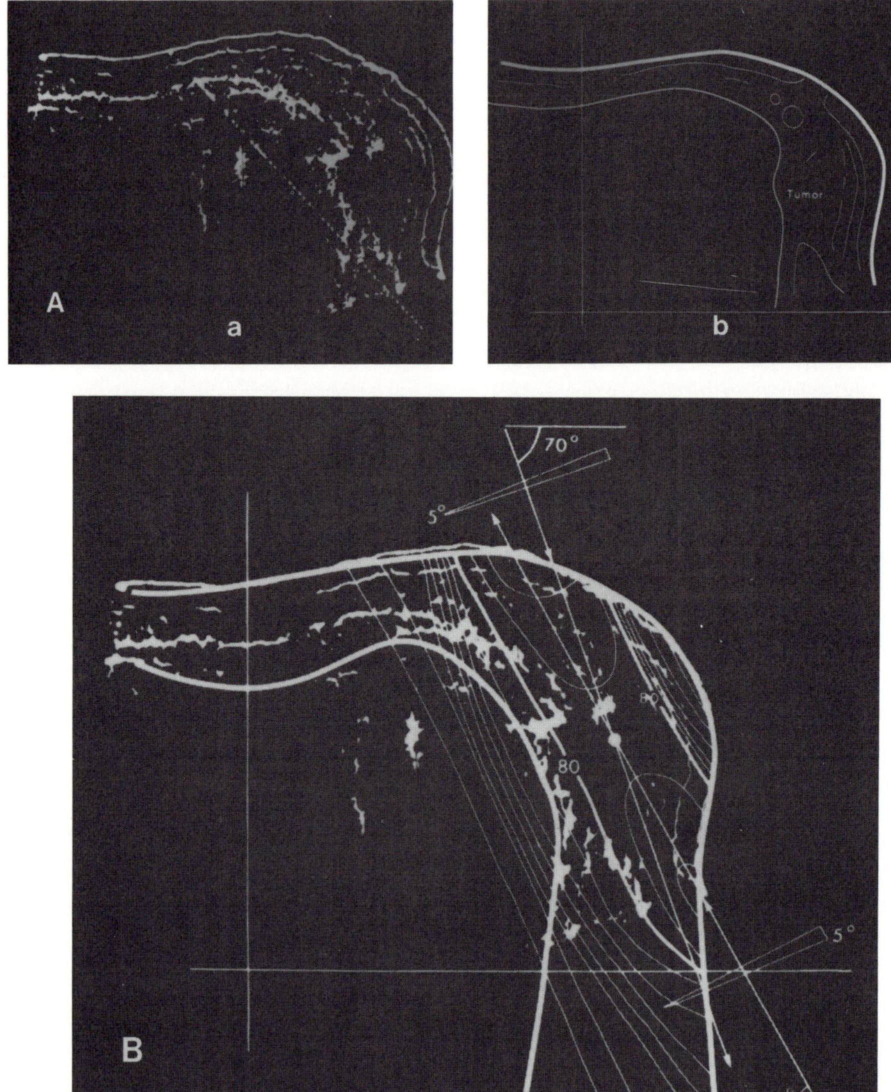

FIGURE 12.9. (a) Treatment planning in breast carcinoma. a = ultrasonic scan evaluating the thickness of the thoracic wall, b = schematic drawing. (b) Treatment planning for this tumor. (Friedrick M, Fiegler W, Scheffler A, Ernst H: Die Ultraschalltomographie und Strahlentherapie. Strahlentherapie 146:298, 1973.)

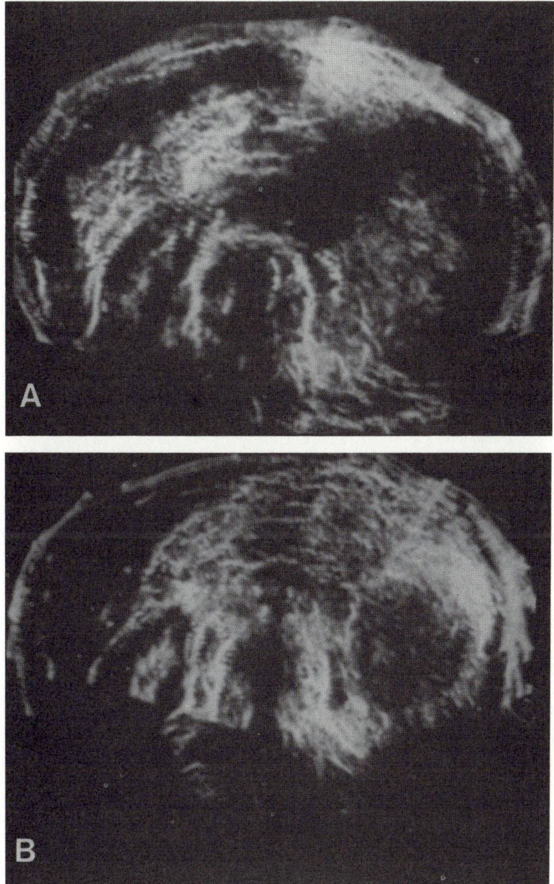

FIGURE 12.10. Response of a left sided Wilms' tumor to X-ray treatment, a = before and b = after treatment.

EVALUATION OF THERAPEUTIC RESPONSE

Tumor regression due to radiation or chemotherapy can easily be followed by ultrasonic examination.[31, 39, 49-52] To record this effect, images obtained at the beginning of therapy can be compared with those taken at appropriate intervals during the course of treatment. Comparison of tumor size and volume provides exact data in this connection. A favorable result could be observed in Wilms tumors, which showed a remarkable reduction in size after irradiation so that operation became possible (Fig. 12.10). This technique is very important in the irradiation of very sensitive tumors, such as lymphomas. According to tumor regression, the radiation fields may be sequentially decreased, thus avoiding unfavorable side effects and latent complications.

A further sign of excellent response to therapy is structural change within

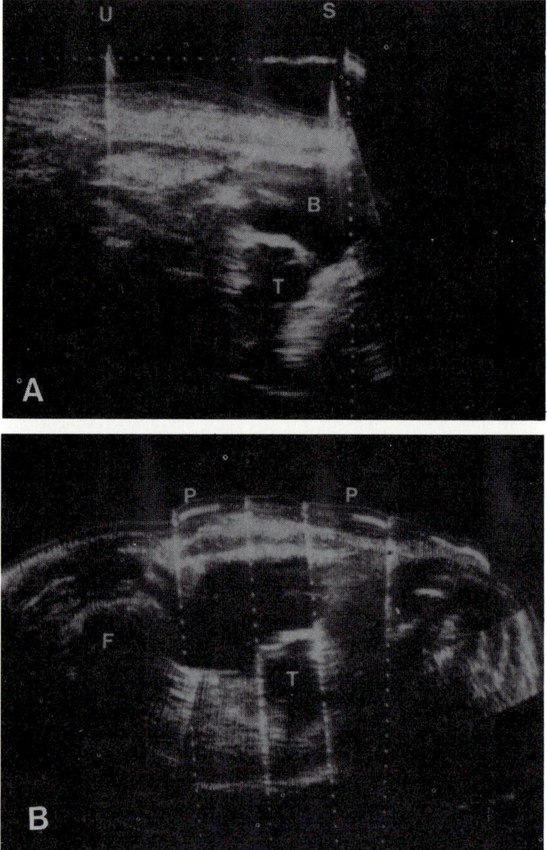

FIGURE 12.11. Recurrence at the left pelvic wall after radical surgery of a cervical carcinoma. a = longitudinal scan, b = transverse scan. Ports of irradiation are marked. U = umbilicus; S = symphysis; B = bladder; T = tumor; F = femoral head.

the mass. Inhomogeneities in primarily weakly echogenic tumors can be noticed as treatment advances. The development of strongly reflecting areas may be related to fibrotic changes.

Detection of Recurrences

All patients suffering from cancer and submitted to radiotherapy or surgery are thoroughly followed, at least on quarterly intervals, to detect recurrences or metastasis to lymph nodes or organs.[18, 23] This is particularly important in the management of Hodgkin disease to detect enlarged lymph nodes. It is also important in tumors of the testicle and of the genital tract.[24]

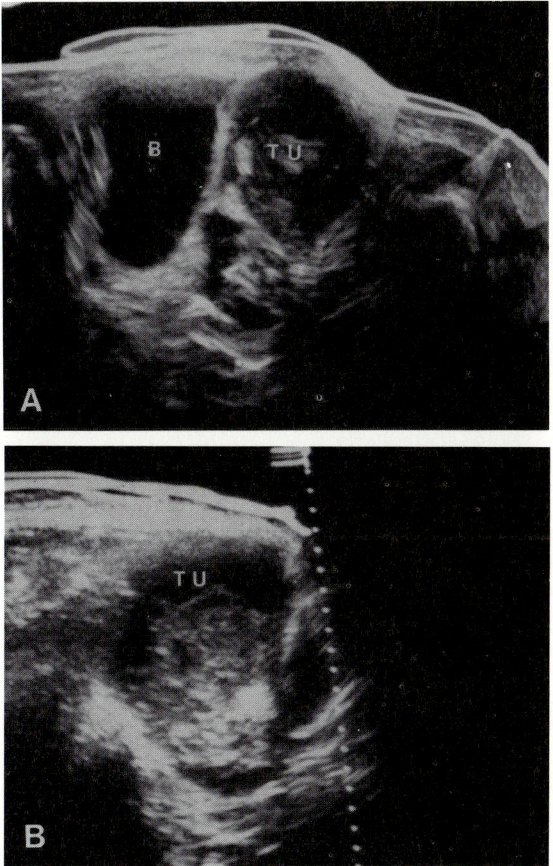

FIGURE 12.12. Recurrence (TU) at the left pelvic wall after cervical cancer impressing the bladder. (a) Transverse and (b) longitudinal scan.

Clinical examination as well as direct and indirect radiologic signs, even arteriography, may not be able to detect recurrences early enough in genital cancer, so that they may be treated. Ultrasonic examination can sometimes be useful in the evaluation of these patients.[53] The examination, in these cases, is always performed using the full-bladder technique to displace the gas-filled bowel cranially to provide an acoustic window to the true pelvis. When searching for such recurrences at the pelvic wall, the transducer must be moved from one wall to the other, encircling the pelvis by at least 180°. By using this technique, not only the genital organs but the pelvic wall and its relation to these organs can be demonstrated (Figs. 12.11 and 12.12).

Suspected tumors after radical hysterectomy may turn out to be sharply demarcated cystic areas corresponding to lymphocysts (Fig. 12.13).

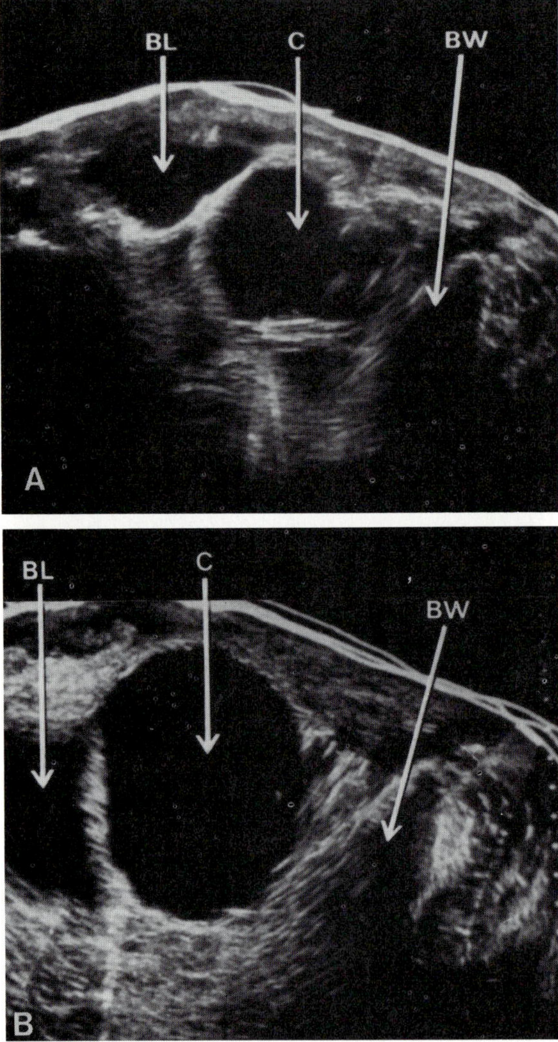

FIGURE 12.13. Lymph cyst at the left pelvic wall after radical surgery for cervical cancer, clinically interpreted as recurrence. BL = bladder, C = lymphcyst, BW = pelvic wall.

In conclusion, ultrasound has proved useful for individual treatment planning. Further improvements may be expected with advancing technology.

References

1. Kärcher KH: Die Anwendung des Ultraschalls in der Strahlentherapie. Strahlentherapie 146:666–668, 1971.

2. Binder W: Anleitung zur Bestrahlungsplanung. In: Physik, Kärcher, KH Eigenverlag Siemens.
3. Heckemann R, Quast U, Glaeser L, Schmitt G: Die Bedeutung der Sonotomographie in der Strahlentherapie. Radiologe 16:342–349, 1976.
4. Lowy RO: The application of ultrasound tomography in radiation therapy. J Can Assoc Radiol 24:301–308, 1973.
5. Friedrich M, Fiegler W, Scheffler A, Ernst H: Die Ultraschalltomographie and Strahlentherapie. Strahlentherapie 146:296–312, 1973.
6. Brascho DJ: Diagnostic ultrasound in radiation treatment planning. J Clin Ultrasound 1: 320–329, 1973.
7. Brascho DJ: Computerized radiation treatment planning with ultrasound. Am J Roentgenol 120:213–223, 1974.
8. Sanders RC, Hughes B, Hazra TA: Ultrasound localization of the kidneys for radiation therapy. Br J Radiol 47:196–197, 1974.
9. Tolbert DD, Zazgebski JA, Banjavic RA, Wiley AL: Quantitation of tumor volumes and response to therapy with ultrasound B-scan. Radiology 113:705–708, 1974.
10. Alth G, Kratochwil A, Hofner W: Zur Herdsuche in der gynäkologischen Strahlentherapie. Strahlentherapie 142:303–307, 1971.
11. Kratochwil A: Ultrasonic diagnosis in pelvic malignancy. Clin Obstet Gynecol 13: 898–909, 1970.
12. Badock PC: Ultrasonic scanning in the radiotherapy department. Clin Radiol 28: 287–293, 1977.
13. Hughes M, Sternick ES: A method for obtaining body contours using ultrasonic scanner and transverse tomograms. Med Phys 1:72–73, 1974.
14. Weyrauch U, Schoknecht G: Die Anwendung von Ultraschall zur Bestrahlungsplanung. Strahlentherapie 139:544–547, 1970.
15. Slater JM, Neilsen JR, Chu WT, et al: Radiotherapy treatment planning using ultrasound. Cancer 34:96–99, 1974.
16. Brascho DJ: Radiation therapy planning with ultrasound. Radiol Clin N Am 13:505, 1975.
17. Goldberg BB, Kother MN, Ziskin MC, Waxham RD: Diagnostic Uses of Ultrasound. New York, Grune and Stratton, 1975, p 329.
18. Kratochwil A, Hofner W, Alth G: Zur Herdsuche in der gynäkologischen Strahlentherapie. Geburtsh Frauenheilk 31:833–841, 1971.
19. Wenzel WW: Improved radiotherapy dose calculations using ultrasound uterine localization. J Clin Ultrasound 3:311–312, 1975.
20. Asher MW, Freimanis A: Echographic diagnosis of retroperitoneal lymphnode enlargement. Am J Roentgenol Rad Ther Nucl Med 105:438–445, 1960.
21. Brascho DJ, Green I, Durant JR: The accuracy of diagnostic ultrasound in detecting retroperitoneal lymph node enlargement in malignant lymphoma and Hodgkin's disease. Ultrasound Med Biol 1:184, 1975.
22. Brascho DJ: Tumor localization and treatment planning with ultrasound. Cancer 39: Suppl 2:697–705, 1977.
23. Kratochwil A: Möglichkeiten und Grenzen der Ultraschalldiagnostik in der Nachsorge urologischer Tumorpatienten. Rö Fo 122:95–99, 1975.
24. Kratochwil A, Pulitzer B: Indication and achievements of after care examinations in Hodgkin's disease. Rö Fo Suppl 123:1973.
25. Kratochwil A: Ultraschalldiagnostik in der Bestrahlungsplanung. In: Anleitung zur Bestrahlungsplanung, ed. Kärcher KH. Eigenverlag Siemens.
26. Heckemann R, Wiechert HC, Rottinger EM, Hossfeld DK: Ultrasound progress control of retroperitoneal tumors during chemotherapy. Fortschr Rö Nukl Med 126:236–240, 1977.

27. Heckemann R, Schmitt G: Sonografische und röntgenologische Verlaufskontrollen nach Strahlentherapie retroperitonealer Tumoren. Strahlentherapie 152:149–154, 1976.

28. Kratochwil A, Stöger H, Zeibekis N: Darstellung von Beckenwandrezidiven im Ultraschalltomogramm. Geburtsh Frauenheilk 34:742–752, 1974.

29. J Eule JR, Bockenstedt F, Salzmann E: Diagnostic ultrasound scanning: A valuable aid in radiation therapy planning. Am J Roentgenol 117:139–145, 1973.

30. Mayer EG, Galindo J, Connor WG, et al: Evaluation of B-mode ultrasound as a means of improving radium dosimetry in the treatment of gynecological cancer. Radiology 117: 141–147, 1975.

31. Freimanis AK: Ultrasonic imaging of neoplasms. Cancer 37:Suppl 1:496–502, 1976.

32. Fry FJ, Sanghvin NT, Eggleton RC: Ultrasonic visualization and therapeutic computer controlled system. Ultrasound Med Biol 2:481–482, 1976.

33. Jentzsch K, Kärcher KH, Böhm B: Ultraschall in der Strahlentherapie, bei der Bestrahlungs planung und Überwachung der Therapieerfolge. Ultrasound Med Biol 1:149–159, 1974.

34. Nieminen U, Jööskelöinen Y: Ultrasonic tomography in the planning of external radiotherapy for gynaecologic tumors. Strahlentherapie 140:400–402, 1970.

35. Sager WD, Hackl A, Schmiedberger H, Gell C: Optimized cross-section determination for treatment planning in radiotherapy. Strahlentherapie 153:660–663, 1977.

36. Jentzsch K: Ultraschalldiagnostik in der Strahlentherapie. Wien Klin Wochenschr 87: 378–381, 1975.

37. Carson PL, Wenzel WW, Avery P, Hendee WR: Ultrasound imaging as an aid to cancer therapy. J Diag Oncol Radiol 1:119–132, 1975.

38. Schulze K, Meudt R, Benz EF: Ultraschalldiagnostik im Rahmen der Abklärung und Verlaufsbeurteilung onkologischer Patienten. Strahlentherapie 154:471–475, 1978.

39. Heckenthaler W: Zur Tumorlikalisation und Bestrahlungsplanung mittels Ultraschall-Echotomographie. Strahlentherapie 146:60–64, 1973.

40. Banjavic RA, Zazgebski JA, Wiley AL, Tolbert DD: A projection system for effective utilization of ultrasound echogram information in radiation therapy. Radiology 116: 731–733, 1975.

41. Slater JM, Neilsen IR, Chu WT, et al: Radiotherapy treatment planning using ultrasound graph pen computer system. Cancer 34:96–99, 1974.

42. Cohen W, Haas W: The application of B-scan ultrasound in the planning of radiation therapy treatment parts. Am J Roentgenol 111:184–188, 1971.

43. Carter SJ, Denney JD, Tesch DW, et al: Ultrasonic evaluation of radiation therapy ports. J Clin Ultrasound 5:103–106, 1977.

44. Ekstrand KE, Dixon RL, Blake DD, Ruben M: The calculation dose distribution for chest wall irradiation using B-mode ultrasonography. Radiology 111:185–187, 1974.

45. Jackson SM, Naylor GP, Kerby IJ: Ultrasonic measurement of post mastectomy chestwall thickness. Br J Radiol 43:458–461, 1970.

46. Porrath S, Avallone LT: Radiation therapy treatment planning using ultrasound. Ultrasound Med Biol 2:165–172, 1976.

47. Reisner K, Heckenrodt J: Use of ultrasonics in radiotherapy. Rö Fo suppl 83:1972.

48. Reisner K, Heckroth J, Ay R: Die Verwendung des Ultraschall B-Bildvrfahrens bei der Bestrehlungsplanung. Strahlentherapie 140:639–646, 1970.

49. Kobayashi T, Takatani O, Kimura K: Clinical investigation of ultrasonotomographic patterns of malignant abdominal tumors in special reference to changes of their patterns after irradiation of chemotherapy. Preliminary report. Jap. J Med Ultrasound 10:18–22, 1971.

50. Kobayashi T, Takatani O, Hattori N, Kimura K: Clinical investigation of ultrasonoto-

mographic patterns of malignant abdominal tumors in special reference to changes of their pattern after irradiation or chemotherapy. Jap J Med Ultrasound 10:132 – 135, 1972.

51. Herring DF, Compton DM: Degree of precision required in radiation dose delivered in cancertherapy. British Journal of Radiology, Special Report Series 5, Proceedings of the First International Conference on Computerized Radiology, 1971, p 51.

52. Kobayashi T, Takatani O, Hattori N, Kimura K: Echographic evaluation of abdominal tumor regression during antineoplastic treatment. J Clin Ultrasound 2:131 – 141, 1972.

53. Kratochwil A, Kärcher KH, Jentzsch K, Wolf G: Die Wertigkeit und Grenzen der Echographie Für die Diagnostik abdomineller Lymphome bei malignen Erkrankungen. Rö Fo 122:410 – 417, 1975.

13 Therapy

FREDERICK W. KREMKAU

Research on the effects of ultrasound on malignancies has been in progress for approximately 50 years. The first mention of this work in the scientific literature[1] appeared just 6 years after the first literature report on the biologic effects of ultrasound.[2] Since then, much work has been done on the effects of ultrasound on malignant cell suspensions, experimental and spontaneous animal tumors, and on human tumors. Approximately 150 articles on the subject have been published.[3] The three approaches to cancer therapy with ultrasound (Fig. 13.1) are: (1) ultrasound alone, (2) ultrasound plus radiotherapy, and (3) ultrasound plus chemotherapy.

Ultrasound combined with radiotherapy was introduced in 1946,[4] and ultrasound in connection with chemotherapy was introduced in 1967.[5] In this chapter, the early work reported during the years 1933–1974, is summarized while the recent work reported during the years 1975–1979, is considered in greater detail.

EARLY WORK (1933–1974)

The first 40 years in which the effects of ultrasound on malignancies were studied were characterized by periods of initiation, enthusiasm, and pessimism.[3] In this early work, the frequencies used ranged from 0.3 to 9 MHz. Often, no intensities were quoted, and even when they were, the method of measurement was seldom described. It is likely that in many cases the intensity values reported were those read off output meters of the physical therapy units commonly used to supply the ultrasound. The reliability of such values is questionable; the values reported ranged from 0.1 to 20 W/cm^2. Exposure times ranged from 60 to 1,500 seconds. In a less common regime, high intensity (150 to 1000 W/cm^2) and short time (1 to 5 seconds) exposures were made. In each regime, on the order of 500 J/cm^2 energy density was delivered by the exposure system.

The first report[1] concerning ultrasound and a malignancy stated that ultrasound had no specific effect on Ehrlich carcinoma. About a year later, the first

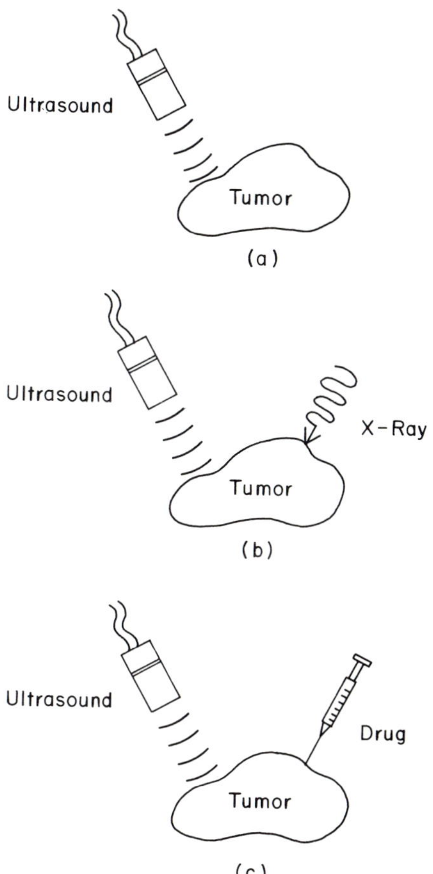

FIGURE 13.1. Three approaches to cancer therapy with ultrasound. (a) Ultrasound alone applied to the tumor through coupling gel or a water path. (b) Ultrasound applied before, during, or after X-ray. (c) Ultrasound applied before, during, or after administration of chemotherapy. (Kremkau FW: Cancer therapy with ultrasound: A historical review. J Clin Ultrasound 7:287–300, 1979. Reprinted by permission of John Wiley & Sons, Inc.)

report of an effect of ultrasound on a tumor appeared.[6] This, and subsequent reports dealing with a mouse adenocarcinoma, indicated that shorter treatment times (approximately 1 minute) enhanced tumor growth, whereas longer treatment times (several minutes) resulted in growth inhibition or tumor resorption. A report on the inhibition of Walker sarcoma 319 tumor growth[7] proposed a thermal mechanism of action (the first report of mechanism considerations).

The clinical use of ultrasound began[8] in 1944 and continued for several years, with little concurrent supporting work in animal experimental tumors. Ultrasound was applied to several human tumors, mostly skin carcinomas and sarcomas. Reduced tumor growth and some resorptions were observed.[9-12] Often, however, the lesions returned in a few months.

Following these initial reports, there was a particularly enthusiastic and active 10-year period of study during which about 60 publications on the subject appeared. Several reports indicated that ultrasound applied to human tumors resulted in beneficial effects.[3] Most of these studies were done with skin carcinomas and sarcomas. Some investigators observed no effects of ultrasound on human tumors, whereas others observed stimulation of tumor growth. A summary of 133 clinical cases reported in the literature[13] indicated that 17 percent improved, 76 percent were unchanged, and 7 percent were made worse. This was not a particularly encouraging summary of clinical data. As a result of this experience and excess enthusiasm for this new mode of treatment in various clinical areas,[14] a resolution was formulated at the Congress on Ultrasound in Medicine at Erlangen, Germany in 1949. This resolution stated that ultrasound was not suited for tumor therapy and that its clinical use should be discontinued.[13, 15]

Following the cessation of clinical studies, much activity continued with experimental animals. Several publications reported the effects of ultrasound on various endpoints in several tumor systems. One rather thorough study[16] considered mouse carcinoma, sarcoma MA387, Ridgeway osteogenic sarcoma, Ak-4 leukemia, sarcoma 180, and sarcoma T241. There was no indication, from this study, that any of the tumors were significantly inhibited by the maximum dosage of ultrasound the mice were able to tolerate. The approach differed from previous studies in that the entire trunk area of each mouse was exposed to ultrasound. The investigators noted that the large body area that was treated might constitute an overly stringent test, since it resulted in exposure of sensitive normal tissues that might be avoided in larger animals. Others[17-20] studied the effects of ultrasound on several tumors in mice, rats, chickens, and dogs. Tumor necrosis was observed but was not accompanied by resorption. There was some consensus in the reports up to this time that ultrasound produced tumor inhibition through heating and that the treatment had to be localized to the tumor area in order to produce a differential effect with respect to normal tissues.

The high-intensity short-time approach[21, 22] was introduced in 1956. It was proposed that this approach might produce nonthermal antitumor effects. Exposure of this type produced resorption of Brown-Pearce rabbit carcinomas.[23-27] In addition to first reporting this type of treatment, these investigators reported two very interesting phenomena: metastases that were not exposed to ultrasound resorbed in addition to the treated tumor, and the cured hosts developed a high resistance to subsequent inoculation of tumor cells. In the first clinical report[22] to have appeared in several years, resorption of human malignant melanoma primary tumors was observed. However, unlike rabbit carcinomas, untreated metastases were not affected. Other investigators reported successful application of the high-intensity short-time approach to treatment of human breast and brain tumors[28] and of Horie's sarcoma in rats.[29]

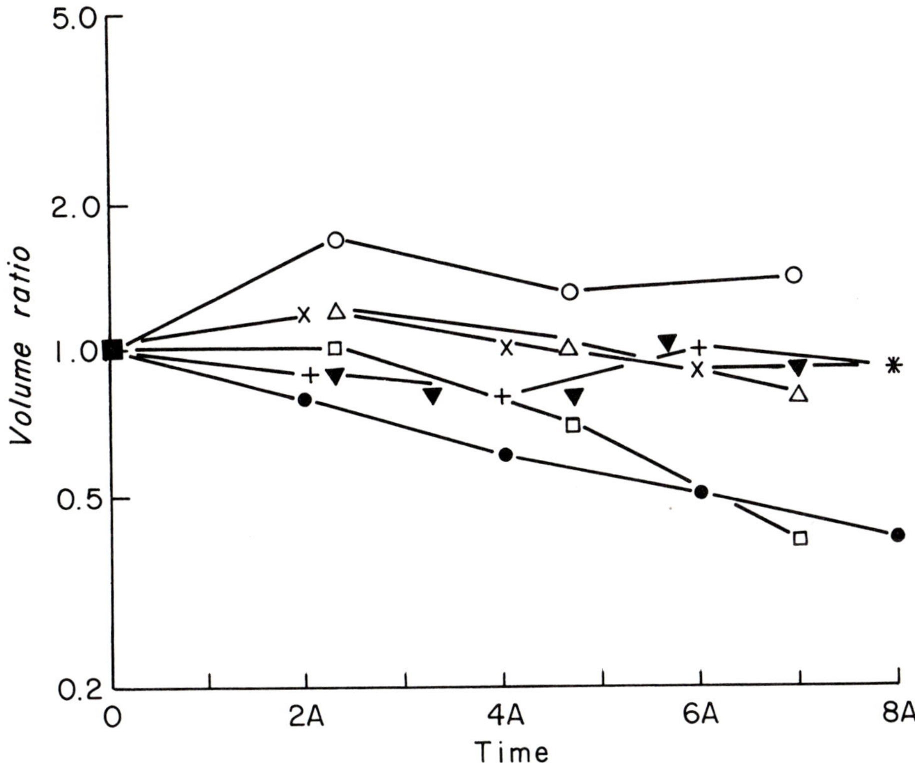

FIGURE 13.2. Tumor growth versus time after ultrasound treatment. Volume ratio is tumor volume (weight for case c) for treated animals divided by mean tumor volume (weight for case c) for controls. Mean volumes or weights are estamated from graphs published in the references cited below. Time axis is days after ultrasound treatment: A = 3 days for cases a and d and A = 1 for cases b, c, and e. Treatment was on day zero except for case e where it was on days zero and two. Case a: mouse glioma (○, △, □),[41] Case b: rat Walker carcinoma (×),[28] Case c: rat BICR/M1 tumor (+),[29] Case d: mouse sarcoma 37 (▼),[44] and Case e: rat Wilms' tumor (•).[32] (Kremkau FW: Cancer therapy with ultrasound: A historical review. J Clin Ultrasound 7:287–300, 1979. Reprinted by permission of John Wiley & Sons, Inc.)

Studies with Walker 256 carcinoma in rats indicated that ultrasound alone produced only a slight reduction in growth rate, but that application of ultrasound in combination with X-ray resulted in approximately a 50 percent reduction in the X-ray dose required to achieve the same effect as with X-ray alone.[30] On the other hand, studies in BICR/M1 rat tumors indicated that ultrasound did not enhance X-ray damage.[31]

The first report concerning ultrasound in combination with chemotherapy[5] appeared in 1967. When Walker 256 rat carcinoma was treated with ultrasound and mechlorethamine, the drug's effectiveness was not enhanced.

Thus, during the first 40 years of study of the effects of ultrasound on human and experimental animal malignancies, several reports, some positive and some negative, appeared. Effects were generally attributed to a thermal mechanism. Attempts at combination therapy were somewhat successful with X-ray but not with chemotherapy. Increased, unchanged, and decreased tumor growth rates have been observed during this period, as well as in subsequent years (Fig. 13.2).

RECENT WORK (1975 – 1980)

Interest and activity in this area of research has increased in the last 5 years, compared to the previous 15. Most reports have been concerned with studies in animal models, but some clinical studies have also been done.

Animal Tumors

Animal studies have been carried out using all three approaches shown in Figure 13.1.

Ultrasound Alone

Several literature reports have described the use of ultrasound alone in the treatment of animal tumors (Fig. 13.2). In the Furth-Columbia rat Wilms' tumor, reductions of mean tumor weight and size (Fig. 13.2), and increases in median survival were observed after 1 MHz ultrasound treatment.[32-37] Ultrasound was applied to the shaved skin surface, using coupling gel as a contact medium. The results were attributed to a thermal mechanism of action. The effect on tumor growth was a local phenomenon, and systemic changes that occurred were not involved in tumor inhibition. The threshold for growth control was reported to be approximately 1.5 W/cm.[2] Rechallenge with untreated tumor in hosts that previously had tumors treated with ultrasound resulted in 100 percent take, thus indicating no host response from the initial implant and treatment.

In a study with EMT6 and KHJJ mouse tumors,[38] application of 5.2 MHz ultrasound produced tumor temperatures of 43° to 44°C for 15 to 45 minutes. Cure rates and growth delay increased with increasing temperature or exposure time. The number of cells required for a 50-percent take when cured animals were rechallenged was ten times higher for ultrasound-cured mice than for untreated controls. Heat and immune recognition were considered to be major factors in the antitumor effect.[39]

Metastases induction was studied in hamster fibrosarcoma HTC-3049-91TC. Five MHz ultrasound at 3 W/cm^2, applied for 6 to 8 minutes, eradicated the 58 tumors treated, with only one tumor recurrence.[40] There was no indication that this treatment induced metastases.

High intensity short-time treatment, initiated several years earlier,[21] has recently been applied. The growth of murine gliomas implanted in the abdominal wall was enhanced following treatment with 0.9 MHz, 100 W/cm^2 ultrasound for 10 seconds.[41] Treatment with 1,000 W/cm^2 for 1 second did not alter growth, whereas 1,000 W/cm² for 2 seconds inhibited tumor growth (Fig. 13.2). The latter treatment increased survival time for recipient hosts. Reimplantation with untreated glioma resulted in over 80 percent rejection for all treatments.

High-intensity treatment was applied to hamster HM medulloblastoma inoculated subcutaneously in the flank. One MHz, 907 W/cm², applied for 7 seconds, resulted in tumor extinction, with a 29 percent cure rate.[42] In these experiments a focused ultrasound regime was used in which the focal region was smaller than the tumor. The treatment procedure involved a matrix of treatment points arranged so that the entire tumor was covered with the appropriate intensity of ultrasound.

A study of ultrasound hyperthermia treatment of spontaneous malignant tumors in 22 cats and dogs has been reported.[43] Frequencies of 0.75 to 5 MHz were utilized, depending on the depth of heating desired. Various intensities were used to achieve tumor temperatures of 43.0° to 44.5°C for 30 minutes in each treatment. Three complete regressions and nine partial regressions were achieved, giving an overall response rate of 55 percent. Squamous cell carcinomas appeared to be the most responsive. There was no apparent correlation between temperature or duration of treatment and response.

Ultrasound and Radiotherapy

Several investigators have reported on the use of ultrasound in combination with X-ray for the treatment of animal tumors. In a study with sarcoma 37 in mice, it was found that 0.9 MHz, 0.5 W/cm² ultrasound, applied for 15 minutes enhanced the sensitivity of this tumor to ionizing radiation.[44] Twenty-one days after treatment, ultrasound alone produced a 14 percent decrease in growth rate, whereas 350 rads of gamma irradiation produced no change. Combined treatment with a 3-minute interval between ultrasound and irradiation resulted in a 32 percent decrease in growth rate, but a 7-minute interval produced a 64 percent decrease as compared with controls. This latter treatment, in another experiment, resulted in a 28 percent tumor regression incidence (controls, 11 percent) and 90 percent survival at 25 days after treatment (controls, 58 percent).

It has been found that ultrasound treatment can enhance ionizing radiation sensitivity in one tumor type while not changing it in another type. Treatment with 1.9 MHz, 1.5 W/cm² ultrasound, for up to 30 minutes had no effect on subcutaneous tumors treated in a water bath. In combination with X-ray, ultrasound before or after the radiation of C3HBA mouse mammary carcinoma did not alter the TCD_{50} (5,000 rads).[45] For mouse sarcoma S180, 15 minutes of ultrasound, either before or after radiation, reduced the TCD_{50} by 40 percent. Water-bath heating (44.5°C for 15 minutes) after radiation reduced the TCD_{50} for both tumors. These results were reported to be consistent with a thermal mechanism of action. The lack of effect of ultrasound on the C3H mammary tumor was considered to be caused by inadequate heating of the tumor periphery. Fractionating X-ray into three equal doses, delivered on alternate days with ultrasound following each X-ray dose, reduced the TCD_{50} 26 percent.[46] Pulsed ultrasound (3 W/cm^2 spatial average temporal peak intensity, 1.5 W/cm^2 spatial average temporal average intensity, 50 percent duty factor) following single-dose X-ray resulted in the same TCD_{50} reduction as with continuous wave ultrasound. Since both ultrasound treatments produce the same tumor temperature rise, the lack of significant difference in results supports the hypothesis that ultrasonic enhancement of radiation effects is a result of absorption heating.

A study of combined ultrasound and X-ray on growth of Walker 256 sarcoma was conducted[47] with results similar to those reported earlier.[30] No effect of ultrasound alone on tumor growth was observed. However, the addition of ultrasound to X-ray treatment produced a growth and cure rate similar to half the X-ray dose alone. In these studies as well as in others,[45] no difference was observed when the X-ray ultrasound treatment sequence was reversed.

Ultrasound and Chemotherapy

It has been shown that *in vitro* ultrasound treatment of L1210 mouse leukemia cells results in no change in the survival of host mice subsequently inoculated with these cells.[48] However, for 5 of 10 anticancer agents studied (arabinosyl cytosine, bis-chloroethyl nitrosourea, the active metabolite of cyclophosphamide, mechlorethamine, melphalan), ultrasound treatment (1.9 MHz, 10 W/cm^2, 10 minutes) of the cell suspension resulted in host survival greater (by at least 20 percent) than that for cells treated with drugs alone.[48-53] It appears that the enhanced cytotoxicity observed in L1210 leukemia is not due to any increased accumulation of drug in the cells. It is possible that the cellular damage inflicted by ultrasound treatment which is normally repaired by the cells, experiences repair inhibition by the presence of cytotoxic agents. In this way, the combined treatment may be more effective against the tumor cells than either treatment alone. Rechallenge of cured hosts with standard inocula of untreated cells resulted in the usual median survival for normal hosts, thus indicating no host response to the combined treatment. It has been shown that in the case of mechlorethamine the drug must be available to the cells at the time of exposure, or within 3 or 4 minutes following, for ultrasound enhancement to occur.

Melanoma cells in culture have been shown[54] to experience preferential loss of viability in melanin-containing cells exposed to ultrasound (1 MHz, 2 W/cm^2, 35 seconds). The amount of damage was dependent on the intracellular melanin concentration. Combined treatment of melanoma cells in culture with ultrasound and the drugs chlorpromazine and kanamycin (which cause preferential damage to melanoma cells) results in enhanced damage in lightly pigmented cells.

Studies in hamster medulloblastoma HM, referred to earlier,[42] showed combined action with a chemotherapeutic agent as well. Bis-chloroethyl nitrosourea administration 24 hours following ultrasound resulted in the same mean survival time in the noncured animals as for those receiving chemotherapy but no ultrasound. However, the cure rate for the combined treatment was 40 percent as compared to zero percent for drug alone.

Clinical Research

Ultrasound has good potential as a clinical hyperthermia tool because of its capability for localization and depth of penetration in tissues.[39, 55-58] Clinical studies have been initiated. A study of 21 patients with the following superficial neoplasms has been reported:[59] squamous cell carcinoma of head, neck, lung; adenocarcinoma of ovary, breast, uterus, nose; medullary carcinoma of thyroid; melanoma; neurofibrosarcoma; diffuse histiocytic lymphoma; mycosis fungoides. The treatment system was designed to raise the tumor temperature to 43° to 45°C. Intensities of 0.5 to 1.2 W/cm^2 at frequencies 1 to 3 MHz were used. Six 30-minute treatments were given to each lesion over a 2 week period. Twenty-six courses of treatment were given to the 21 patients. Three of the courses (12 percent) resulted in complete responses (clinical disappearance of tumor within the heated area), 11 (42 percent) resulted in partial responses (greater than 50 percent decrease in tumor volume within the heated area for greater than 2 weeks), and 12 (46 percent) produced no effect. Response rate did not correlate with tumor temperature. In some cases local pain was experienced by the patient during treatment. In a few cases, small cutaneous burns occured at thermocouple implant sites. These healed in a week. It was concluded that ultrasound could safely and effectively heat superficial tumors and that this heating appeared to have some antitumor effect, especially on squamous cell carcinomas of the head and neck (67 percent response).

Sixteen patients who had previously been irradiated with 4,400 to 11,000 rad were treated with the system used above.[60] Tumors included squamous cell carcinoma, adenocarcinoma, and diffuse histiocytic lymphoma, in most cases, of the head and neck. Three to 25 treatments of 30 minutes duration raised tumor temperatures 43.5° to 45°C. Eighteen courses of treatment were given. Two resulted in complete and 9 in partial responses, while 7 had no effect. Small superficial burns occurred at the thermocouple implant site in three of the 18 treatment courses. In this study five additional patients were given six courses of treatment in combination with low-dose (1,200 to 2,400 rad) irradiation. Three complete responses, two partial responses, and one case of no effect were observed. These results suggest that ultrasound can be combined safely with low-dose irradiation in patients who have recurrent tumor in previously irradiated sites.

A clinical study with combined X-ray and ultrasound has been reported.[61] Matched tumor sites were used in 12 patients, with both sites treated identically with X-ray and one site receiving ultrasound. In 4 of 12 patients the combined treatment resulted in a complete response, compared to a partial response to X-ray alone. In 2 of these, an increased radiation skin reaction

TABLE 13.1. Summary of observations on ultrasound treatment of tumors (1975–1980).

References	Reduced Tumor Growth	Enhanced Radiation Effects	Enhanced Chemotherapy Effects	Human Study
32–37	yes	–	–	no
38–39	yes	–	–	no
40	yes	–	–	no
41	yes	–	–	no
42	yes	–	yes	no
43	yes	–	–	no
44	yes	yes	–	no
45–46	no	yes	–	no
47	no	yes	–	no
48–53	no	–	yes	no
54	yes	–	yes	no
59–61	yes	yes	–	yes
62	–	–	yes	yes
63	–	–	yes	yes

was observed at the site where the combined treatment had been applied. This study suggests that ultrasound may improve the X-ray response in some human tumors but that it appears to sensitize skin to X-ray damage as well.

Some clinical studies have been done with ultrasound in combination with chemotherapy. Four patients with brain malignancies[62] were treated with methyl cyclohexyl-chloroethyl nitrosourea and twice daily with 1 MHz, 3 W/cm^2 ultrasound. There was some indication that ultrasound improved the effectiveness of the chemotherapy. Encouraging results have been observed in recent studies with ultrasound and cis-platinum in a small number of patients with superficial tumors.[63]

An approach to the clinical application of chemotherapy and ultrasound has been described.[58] The rationale for the approach is that localized heating leads to "thermal focusing" of the drug into the selected region by a local increase in blood flow. Ultrasound is to be used to increase local tumoricidal cytotoxicity by producing local tumor hyperthermia, while reducing systemic toxicity by inducing whole body hypothermia. Preliminary experiments using this approach in mice show considerable promise.[58]

A summary of the results reported during 1975–1980 for ultrasound tumor therapy in animals and humans is given in Table 13.1.

SUMMARY

The potential of ultrasound as a cancer therapy tool has been studied for about 50 years. During the period of early work (1933–1974) many reports on the subject appeared. Clinical use became popular and then declined following the Erlangen resolution. Animal studies yielded variable results, producing reports of decreased tumor growth, no effect, and growth enhancement. Two approaches have been used: low intensity-long time and high intensity-short time. During the years 1975–1980, studies with ultrasound alone and in combination with radiotherapy and chemotherapy have been conducted. A revival in clinical studies, based primarily on a hyperthermia rationale, has occurred. The potential of ultrasound as a clinical tool for local tumor control or local enhancement of radiotherapy or chemotherapy motivates the several research groups who are continuing their studies of the subject.

References

1. Szent-Gyorgyi A: Chemical and biological effects of ultrasonic radiation. Nature 131: 278, 1933.
2. Wood RW, Loomis AL: The physical and biological effects of high-frequency sound waves of great intensity. Phil Mag S, Series 7, 4:417–436, 1927.
3. Kremkau FW: Cancer therapy with ultrasound: A historical review. J Clin Ultrasound 7: 287–300, 1979.
4. Horvath J: Uber die Wirkung der Ultraschallwellen auf das menschliche Karzinom. Klin Prax 1:10–14, 1946.
5. Hill CR: Changes in tissue permeability produced by ultrasound. Br J Radiol 40:317–318, 1967.
6. Nakahara W, Kobayashi R: Biological effects of short exposure to supersonic waves: Local effect on the skin. Jap J Exp Med 12:137–142, 1934.
7. Beck FF, Krantz JC: Glycolysis in tumor tissue. III. The effect of ultrasonic vibrations on the growth and glycolysis of Walker sarcoma 319. Am J Cancer 39:245–250, 1940.
8. Horvath J: Ultraschallwirkung beim menschlichen Sarkom. Strahlentherapie 75:119–125, 1944.
9. Dyroff R, Horvath R: Ultraschallwirkung beim menschlichen Sardom. Strahlentherapie 75:126–130, 1944.
10. Horvath J: Weitere Erfahrungen uber die Wirkung der Ultraschallwellen auf das menschilelhe Karzinom. Klin Prax 1:108–110, 1946.
11. Horvath J: Uber den Einfluss von Ultraschallwellen auf das Karzinom. Asklepios 1:1–14, 1947.
12. Horvath J: Die morphologischen Veränderungen der Karzinomzellen nach Ultraschalleinwirkung. Dtsch Med Wochenschr 74:392–399, 1947.
13. Pohlman R: Die Ultraschalltherapie, Praktisch Anwendung der Ultraschalls in der Medizin. Bern, Verlag Hans Huber, 1951.
14. Hill CR: Medical ultrasonics: An historical review. Br J Radiol 46:899–905, 1973.
15. Licht S: Therapeutic Heat. New Haven, Licht, 1958, p 303.
16. Southam CM, Beyer H, Allen AC: The effects of ultrasonic irradiation upon normal and neoplastic tissues in the intact mouse. Cancer 6:390–396, 1953.
17. Schroder JD, Herrick JR, Karlson AG: The effect of ultrasound on the transmissible Walker rat carcinoma. Arch Phys Med 33:660–667, 1952.
18. Lehmann JF, Krusen FH: Biophysical effects of ultrasonic energy on carcinoma and their possible significance. Arch Phys Med Rehabil 36:452–459, 1955.
19. Herrick JF: Temperatures produced in tissues by ultrasound: Experimental study using various technics. J Acoust Soc Am 25:12–16, 1953.

20. Herrick JF: Am Ind Hyg Assoc Q 14:168–169, 1953.
21. Burov AK: High intensity ultrasonic oscillation for treatment of malignant tumors in animals and man. Dokl Akad Nauk SSSR 106:239–241, 1956.
22. Burov AK, Andreevskaya GD: The effect of ultra-acoustic oscillation of high intensity on malignant tumors in animals and man. Dokl Akad Nauk SSSR 106:445–448, 1956.
23. Dmitrieva NP: Influence of ultrasonics of great intensity on the growth and metastasization of Brown-Pearce tumour in rabbits. Dissertation, Moscow, 1956.
24. Dmitrieva NP: Biull Eksp Biol Med 6:60–62, 1957.
25. Dmitrieva NP: Biull Eksp Biol Med, 11:81–85, 1957.
26. Dmitrieva NP: Histological changes in the Brown-Pearce tumor after exposure to ultrasound of high intensity. Vopr Onkol 3:688–692, 1957.
27. Dmitrieva NP: The action of ultrasonics on spontaneous and transplantable tumors in animals and on malignant tumours of humans. Probl Oncol 6:1379–1386, 1960.
28. Oka M: Surgical application of high-intensity focused ultrasound. Clinic All-Round (Japan) 13:1514–1523, 1960.
29. Saigusa K: Destruction of malignant tumor by intense focused ultrasound. Annual report (1970) of the Medical Ultrasonics Research Center, Juntendo University School of Medicine, Tokyo, 1971.
30. Woeber K: The effect of ultrasound in the treatment of cancer. In: Ultrasonic Energy, ed. Kelly E. Urbana, University of Illinois Press, 1965, pp 135–149.
31. Clarke PR, Hill CR, Adams K: Synergism between ultrasound and x-rays in tumour therapy. Br J Radiol 43:97–99, 1970.
32. Longo FW, Tomashefsky P, Rivin BD, et al: Interaction of ultrasound with neoplastic tissue. I. Local effect upon subcutaneously implanted Furth-Columbia rat Wilms' tumor. Urology 6:631–634, 1975.
33. Longo FW, Tomashefsky P, Rivin BD, et al: Interaction of ultrasound with neoplastic tissue. II. Systemic effects after local sonic irradiation. Urology 7:80–84, 1976.
34. Longo FW, Tomashefsky P, Rivin BD, et al: Interaction of ultrasound with neoplastic tissue. III. Electron microscopic demonstration of ultrasonic destruction of Wilms' tumor and its cellular membranes. Trans Am Assoc Genitourin Surg 68:121–124, 1976.
35. Longo FW, Tomashefsky P, Willhite M, et al: Interaction of ultrasound with neoplastic tissue. IV. Alteration of biologic activity in cells derived from rat Wilms' tumor sonicated in vivo. Urology 8:177–179, 1976.
36. Tomashefsky P, Longo FW, Rivin BD, et al: The reaction of a transplantable rat Wilms' tumor to ultrasound. In: Ultrasound in Medicine, vol 3B, eds. White D, Brown RE. New York, Plenum, 1977, pp 2051–2061.
37. Longo FW, Tomashefsky P, Rivin BD, et al: The direct effect of ultrasound upon Wilms' tumor in the rat. Invest Urol 15:87–89, 1977.
38. Marmor JB, Hilerio FJ, Hahn GM: Tumor eradication and cell survival after localized hyperthermia induced by ultrasound. Cancer Res, in press.
39. Hahn GM, Pounds D: Heat treatment of solid tumors: Why and how. Appl Radiol 5: 131–144, 1976.
40. Smachlo K, Fridd CW, Child SZ, et al: Ultrasonic treatment of tumors: I. Absence of metastases following treatment of a hamster fibrosarcoma. Ultrasound Med Biol 5:45–49, 1979.
41. Kishi M, Mishima T, Itakura T, et al: Experimental studies of effects of intense ultrasound on implantable murine glioma. In: Proceedings of the Second European Congress on Ultrasonics in Medicine, eds. Kazner E, et al. Amsterdam, Exerpta Medica, 1975, pp 28–33.
42. Fry FJ, Johnson LK: Tumor irradiation with intense ultrasound. Ultrasound Med Biol 4:337–339, 1978.

43. Marmor JB, Pounds D, Hahn N, Hahn GM: Treating spontaneous tumors in dogs and cats by ultrasound-induced hyperthermia. Int J Radiat Oncol Biol Phys 4:967–973, 1978.

44. Gavrilov LR, Kalendo GS, Ryabukhin VV, et al: Ultrasonic enhancement of the gamma radiation of malignant tumors. Sov Phys Acoust 21:119–121, 1975.

45. Witcofski RL, Kremkau FW: Ultrasonic enhancement of cancer radiotherapy. Radiology 127:793–797, 1978.

46. Kremkau FW, Witcofski RL: Enhanced tumor radiosensitivity by ultrasonic heating. Proceedings of the 24th Annual Meeting of the American Institute of Ultrasound in Medicine, vol 1. 1979, p 44.

47. Ishigaki T, Makino N, Mizertani H, et al: Effect of ultrasound on ionizing radiation effects. IV. Effect on growth of transplanted tumors. Nippon Igaku Hoshasen Gakkai Zasshi 38:1137–1144, 1978.

48. Kremkau FW, Kaufmann JS, Walker MM, et al: Ultrasonic enhancement of nitrogen mustard cytotoxicity in mouse leukemia. Cancer 37:1643–1647, 1976.

49. Kremkau FW: Enhanced action of chemotherapeutic drugs by using ultrasound. In: Proceedings of the International Symposium on Cancer Therapy by Hyperthermia and Radiation, eds. Wizenberg MJ, Robinson JE. Chicago, American College of Radiology, 1975, p 224.

50. Kremkau FW, Kaufmann JS: Time/intensity studies of mechlorethamine enhancement by ultrasound. In: Proceedings of the 29th Annual Conference on Engineering in Medicine and Biology. Alliance for Engineering in Medicine and Biology, Chevy Chase, Md, 1976, p 70.

51. Kremkau FW, Kaufmann JS, Burch PG, et al: Ultrasonic enhancement of anticancer agents. In: Ultrasound in Medicine, vol 3B, eds. White D, Brown RE. New York, Plenum Press, 1977, pp 2109–2110.

52. Kaufmann JS, Kremkau FW: Influence of ultrasound on mouse leukemia cell DNA synthesis, membrane intergity, and uptake of anticancer drugs in vitro. In: Ultrasound in Medicine, vol 4, eds. White D, Lyons EA. New York, Plenum Press, 1978, pp 589–590.

53. Kremkau FW: Research in cancer therapy with ultrasound. In: 1977 Ultrasonics Symposium Proceedings, IEEE catalog 77CR:264-1SU eds. de Klerk J, McAvoy BB. New York, Inst Elec Electron Eng, 1977, pp 142–146.

54. Armour E, Corry P, McGinness J: Preferential cytotoxicity of cultured melanoma cells by ultrasound and melanin binding drugs. Radiat Res 70:690–691, 1977.

55. Har-Kedar I, Bleehen NM: Experimental and clinical aspects of hyperthermia applied to the treatment of cancer with special reference to the role of ultrasonic and microwave heating. In: Advances in Radiation Biology, vol 6, eds. Lett JT, Adler H. New York, Academic Press, 1976, pp 228–266.

56. Lele PP: In Proceedings of the International Symposium on Cancer Therapy by Hyperthermia and Radiation, eds. Wizenburg MJ, Robinson JE. Chicago, American College of Radiology, 1975, pp 168–178.

57. Hahn GM: Ultrasound for the induction of localized hyperthermia. Int J Radiat Oncol Biol Phys 4:1117–1118, 1978.

58. Lele PP: A strategy for localized chemotherapy of tumors using ultrasonic hyperthermia. Ultrasound Med Biol 5:95–96, 1979.

59. Marmor JB, Pounds D, Postic TB, Hahn GM: Treatment of superficial human neoplasms by local hyperthermia induced by ultrasound. Cancer 43:188–197, 1979.

60. Marmor JB, Hahn GM: Ultrasound heating in previously irradiated sites. Int J Oncol Biol Phys 4:1029–1031, 1978.

61. Marmor JB, Hahn GM: Radiation with ultrasound induced hyperthermia for superficial human neoplasms. Presented at the 15th Annual Meeting of the American Society of Clinical Oncology, New Orleans, 1979.

62. Heimburger RF, Fry FJ, Franklin TD, et al: Ultrasound potentiation of chemotherapy for brain malignancy. In Ultrasound in Medicine, vol 1 ed. White D. New York, Plenum Press, 1975, pp 273–281.

63. Systemic Hyperthermia at MDAH, The University of Texas System Cancer Center Newsletter 24:4–7, 1979.

CASE NO. 1

S. J. Pussell
D. O. Cosgrove

Liver Cyst in a Woman with Carcinoma of the Ovary

A 51-year-old woman, who had had a mastectomy in 1973 for carcinoma, presented in February 1977 with a pelvic mass and ascites. Stage IV carcinoma of the ovary was diagnosed at laparotomy and she received eight courses of chemotherapy consisting of cis-platinum, doxorubicin (adriamycin), and chlorambucil. She responded very well and had a second laparotomy in August 1977, at which time a total hysterectomy and bilateral salpingoophorectomy were performed. She was left with peritoneal seedlings and small liver metastases. She received further courses of cis-platinum and chlorambucil and then 12 months of maintenance chlorambucil. In February 1979 treatment was stopped as she was clinically and ultrasonically free of disease. Figure 1 shows the liver ultrasound scan taken in April 1979 (sagittal section right midclavicular line). In July 1979 she suddenly developed malignant ascites, which was drained, and tender hepatomegaly. Figure 2 shows the liver ultrasound scan taken at that time. Her hemoglobin, which had been steady at 12.5 g percent throughout, suddenly dropped to 12.0 g percent. In August 1979 she commenced high dose cis-platinum. Her hemoglobin returned to 12.9 g percent by September 1979. What do A and B represent in Figure 1?

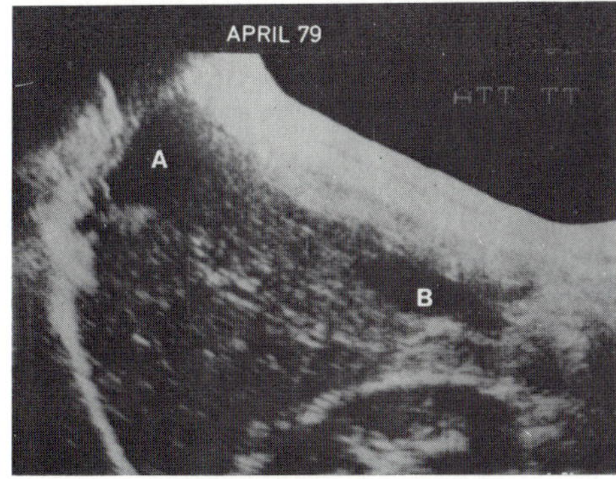

FIGURE 1.

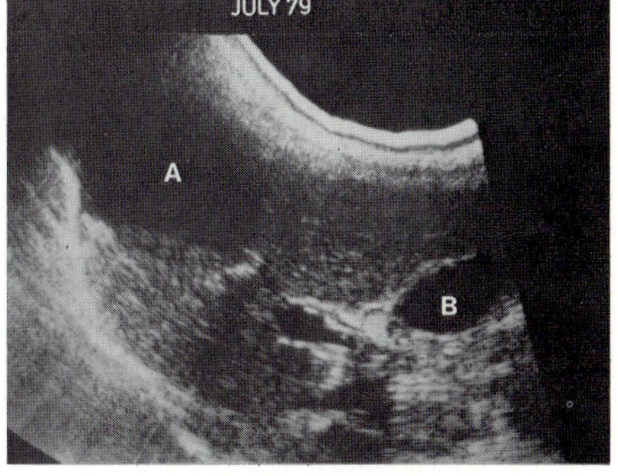

FIGURE 2.

DISCUSSION

Figure 1 shows a new 2-cm cystic lesion (A) on the diaphragmatic surface of the liver soon after chemotherapy was stopped (internal echo levels are the same as those reflected from the gallbladder, B). This lesion enlarged about threefold at the time of clinical relapse and, in addition, acquired internal echoes shown as gravitational layering (Fig. 2). Subsequent scans show progressive shrinkage towards the original size (Fig. 3). It seems likely that hemorrhage occurred into the lesion in June 1979, with subsequent resolution. The differential diagnosis of such a lesion rests between a simple cyst, hemangioma and a cystic metastasis. Due to its position against the diaphragm, distal enhancement would not be observed in hemangiomata. It does appear beyond this enlarged lesion. Simple cysts and hemangiomata grow slowly and would have been detected on earlier ultrasound and at the laparotomies. A cystic metastasis in the liver could behave in this way and is not uncommon to originate from the ovary or pancreas.

Final diagnosis: Hemorrhage into a cystic metastasis from an ovarian primary.

REFERENCE Pussell SJ, Cosgrove DO, Wiltshaw E, Barker GH, Hinton J: Carcinoma of the ovary: correlation of ultrasound with 2nd look laparotomy. Unpublished data.

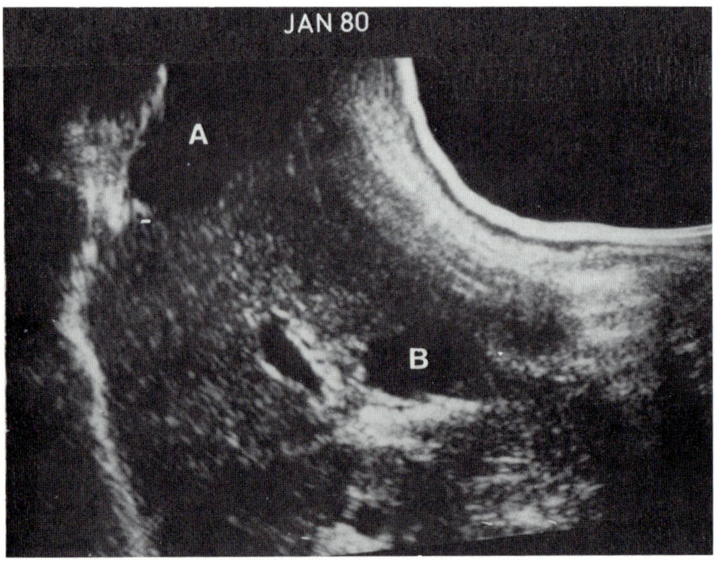

FIGURE 3.

CASE NO. 2

M. Crade
K. Taylor

Carcinoma of the Gallbladder? What is Your Diagnosis?

A 70-year-old male with previous history of recurrent bouts of upper abdominal discomfort underwent an ultrasound examination during such an episode. While other sections demonstrated findings diagnostic of intraluminal gallstones, this longitudinal section is presented for your evaluation (Fig. 1A).

Is the appearance specific for a gallbladder neoplasm? What has been seen on ultrasonic examination of such tumors? If tumor is found at surgery, what are the expectations for survival?

What other diagnoses should be considered?

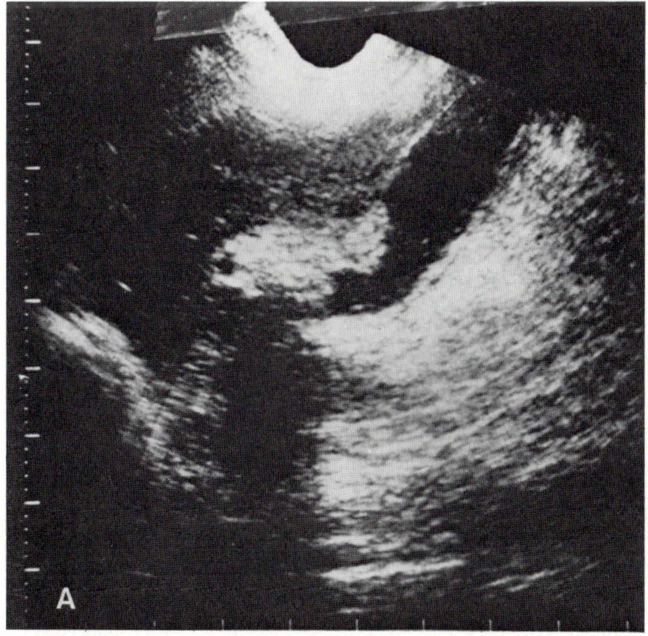

FIGURE 1A.

DISCUSSION

The longitudinal ultrasound shows a densely echogenic region (arrow) associated with the proximal portion of the gallbladder (G). Shadowing (S) distal to this region is noted (Fig. 1B).

Although many authors have described a range of echo appearances for gallbladder tumors, no ultrasonic findings are entirely specific for this diagnosis. However, the possibility of a gallbladder carcinoma should be considered when an intraluminal mass, a greatly thickened wall or an obliterating mass is visualized. Also, it should be remembered that similar changes may be seen with inflammation. As tumor growth virtually always occurs in the presence of inflamed mucosa, ultrasonic differentiation becomes difficult, if not impossible.

Survival after a gallbladder tumor is diagnosed is decidedly poor. Despite innovative surgery and aggressive chemotherapy, only 3 to 4 percent of patients can expect to live 5 years. As yet, there has been no reported case of a curative resection prompted by an early diagnosis using ultrasound.

This particular patient had an inflamed gallbladder with stones (Fig. 2), and an adjacent

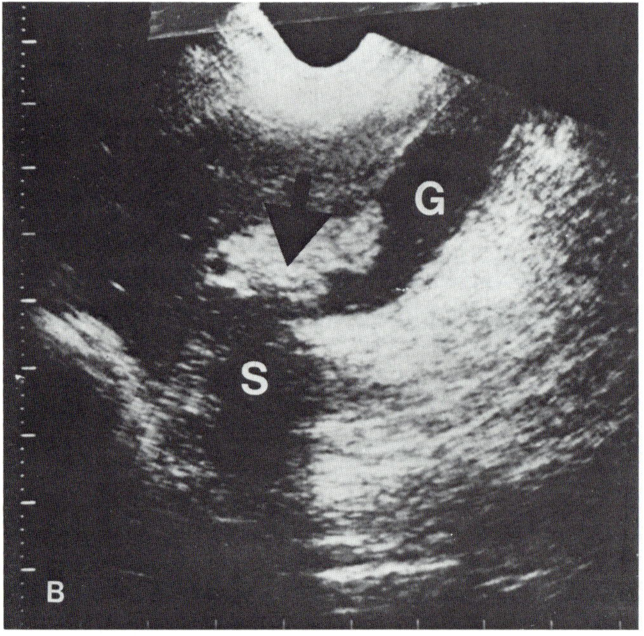

FIGURE 1B.

walled-off abscess, producing the echogenic and shadowing mass seen in the figure. These appearances may be mimicked by tumor growth.

Figure 3 demonstrates an intraluminal protrusion (arrow), again suggestive of a neoplasm, but found to be a chronically inflamed and thickened mucosa.

In conclusion, although the diagnosis of gallbladder tumor may be suggested by scan appearances, similar changes may be seen when the gallbladder is affected only by acute and chronic inflammation.

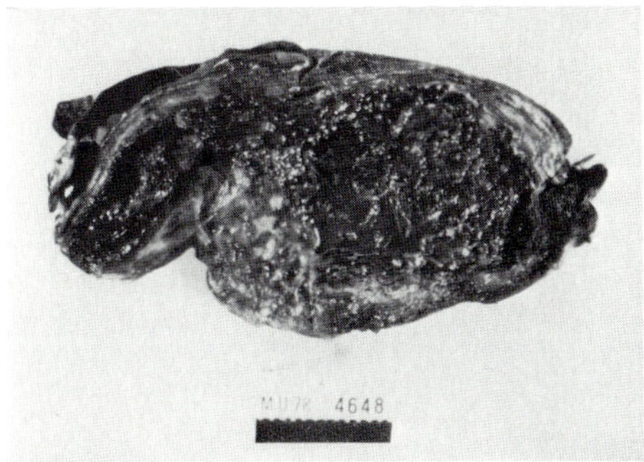

FIGURE 2.

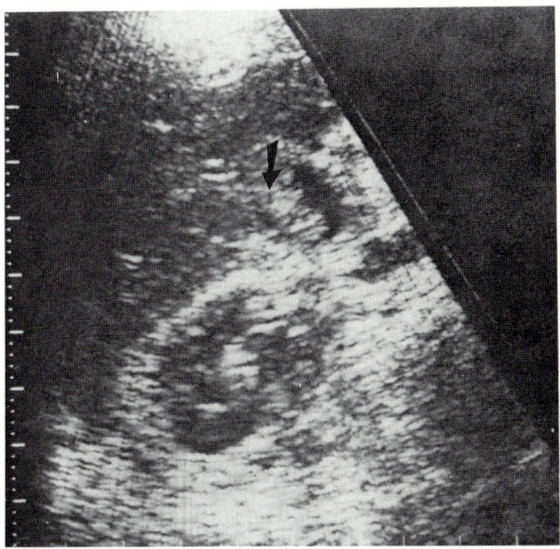

FIGURE 3.

CASE NO. 3

B. J. Weinstein
D. P. Weinstein

Painless Jaundice

A 76-year-old woman was referred for evaluation of painless jaundice. Scans of the liver, gallbladder, biliary tree, pancreas, and paraaortic region were performed. No focal masses were found in the liver. The gallbladder was contracted. Figures 1 and 2 are representative subcostal oblique and longitudinal scans of the porta hepatis to define the biliary tract. Figures 3 and 4 are representative transverse and longitudinal views of the pancreas and paraaortic areas. Is there bile duct dilatation? Is there a mass? If so, describe its location.

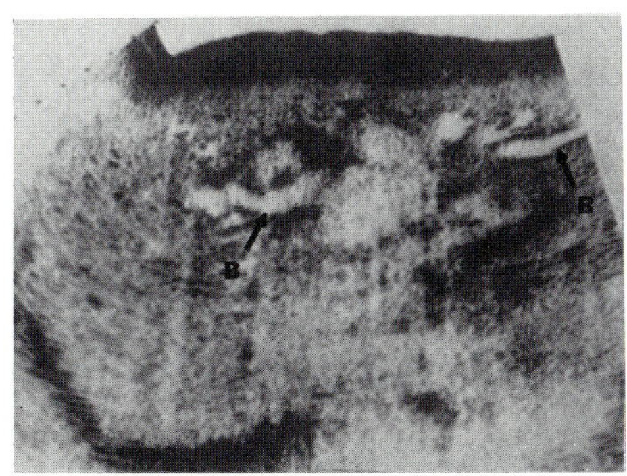

FIGURE 1. Right subcostal oblique scan through porta hepatis. B = bile ducts; PV = portal vein; I = inferior vena cava; SV = splenic vein; A = aorta; SMA = superior mesenteric artery; C = celiac artery.

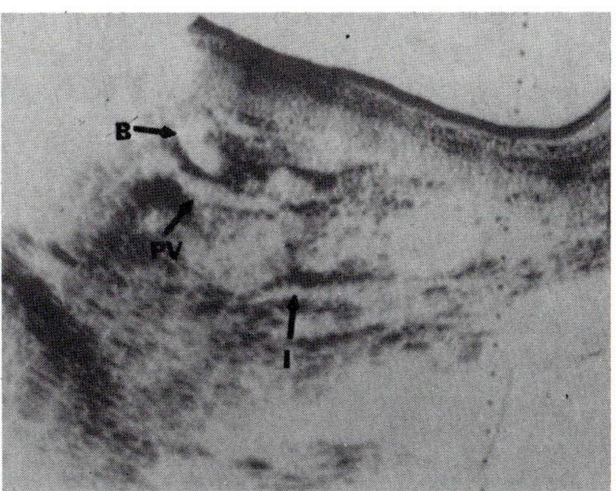

FIGURE 2. Longitudinal scan through porta hepatis.

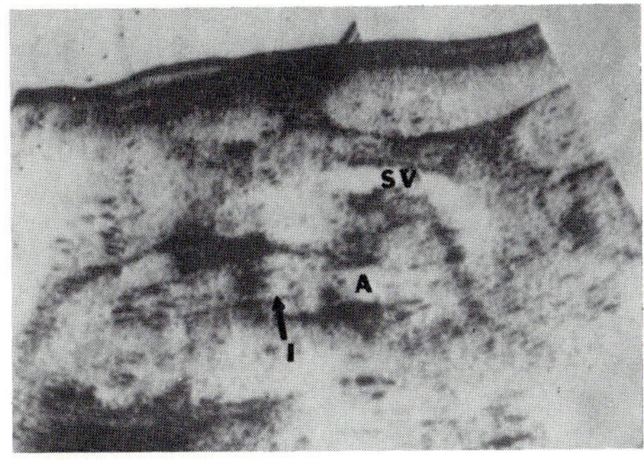

FIGURE 3. Transverse scan through level of pancreas.

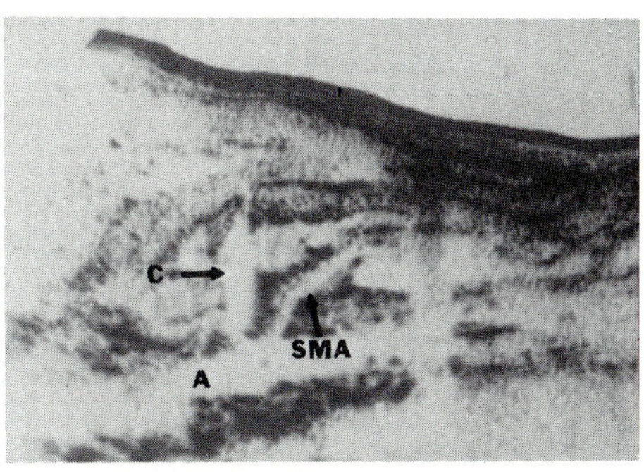

FIGURE 4. Midline longitudinal scan.

DISCUSSION

The scans of the porta hepatis show biliary obstruction at the liver hilum. Dilated intrahepatic ducts can be traced to the porta hepatis where multiple hypoechoic masses are seen. The high level of biliary obstruction was confirmed by cholangiography (Fig. 5). This explains the finding of a small gallbladder. The body of the pancreas blends into a faintly echoing lobulated mass at the pancreatic head. The superior mesenteric and celiac arteries are displaced anteriorly by multiple paraaortic masses. The echo texture, multiplicity, and location of these masses are characteristic of lymphadenopathy.

Extensive lymphadenopathy secondary to pancreatic carcinoma is usually accompanied by liver metastases and none were found in this case. The ultrasonic findings are more compatible with lymphoma than with metastatic pancreatic carcinoma. Since lymphoma is radio-sensitive and has a far more favorable prognosis, it is important to make this distinction. A definitive diagnosis can be established by an ultrasound-guided aspiration biopsy.

In view of the high level of obstruction, temporary biliary drainage would be best accomplished by a percutaneous approach. In addition to the presumptive diagnosis, the sonogram provided significant therapeutic information.

Final diagnosis: Lymphocytic lymphoma.

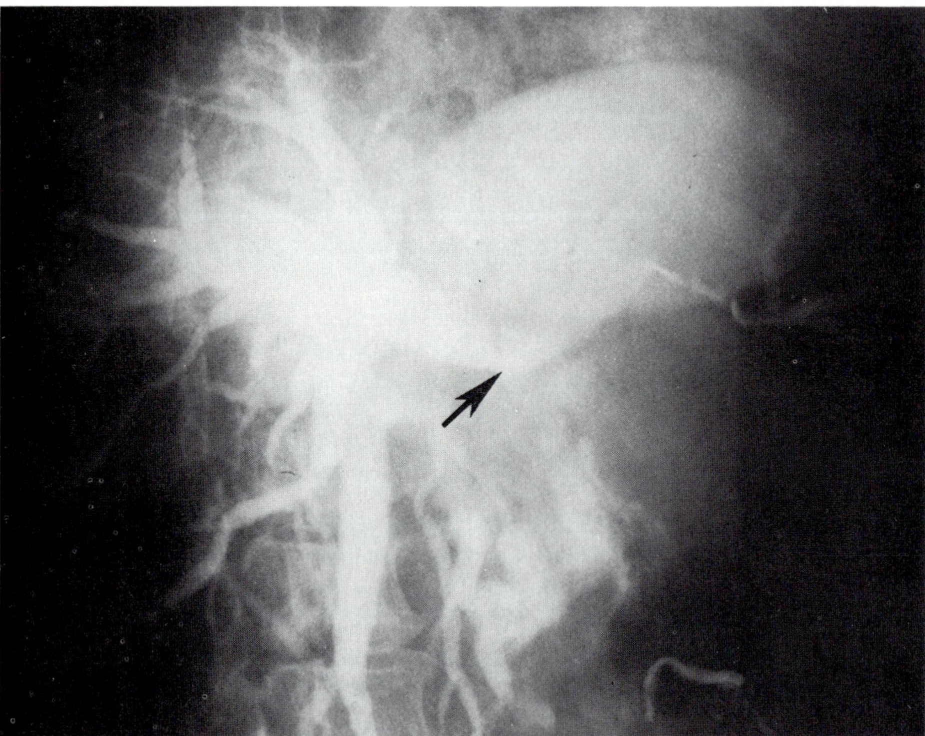

FIGURE 5. Percutaneous transhepatic cholangiogram confirming complete obstruction of the biliary tract high in the porta hepatis. No contrast material was seen distal to the junction of the right and left hepatic ducts (arrow).

CASE NO. 4

B. Carroll

Fever and Right Inguinal Mass in a Young Man

A 34-year-old man, previously treated for lymphoma and considered in remission, was admitted with low-grade fever, malaise, and a right inguinal swelling. Physical examination disclosed right inquinal lymphadenopathy, without other peripheral nodes. A KUB revealed no change in the adequately opacified abdominal lymph nodes, with no evidence of recurrent disease. An abdominal sonogram of the right lower quadrant was requested. Figure 1 is a sagittal supine scan obtained through the right lower quadrant of the abdomen. I = iliac wing; superficial right lower quadrant mass (m); deeper right lower quadrant mass (arrows). Describe the ultrasonic characteristics of the masses.

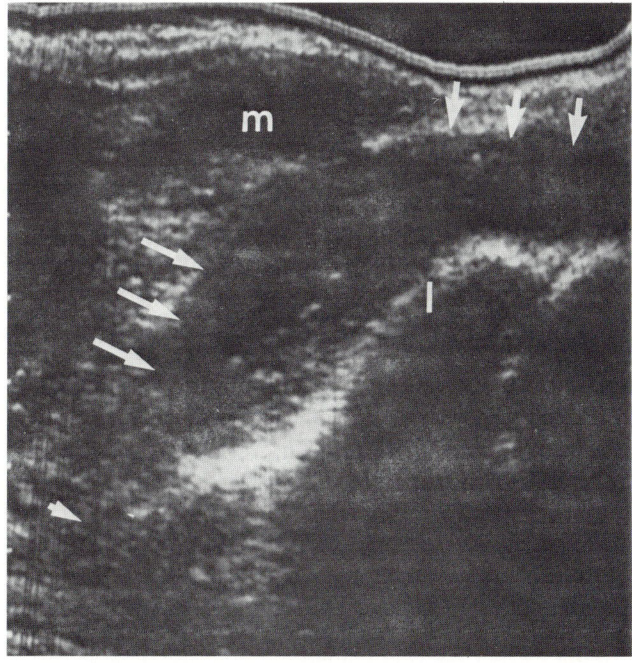

FIGURE 1.

DISCUSSION

The gray-scale sonogram shows a large, anechoic, superficial right lower quadrant mass. The mass, although largely anechoic, does not demonstrate significant posterior acoustic sound tranmission or peripheral refractory shadowing. The contiguous deeper mass corresponds to the position and configuration of the right iliopsoas muscle. The low echo mass appears to consist of enlargement of the entire muscle without well-defined focal masses within the muscle. The findings are compatible with lymphomatous infiltration of the right iliopsoas muscle and associated superficial lymphadenopathy.

The CT scan performed on the patient 1 day later (Fig. 2) confirmed the sonographic findings. The tomographic section reveals enlargement of the right ilipsoas muscle (arrows) and contiguous superficial soft tissue(s). Surgical exploration confirmed infiltration of the right iliospoas muscle and adjacent lymph nodes and superficial soft tissues by diffuse histiocytic lymphoma.

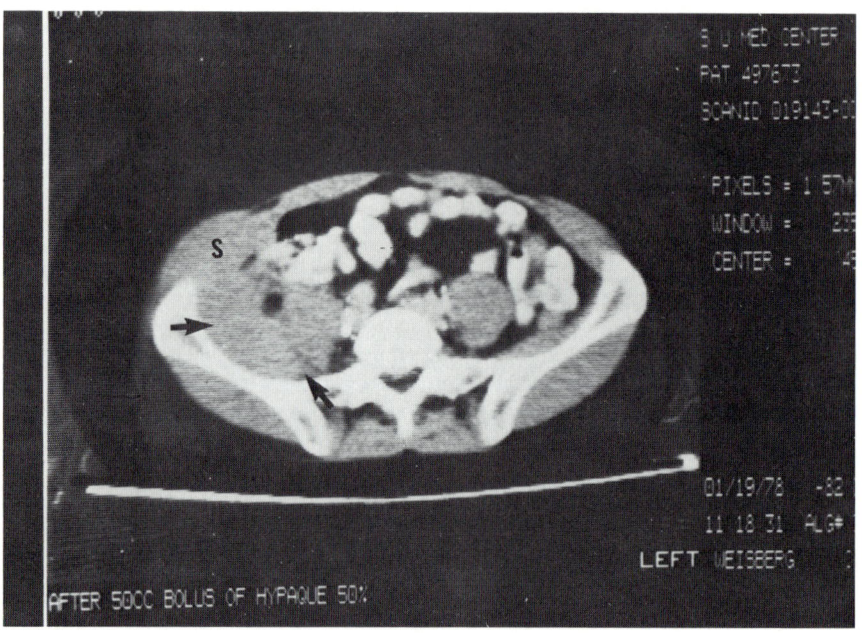

FIGURE 2.

CASE NO. 5

R. Sanders

The Multiple Appearances of Hematomas

An otherwise healthy neonate was examined 3 days after delivery and found to have a mass on the right side. A sonogram was performed. Longitudinal and transverse sections of the right kidney area are shown (Figs. 1 and 2). Describe the ultrasonic characteristics of the area of abnormality.

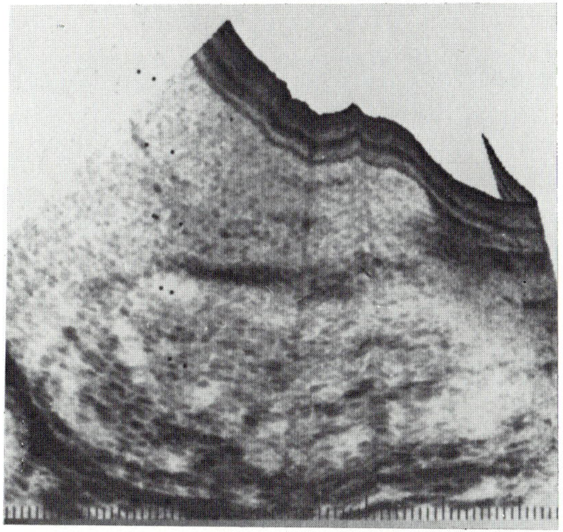

FIGURE 1. Longitudinal section 5 cm to the right of midline in the upper abdomen.

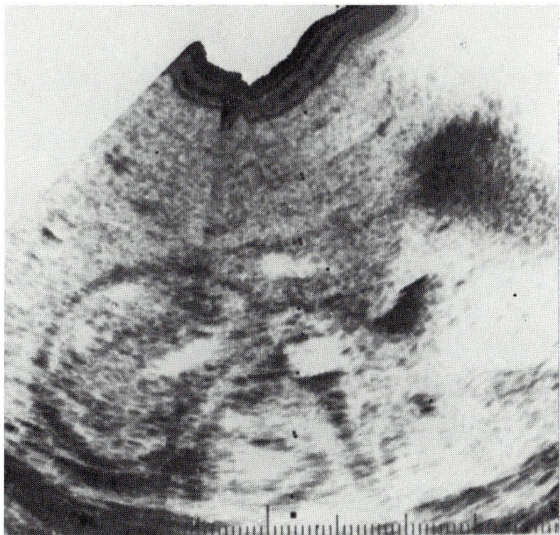

FIGURE 2. Transverse section 1 cm below the xiphisternum.

DISCUSSION

Detailed sonographic examination showed that the mass was superior to the right kidney and posterior to the liver. The mass was densely echogenic apart from two cystic areas (Figs. 3 and 4). Although teratoma or neuroblastoma was thought most likely, an adrenal hematoma was considered possible. A diagnostic laparotomy had been scheduled but it was decided to repeat the sonogram in three days time to see if the appearances changed. A second examination showed that the cystic areas had significantly increased in size (Figs. 5 and 6), making adrenal hematoma the most likely diagnosis. A further examination three weeks later showed a much smaller totally cystic lesion (Fig. 7). Eventually a calcified rim was seen on x-ray. A helpful study which supported the sonographic impression of an adrenal hematoma was a scintigram. There was absence of perfusion of both adrenal areas indicating that there was a smaller adrenal hematoma on the contralateral side which was not visualized on the sonogram (Fig. 8). Bilateral adrenal hematoma are common in neonates.

The case illustrates the multiplicity of appearances that hematomas can adopt. Although Kaplan and Sanders (1973) suggested that the usual progress of a hematoma was a cystic lesion that became echogenic, the reverse may also occur, as this case illustrates.

REFERENCE Kaplan G, Sanders RC: The use of ultrasound in post-operative haematoma. J Clin Ultrasound 1:1973.

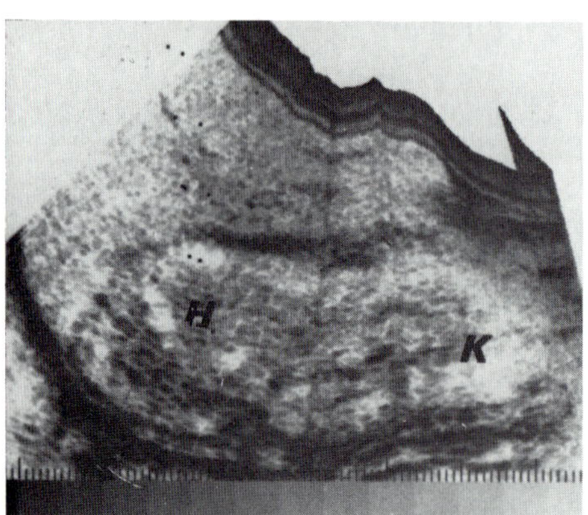

FIGURE 3. Longitudinal section 5 cm to the right of midline in the upper abdomen. H = adrenal hematoma; K = kidney.

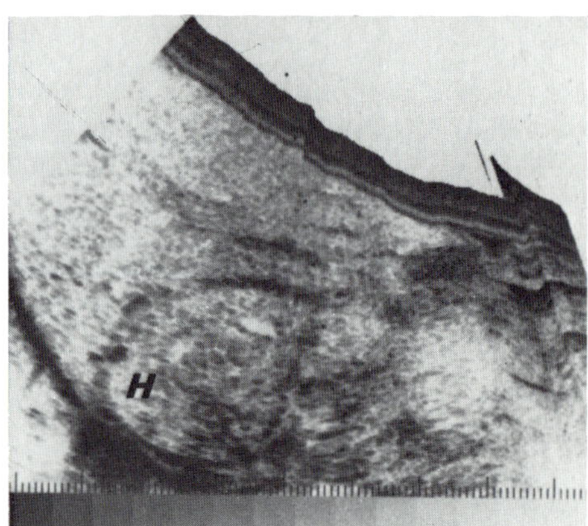

FIGURE 4. Longitudinal section 4 cm to the right of midline. H = adrenal hematoma.

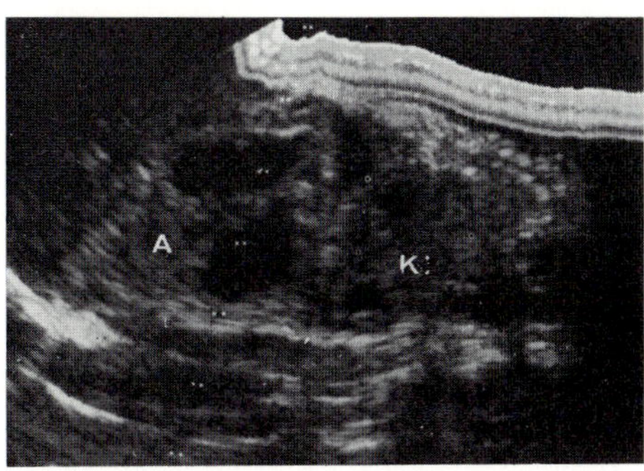

FIGURE 5. Longitudinal section on reexamination of the infant 3 days later. The adrenal hematoma (A) now contains two large cystic areas. K = kidney.

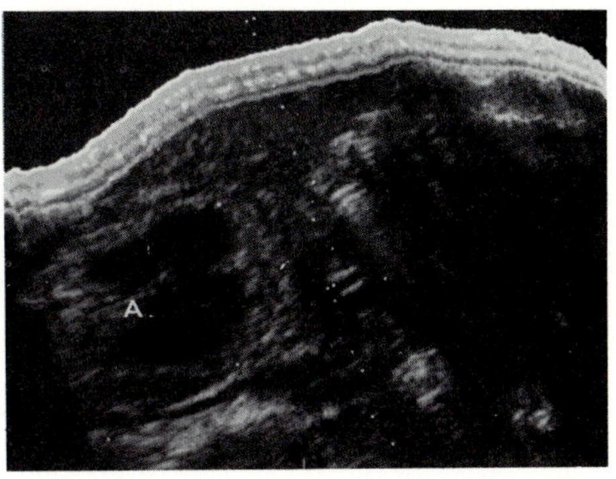

FIGURE 6. Transverse section through the adrenal hematoma (A). The cystic areas are well seen.

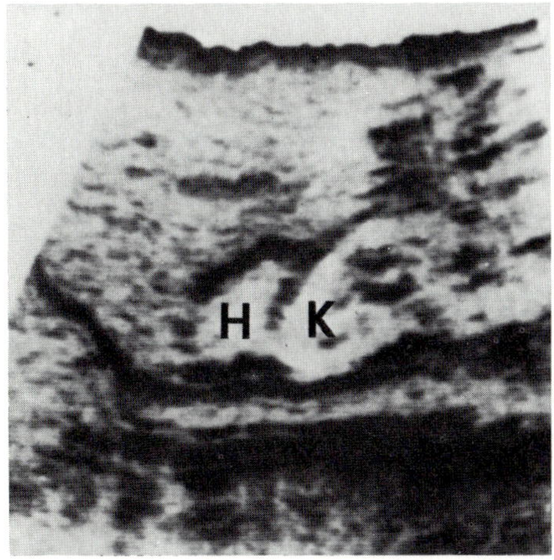

FIGURE 7. Longitudinal section 5 cm to the right of the midline 3 weeks later. The adrenal hematoma (H) is now echo free. K = kidney.

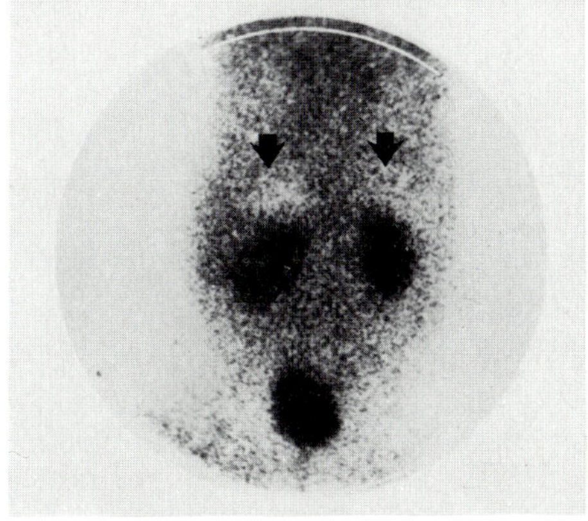

FIGURE 8. Technetium DTPA nuclear medicine study showing photon-deficient areas superior to both kidneys (ar rows).

CASE NO. 6

A. B. Kurtz
J. W. Breckenridge

Increasing Abdominal Girth in a Young Woman

A 29-year-old woman presented with increasing abdominal fullness and weight gain. Physical examination revealed tense ascites. A bimanual pelvic examination detected prominent, slightly enlarged firm ovaries and a suggested fullness within the cul-de-sac. Routine laboratory evaluation was unremarkable. An ultrasound examination was performed, including a transverse ultrasound pelvic scan immediately superior to the urinary bladder (Fig. 1) and a midline longitudinal pelvic and abdominal scan (Fig. 2). Can a specific diagnosis be made? If not, what is the most likely diagnosis?

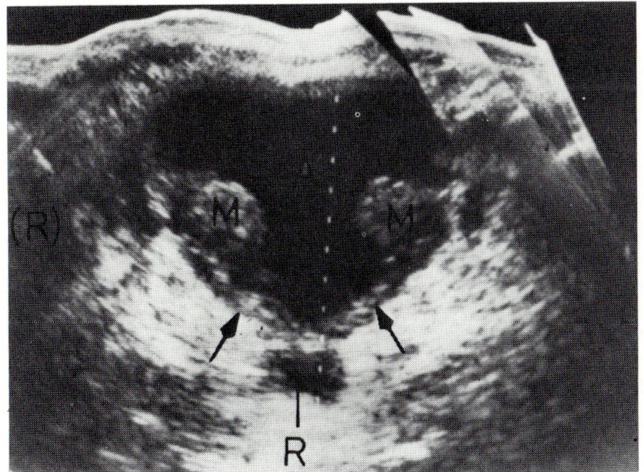

FIGURE 1.

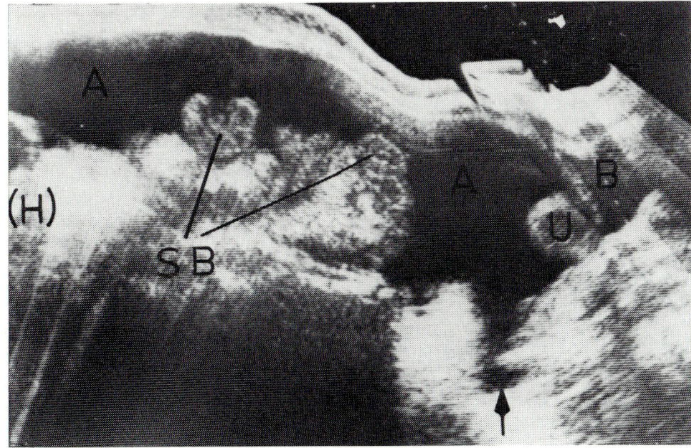

FIGURE 2.

DISCUSSION

Figure 1 revealed marked ascites (A) and two solid ultrasound masses (M) consistent with enlarged ovarian neoplasms. Additional echogenic areas were imaged lining the area of the cul-de-sac (arrows), representing peritoneal tumor seeding. The posterior cystic area was a pseudotumor of the rectum (R), determined by a subsequent water enema. Figure 2 again showed the marked ascites (A) and the cul-de-sac fullness (arrows). Small bowel loops (SB) were imaged, bound down, and not floating freely within the ascites. U = uterus. B = urinary bladder. These findings were felt to be consistent with primary ovarian carcinoma, metastatic to the mesentary and peritoneum.

A subsequent barium enema (Fig. 3) showed persistent narrowing of the sigmoid colon (arrows) with mild irregularity, consistent with extrinsic involvement. Because ovarian metastases could not be excluded, an upper gastrointestinal series was performed (Fig. 4). It revealed a large irregular stomach mass (arrows) with an ulcer crater on the lesser curvature. The final pre-operative diagnosis, confirmed at surgery, was bilateral Kruckenberg tumors of the ovaries from a primary gastric carcinoma with additional extensive invasion of the mesentery, peritoneum, and cul-de-sac.

Kruckenberg tumors of the ovaries are metastatic neoplasms from primary lesions of the gastrointestinal tract, particularly carcinoma of the stomach. These tumors may infrequently also arise from the gallbladder, pancreas and breast. They usually cause bilateral involvement of the ovaries, which are only mildy enlarged and on physical examination are quite firm. Ascites is frequently present. Rarely these tumors cause clinical signs of masculinization. Microscopically, the stroma is usually quite pronounced and mucoproducing carcinoma is present with numerous signet ring cells.

Final diagnosis: Kruckenberg tumors of the ovaries.

REFERENCE Ackerman LV del Regato JA: Cancer of the female genital organs. In *Cancer, Diagnosis, Treatment and Prognosis, Fourth Edition.* St Louis, CV Mosby, 1970, pp 729–737.

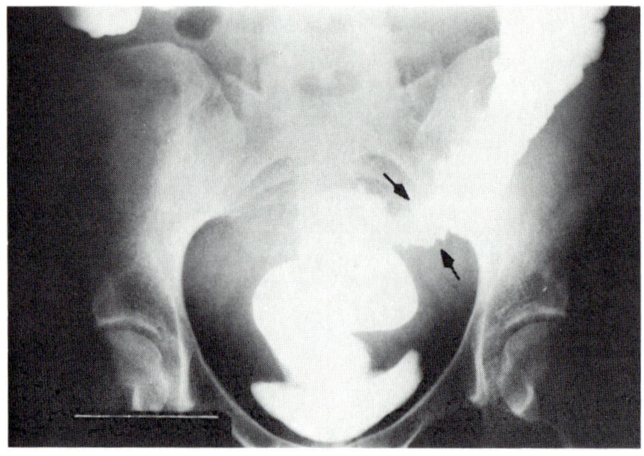

FIGURE 3.

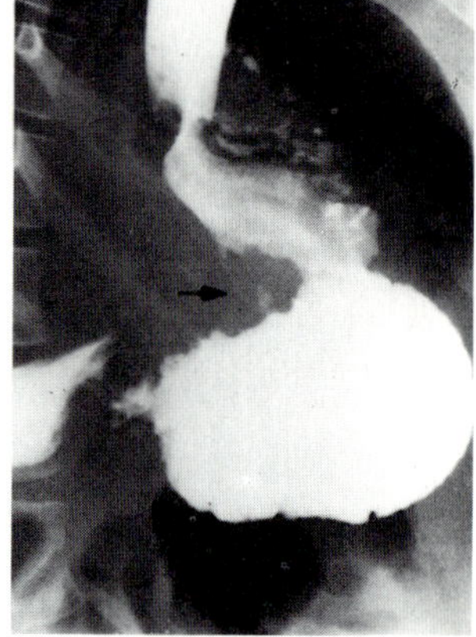

FIGURE 4.

CASE NO. 7

M. Schneider

Palpable Left Flank Mass

This 6-month-old child was discovered to have a large palpable left flank mass. An intravenous urogram revealed a normal right kidney and a distorted left kidney. Ultrasound of the left kidney was performed (Figs. 1 and 2). Can the kidney be identified? Do the cystic areas (a) and solid areas (b) suggest a specific diagnosis?

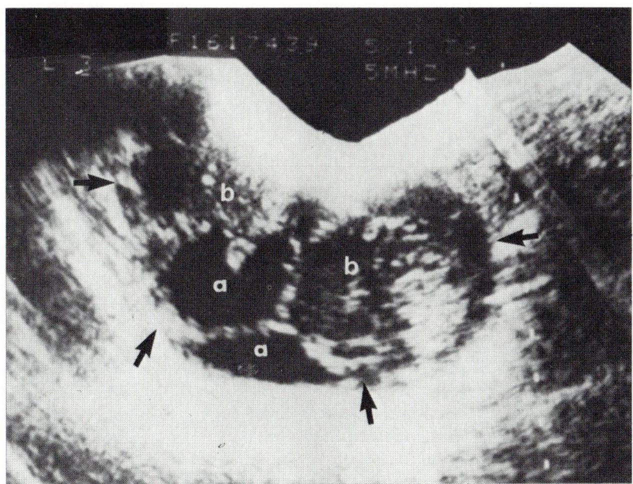

FIGURE 1. Longitudinal prone scan.

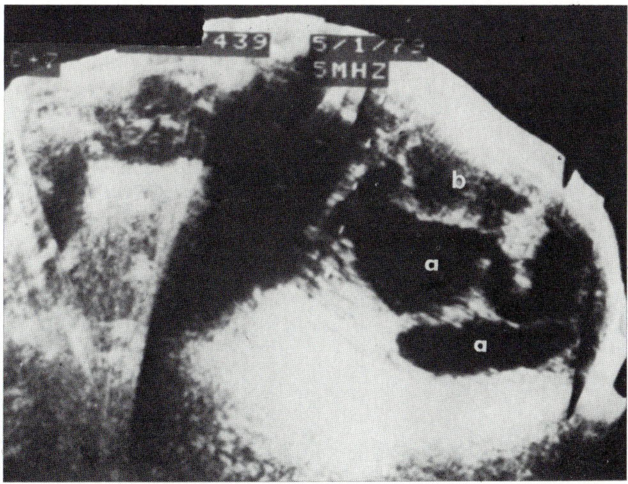

FIGURE 2. Transverse prone scan.

DISCUSSION

Sonogram reveals a complex left flank mass in the retroperitoneum. No normal left kidney can be identified. The mass (arrows) has echo-poor cystic areas (a) and solid echo echogenic areas (b). These findings do not appear to be compatible with simple hydronephrosis. The findings suggest the differential diagnosis of a benign multilocular cystic nephroma, Wilms tumor, or a mesonephric blastoma. This mass was surgically removed, and the final pathology was a mesonephric blastoma.

CASE NO. 8

G. R. Leopold

Thyroid Nodule – Benign or Malignant?

This 45-year-old man was undergoing diagnostic evaluation because he had a previous history of head and neck radiation for acne when he was 13 years old. Physical examination disclosed a small nodule of the left lobe of the thyroid. An ultrasonographic study was ordered (Fig. 1). Following this, a nuclear medicine study was performed and demonstrated that the lesion in question did not take up radioiodine. What is your diagnosis, and how should the patient be managed?

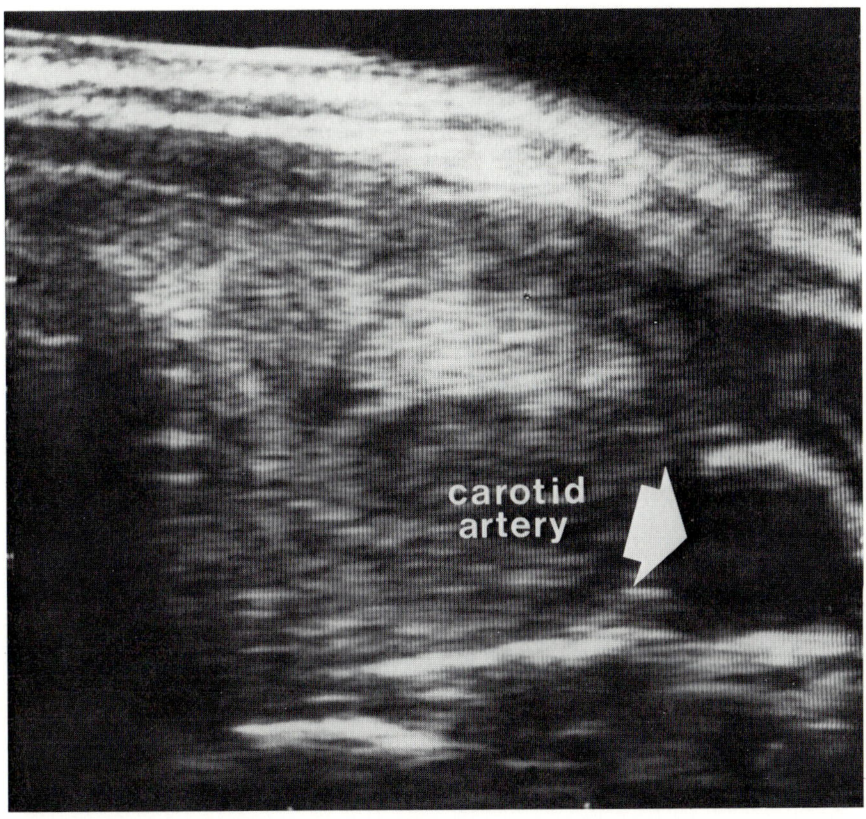

FIGURE 1.

DISCUSSION

The ultrasound study shows a solid mass within the substance of the left lobe of the thyroid. An obvious "halo" separates the lesion from normal gland. This finding is most compatible with a benign adenoma, although there is also the remote possibility that the nodule is a pure follicular carcinoma. If a history of prior radiation exposure had not been present, such a patient might be placed on thyroxine and restudied in 3 months. If the tumor shrinks under this regimen of TSH suppression, many would feel that this is strong evidence for a benign lesion and treat the patient conservatively.

In patients with previous head and neck irradiation, the incidence of both benign and malignant tumors is increased. "Cold" lesions on radionuclide examination have a 50 percent chance of being malignant, so that most would wish to obtain a tissue diagnosis under these circumstances. Aspiration biopsy with cytology might be performed to clarify its nature. In this case, however, surgery was elected. The lesion proved to be a benign adenoma. No additional lesions were discovered and the patient remains well 1 year after surgery. Serial studies at yearly intervals are planned to detect new nodules in the remaining right lobe of the gland.

Final diagnosis: Benign thyroid adenoma.

Index

Page numbers followed by f represent figures; page numbers followed by t represent tables.

A-scan for eyes, 137
Abdomen
  girth of, increasing, 212–214, 212f–213f
  lymphoma and, 64–66, 66t
  tumors of, pediatric, 115–118
    adrenal neuroblastoma as, 116–117, 117f
    excretory urogram in, 115
    hepatoblastoma as, 117–118
    liver metastases in, 118, 117f
    Wilms tumor as, 115–116, 116f
Accuracy of ultrasound
  liver malignancy and, 14–16, 15t
  pancreas and, 49–50
Adenocarcinoma, pancreatic, 35–44
  associated ultrasound findings in, 43–44, 38f
  biliary obstruction and dilatation in, 41, 39f, 40f
  body masses in, 41–43, 42f
  clinical and pathologic features of, 36t
  early diagnosis of, 44
  echogenesis in, 35, 38f
  gas artefact in, 39, 39f
  liver metastases and, 44, 42f, 43f
  longitudinal scan in, 41, 39f
  mesenteric vessel displacement in, 44, 38f
  pancreatic duct dilatation in, 41, 40f
  survival in, 41
  tail masses in, 43, 43f
  ultrasound features of, 37t, 38t
Adenoma
  liver, 2
  thyroid, 127, 128f–129f
Adrenal gland, 97–100
  CT scan vs ultrasound in, 97
  echo-architecture enlargement and, 99, 98f
  inferior vena cava in carcinoma of, 99–100, 99f
  optimum views of, 97
  pediatric, neuroblastoma of, 116–117, 117f
  pseudocysts of, 100
Ampullary carcinoma, 46, 47f
Angiomyolipoma, kidney, 74, 76f–77f
Arteriography in liver malignancy, 17

B-scanning
  contact, breast and, 157
  eye and, 137
  real-time, breast and, 158
Bi-axial pendulum treatment, 173f
Bile duct tumors, 24–30
  anatomic distribution of, 25
  bile in, 25
  classification of, 25–27
  early misdiagnosis of, 25
  populations at risk for, 25
  prevalence of, 24–25
  surgery in, 27
  survival rate in, 27
Biliary tract, 21–34
  bile duct tumors in, 24–30
  gallbladder carcinoma in, 21–24
  tumors of
    early diagnosis of, 31–32
    ultrasound in, 30–32
Bladder
  neoplasms of, 84–85
  urinary, 100–102, 100f
Body contour and circumference, 169–170
Brachytherapy in carcinoma of cervix, 173f
Breast, 157–166
  abnormal ultrasound patterns in, 160
  carcinoma of, treatment planning in, 178f
  contact B-scanning of, 157
  disease of, flow chart for diagnosis and treatment in, 164, 162f–163f
  fibroadenomas of, 164, 164f
  fluid-filled cyst in, 160, 160f
  infiltrating duct carcinoma of, 164, 165f
  normal postmenopausal, 158, 158f
  normal premenopausal, 158, 159f
  real-time B-scanning of, 158
  tumor shadowing in, 160–161, 161f
  ultrasound criteria for, 160, 159t
  water path techniques for, 157
  x-ray mammography of, 161, 164
Bulls-eye lesion, 7, 10f

Cancer therapy, three approaches to, 187f
Carotid artery, 124, 125f
Cellulitis, 152
Cervix
  cancer of, 107f
  carcinoma of
    brachytherapy in, 173f
    recurrence of, 180f–182f
Chemotherapy plus ultrasound, 189, 192–193
Chest wall thickness, 177, 178f

Children. *See* Pediatrics.
Cholangiocarcinomas, 24–30. *See also* Bile duct tumors.
Cirrhosis, macronodular, 3
Column of Bertini, 83–84, 86f
Computer interface in dose calculation, 174, 174f–176f
CT scan
  adrenal gland and, 97
  gynecology and, 104
  liver malignancy and, 16–17
  lymphadenopathy and, 91
  orbit and, 155
Cul-de-sac
  pseudotumors and, 108, 108f
  secondary masses of, 109, 108f
  tumors of, 108–109
Cysts
  liver, 1–2, 4f
  neoplasms vs, 68, 76–77, 69f, 81f
  ocular tumors vs, 144, 145f
  ovarian, 109–110, 109f
  paraovarian, 110
  serous and mucinous cystadenoma, 111, 110f
  theca lutein, 111
  thyroid, 126–127, 126f
Cystadenocarcinoma, pancreatic, 45, 46f, 36t, 37t
Cystadenoma vs cystadenocarcinoma, 111, 110f
Cystic teratoma, pediatric, 118–120, 120f

Dermoids
  differential diagnosis of, 112–113
  ovarian, 111, 111f
Dosimetry, 172–174, 171f–176f
Dysgerminomas, pediatric, 120
Dysthyroid exophthalmos, 152–153, 153f

Epididymis, 133, 133f
Eye and orbit, 136–155
  ocular tumors of, 138–144
  orbital tumors of, 144–155
  technical requirements for, 136–138
    A-scan in, 137
    B-scan in, 137
Exophthalmos, dysthyroid, 152–153, 153f
Extranodal lymphoma, 58–64
Extraperitoneal space, 90

Fibroadenoma, breast, 164, 164f

Gallbladder carcinoma, 21–24, 201–203, 201f–203f
  diagnosis of, 22–23
  fungating tumor in, 22
  gallstones and, 21–22
  histology in, 22
  infiltrating tumor in, 22
  metastasis from, 22
  prevalence of, 21
  survival in, 22
  ultrasound in, 23–24, 24f, 26f–27f
Gallium studies in liver malignancy, 16
Gallstones, 21–22
Gastric carcinoma, 47, 49f
Gastrointestinal tract and lymphoma, 60–62, 63f
Gynecology, 104–114
  CT scan vs ultrasound and, 104
  cul-de-sac tumors and, 108–109
  differential diagnosis in, 112–113
  full-bladder technique in, 104
  normal anatomy in, 105–106, 105f
  ovarian tumors and, 109–112
  uterine corpus tumors and, 106

Hamartoma, liver, 1
Hemangioma
  liver, 1, 7, 3f, 2t
  ocular, 141–142
Hematoma(ta)
  liver, 7
  multiple appearance of, 209–211, 209f–211f
Hemorrhage
  subretinal, 143–144
  vitreous, 140, 142f
Hepatoblastoma, pediatric, 5, 117–118
Hepatocellular carcinoma, 5
High-intensity short-time ultrasound therapy, 188
Hodgkin disease
  hypoechoic mass in, 92f
  large solitary abdominal mass in, 94f
  liver metastases in, 12, 12f
  multiple discrete lymph node masses in, 93f
Hypernephroma, kidney, 68–70, 70f, 71f
  calcification of, 83
  metastases of, 81–83, 84f
  renal vein invasion by, 80–81, 83f
  treatment planning in, 171f
  liver, 2–3
  sinus, 13

Infiltrating duct carcinoma of breast, 164, 165f
Infrahepatic nodes, lymphoma of, 57–58, 56f
Inguinal mass with fever, 207–208, 207f–208f
Intracavitary treatment planning, 177
Islet cell carcinoma, 44–45, 45f, 36t, 37t

Jaundice, 205–206, 205f–206f
Jugular vein, 124

Kidneys, 68–89
  ancillary ultrasonic views of, 80
  angiomyolipoma of, 74, 76f–77f
  benign mesoblastic nephroma of, 73, 74f

benign multilocular cyst of, 77, 82f
column of Bertini and, 83–84, 86f
cysts vs neoplasms of, 68, 76–77, 69f, 81f
hematoma and abscess of, 77
hypernephroma of, 68–70, 70f, 71f
calcification of, 83
metastases of, 81–83, 84f
renal vein invasion by, 80–81, 83f
lymphoma of, 60, 75–76, 61f, 62f, 78f–79f
metastatic lesions of, 76, 80f
neoplastic invasion of, 83, 85f
small neoplasms in, 70–72
transitional cell carcinoma of, 73–74, 75f
tumors of, bi-axial pendulum treatment in, 173f
Wilms' tumor of, 72, 72f, 73f

Left flank mass, 215–216, 215f–216f
Leukemia, pediatric, 118, 119f
Liver, 1–20
adenocarcinoma metastases to, 44, 42f, 43f
cyst of, ovarian carcinoma and, 199–200, 199f–200f
hemangiomata of, 7
hematomata of, 7
hypernephroma metastases to, 81–83, 84f
lymphoma of, 58–59, 60f
normal structures of, 3, 4f
pesudotumors of, 3
tumors of, 1–17
algorithm for, 17f
benign, 1–3, 3f–4f, 2t
adenoma, 2
cysts, 1–2, 4f
focal nodular hyperplasia, 2–3
hemangioma, 1, 3f, 2t
mesenchymal hamartoma, 1
solid, 2–3
clinical role of ultrasound in, 17–18, 17f
malignant, 5–17
arteriography in, 17
carcinomata as, 13
CT scan in, 16–17
cystic, 7, 10f
cystic metastases in, 13
echogenic metastases as, 6–7, 7f
echo-poor metastases as, 6–7, 8f–9f
gallium studies in, 16
hepatocellular carcinoma, 5
histologic correlation in, 12–14
lymphocyte infiltration and, 12, 12f
lymphoma as, 13
metastatic, 5, 5t
miliary metastases in, 12
necrosis of, 14
necrotic metastasis in, 7, 11f
ovarian metastases in, 13
sarcomata, 9, 13
scintigraphy in, 16
serum biochemistry in, 17
sinus hyperplasia and, 13
target or bulls-eye, 7, 10f
treatment response of, 14
ultrasound accuracy in, 14–16, 15t
ultrasound appearance of, 6–12
ultrasound vs other investigations in, 16–17
widespread, 12, 11f
Lymph nodes, seminoma of, 170f
Lymphadenopathy, 91–97
CT scan and ultrasound in, 91
hypoechoic mass in, 94, 92f
individual node size in, 95, 93f
large solitary abdominal masses in, 95, 94f
left renal collecting system in, 96f
lymphangiography in, 91
metastatic neoplasms in, 95–97, 95f
silhouette sign in, 94–95, 92f
Lymphangiography, 65, 66t
Lymphatic system, tumor extension into, 168–169
Lymphoma, 52–67
abdominal, 64–66, 66t
extranodal, 58–64
gastrointestinal, 60–62, 63f
infrahepatic nodal, 57–58, 56f
kidney, 60, 75–76, 61f, 62f, 78f, 79f
liver, 58–59, 60f
lymphangiography in, 65, 66t
mesenteric nodal, 55–57
metastases to liver of, 13
muscular involvement in, 63, 65f
non-Hodgkin
hypoechoic mantle in, 92f
urinary bladder displacement in, 96f
pancreatic, 46–47, 62–63, 48f, 64f
paraaortic lymph nodes and, 52–55
pediatric, 118, 119f
portal nodal, 58, 57f
retroperitoneal nodal, 58, 56f
splenic, 58, 59f

Melanoma, malignant, 138–140
Meningioma, sphenoid wing, 150
Mesenteric node, lymphoma of, 55–57, 55f
Mesoblastic nephroma, kidney, 73, 74f
Multilocular cyst, kidney, 77, 82f
Muscle and lymphoma, 63, 65f
Myoma, uterine, 106, 107f

Neoplasms vs cysts, 68, 76–77, 69f, 81f
Neuroblastoma, adrenal, 116–117, 117f
Nonpancreatic periampullary tumors, 46, 47f

Ocular tumors, 138–144
cysts vs, 144, 145f
hemangiomas, 141–142
malignant melanoma, 138–140
B-scan of, 138, 139f
excavation in, 138
high lead echo in, 140, 141f
internal echo pattern of, 138

Ocular tumors, *(continued)*
retinal detachment vs, 140, 143f
shadowing artifact in, 138, 140f
size and growth of, 140
topographic pattern variations of, 138
ultrasonographic features of, 144t
vitreous hemorrhage vs, 140, 142f
metastatic, 141, 145f
most common, 138
retinoblastoma, 142
subretinal hemorrhage vs, 143–144
Orbit
CAT-scan for, 155
foreign bodies in, 154
hematoma of, 154
inflammation of, 151–153
cellulitis, 152
dysthyroid exophthalmos, 152–153, 153f
idiopathic, 152
normal, B-scan of, 146, 146f
proptosis of, 153–154
pseudotumor of, 153
trauma to, 153–154
tumors of, 144–155
A-scan vs B-scan of, 146, 147f
incidence of, 146
mass lesions as, 148–152
angiomatous tumors, 149, 151f
classification of, 150–151
cystic tumors, 149, 148f
infiltrative tumors, 149–150, 152f
solid tumors, 149, 150f
ultrasonic diagnosis of, 154, 154t
vascular communications in, 154
Ovaries
carcinoma of
bilateral primary, 112, 112f
liver cyst and, 199–200, 199f–200f
cysts of, 109–110, 109f
dermoids of, 111, 111f
metastases from, 13
metastases to, 112
normal anatomy of, 106, 105f
tumors of, 109–112

Pancreas, 35–51
accuracy of ultrasound in, 49–50
adenocarcinoma of, 35–44
carcinoma of, 174f
cystadenocarcinoma of, 45
focal masses of, 49
islet cell carcinoma of, 44–45
lymphoma of, 46–47, 62–63, 48f, 64f
ultrasound accuracy in, 49–50
Pancreatitis, focal masses in, 49, 50f, 37t
Paraaortic lymph nodes, lymphoma of, 52–55
decubitus projection in, 55, 54f
silhouetting in, 55, 53f
Parathyroid glands, 124
Pediatrics, 115–122
abdominal tumors in, 115–118
hepatoblastoma in, 5
leukemia and lymphoma in, 118
pelvis in, 118–120
retinoblastoma in, 142
testicular sonography in, 121
Pelvis, pediatric, 118–120
cystic teratoma of, 118–120, 120f
dysgerminomas in, 120
rhabdomyosarcoma of, 118, 120f
Periampullary tumors, nonpancreatic, 46, 47f
Peritoneal cavity, 90
Portal node, lymphoma of, 58, 57f
Proptosis, orbital, 153–154
Prostate
cancer of, treatment planning in, 172f
carcinoma of, 102, 101f
neoplasia of, 85–88, 86f, 87f
longitudinal section in, 87, 86f, 87f
transrectal scanners in, 85
Pseudotumors
liver, 3
orbital, 153
rectosigmoid colonal, 108f

Radiation ports and pendulum axis, 177
Radiation target depth, 170
Radiation therapy planning, 167
Radiosensitive organ location, 171–172
Radiotherapy and ultrasound treatment, 191–192
Rectosigmoid colon, pseudotumor of, 108f
Recurrence detection, 180–182, 180f–182f
Research, clinical, 193–194
Retinal detachment, 140, 143f
Retinoblastoma, 142
Retroperitoneum, 90–103
adrenal gland and, 97–100
lymphadenopathy and, 91–97
nodes of, lymphoma of, 58, 56f
scanning techniques for, 90–100
urinary bladder and, 100–102
Rhabdomyosarcoma, pediatric, 118, 120f

Sarcomata
metastases to liver of, 13
liver, 9
Scintigraphy in liver malignancy, 16
Scrotal masses, 132–135
epididymis and, 133, 133f
Seminoma, lymph nodes in, 170f
Serum biochemistry in liver malignancy, 17
Silhouette sign, 94–95, 92f
Sinus hyperplasia, 13
Spleen, lymphoma of, 58, 59f
Stein-Levanthal syndrome, 110
Superficial organs, 123–135
equipment for, 123–124
testicle, 131–135
thyroid, 124–131

Target lesion, 7, 10f
Teratoma, cystic, pediatric, 118–120, 120f
Testicle, 131–135
  cephalad pole of, 132
  chronic abscess of, 135, 134f
  sonography of, 121, 121f
  technique for, 131–132
  tumors of, 133–135, 134f
Therapeutic response evaluation, 179–182, 179f
Therapy, 186–198
  clinical research in, 193–194
  early work in, 186–190
    chemotherapy plus ultrasound in, 189
    clinical trials in, 187–188
    high-intensity short-time approach in, 188
    intensity measurement in, 186
    treatment length in, 187
    X-ray plus ultrasound in, 189
  recent work, 190–194, 194t
    ultrasound alone, 190–191
    ultrasound and chemotherapy, 192–193
    ultrasound and radiotherapy, 191–192
  tumor growth vs time after ultrasound, 189f
Thyroid, 124–131
  common carotid artery and, 124, 125f
  internal jugular vein and, 124
  masses of, 126–131
    adenomas, 127, 128f–129f
    carcinoma, 131, 130f
    cysts, 126–127, *126*
  nodule of, 217–218, 217f
  normal scan of, 124, 125f
  technique for, 124
Tomography and treatment planning, 167–168
Transitional cell carcinoma, kidney, 73–74, 75f
Treatment planning, 167–185
  body contour and circumference in, 169–170
  breast carcinoma and, 178f
  chest wall thickness in, 177, 178f
  compound scanners in, 168
  computer interface in, 174, 174f–176f
  different scan locations in, 169, 170f
  dosimetry in, 172–174, 171f–176f
  essential scan information in, 169
  hypernephroma in, 171f
  intracavitary, 177
  prostatic cancer and, 172f
  radiation ports and pendulum axis in, 177
  radiation target depth in, 170
  radiation therapy planning in, 167
  radiosensitive organ location in, 171–172
  recurrences and, 180–182, 180f–182f
  therapeutic response in, 179–182, 179f
  tomography in, 167–168
  tumor extension evaluation in, 168
  tumor location in, 167
  tumor volume in, 170
Tumors
  abdominal, pediatric, 115–118
  benign, liver, 1–3, 3f–4f, 2t
  cul-de-sac, 108–109
  evaluation of extension of, 168–169
  growth of, time after ultrasound and, 189f
  kidney, 173f
  malignant
    liver, 5–17
    metastatic, liver, 5, 5t
  ocular, 138–144
  orbital, 144–155
  ovarian, 109–112
  uterine, 106
  volume of, 170
  Wilms, 72, 115–116, 72f, 73f, 116f, 179f

Urinary bladder, 100–102, 100f
Uterus
  cervical cancer and, 106, 107f
  normal anatomy of, 106
  tumors of, 106
    myoma, 106, 107f

Water path techniques, 157
White bile, 22
Wilms tumors, 72, 115–116, 72f, 73f, 116f, 179f

X-ray and ultrasound treatment, 189, 191–192